Encyclopedia of Neuroimaging: Clinical Relevance

Volume V

Encyclopedia of Neuroimaging: Clinical Relevance

Volume V

Edited by **Miles Scott**

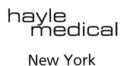

New York

Published by Hayle Medical,
30 West, 37th Street, Suite 612,
New York, NY 10018, USA
www.haylemedical.com

Encyclopedia of Neuroimaging: Clinical Relevance
Volume V
Edited by Miles Scott

International Standard Book Number: 978-1-63241-186-0 (Hardback)

Contents

Preface

In my initial years as a student, I used to run to the library at every possible instance to grab a book and learn something new. Books were my primary source of knowledge and I would not have come such a long way without all that I learnt from them. Thus, when I was approached to edit this book; I became understandably nostalgic. It was an absolute honor to be considered worthy of guiding the current generation as well as those to come. I put all my knowledge and hard work into making this book most beneficial for its readers.

Modern neuroimaging tools provide exceptional chances for understanding brain neuroanatomy and its role in health and illness. Each feasible technique carries with it a specific balance of potentials and drawbacks, such that converging evidence formed on multiple methods provides the strongest approach for enhancing our knowledge in the fields of clinical and cognitive neuroscience. The aim of this book is to provide a "snapshot" of present developments using well established and newly emerging techniques. The book includes the role of SPECT in the diagnosis of idiopathic Parkinson's disease, developments in dopamine transporter imaging and the application of non-conventional neuroimaging techniques in neuropsychiatric systemic lupus erythematosus (NPSLE) is discussed in detail.

I wish to thank my publisher for supporting me at every step. I would also like to thank all the authors who have contributed their researches in this book. I hope this book will be a valuable contribution to the progress of the field.

Editor

Pseudotumor Cerebri (Idiopathic Intracranial Hypertension) an Update

Eldar Rosenfeld and Anat Kesler

Neuro-ophthalmology Unit, Department of Ophthalmology, Tel-Aviv Medical Center,
Sackler School of Medicine, Tel Aviv University, Tel Aviv,
Israel

1. Introduction

1.1 History

Historically, several terms have been used to depict pseudotumor cerebri (PTC). In the late 1890's, Quincke (1893, 1897) was the first to describe and name this syndrome - "meningitis serosa" - patients suffering from headache, impaired visual acuity and papilledema. He related the symptoms to a state of elevated intracranial pressure and presumed it was caused by increased secretion of CSF by the autonomic nervous system. In 1904, Nonne (1904) termed this syndrome "pseudotumor cerebri" as the symptoms resembled a suspected intracranial mass. Foley (1955) renamed the condition "benign intracranial hypertension". However, in the late 1980's, Corbett et al (1982) altered the name to idiopathic intracranial hypertension, since the syndrome was not benign as once thought. In some cases, up to 25% of patients may lose their vision if appropriate treatment measures are not taken. At present, idiopathic intracranial hypertension is the accepted designation.

1.2 Demographics and epidemiology

Pseudotumor cerebri (PTC), also known as idiopathic intracranial hypertension (IIH) is a disorder of unknown etiology, predominantly affecting obese women of childbearing age (Ahlskog & O'Neill, 1982). In the general population, the annual incidence of PTC is estimated between 1-2 per 100,000 (Friedman & Jacobson, 2002, 2009). The incidence has been reported to have risen to 3.5 per 100,000 in women aged 20 - 44 years and may reach as high as 19 cases per 100,000 in women who are >20% over the ideal body weight (Durcan, 1988; Kesler et al 2001; Radhakrishnan et al., 1993, 1994).
PTC is uncommon in men, with female to male ratios reported approximately 4.3:1 to 8:1 (Binder et al, 2004; Durcan, 1988). The association between obesity and PTC is well established, >90% of women and >60% of men who suffer from this disorder are obese (Friedman et al., 2002; Radhakrishnan et al, 1994). The syndrome is relatively rare in the pediatric population. In the pre-pubertal population, it seems that obesity is not a risk factor. There is an equal distribution between boys and girls with an estimated incidence of approximately 1 case per 100,000.

1.3 Presenting signs and symptoms

Headaches, the most common presenting symptom in all age groups, occur in >90% of patients (Binder et al., 2004; Lessell, 1992). A PTC-associated headache has no specific characteristics, but is usually more severe and different than previously described headaches. In PTC, the headache is most commonly bifrontal or generalized, usually occurring daily, but may also occur intermittently, worsening in the morning. When cerebral venous pressure is increased by the Valsalva maneuver, the headaches are often exacerbated and accompanied by neck pain.

Transient visual obscurations (TVO), the second most common symptom is more frequently reported in adult patients than in pediatric PTC patients, 72% vs. 2-53% respectively (Lessell, 1992). TVO may be unilateral or bilateral, usually lasting less than a minute and often precipitated by a change in posture. TVO indicate the presence of optic disc edema resulting in transient ischemia to the optic nerve head. Over half (60%) of PTC patients may experience pulsatile tinnitus as the initial complaint. Pulsatile tinnitus is thought to result from a turbulence created by higher to lower venous pressure around the jugular bulb (Binder et al., 2004).

In patients with PTC, focal neurological deficits are extremely uncommon. An alternative diagnosis should be considered when these deficits occur. Nevertheless, isolated 6th cranial nerve paresis, thought to be attributed to nerve traction from increased intracranial pressure has been observed in approximately 20% of adult cases (Binder et al., 2004). However, in children, the incidence was found to be as high as 50% (Cinciripini et al 1999; Lessell, 1992; Rangwala & Liu, 2007). Paresis of the 3rd, 4th, 7th or 12th nerve is extremely rare, occurring mostly in the pediatric population. Young children with PTC may present with irritability rather than headaches (Lessell, 1992), and may consequently develop signs of a posterior

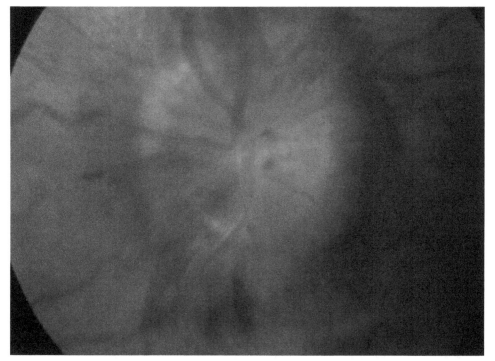

Fig. 1. Papilledema in a 26 year old PTC female patient.

fossa lesion, including ataxia, facial palsy, nuchal rigidity, malaise, torticollis (Lessell, 1992; Rangwala & Liu, 2007).

Papilledema is the diagnostic hallmark of PTC and is present in almost all patients (Mathew, 1996) (Figure 1). To note, although, unilateral cases may be encountered in approximately 10% of cases (Maxner et al., 1997; Wall & White, 1998) and a small number of patients may not have papilledema at all (Mathew, 1996; Wang et al., 1998; Winner & Bello, 1996), most cases occur either in very young infants with unfused sutures or in patients with anatomical variants of the endings of the optic nerve sheath (Hayreh, 1977; Killer et al., 1999).

Post-papilledema optic atrophy can occurs in untreated or inadequately treated patients after variable periods of time, usually over several months; in rare cases of fulminant PTC it can appear within weeks of the onset of symptoms. Some patients have persistent chronic papilledema without obvious visual deterioration. Visual field testing is the most sensitive method for detecting visual dysfunction. The most common abnormalities are an enlarged blind spot, generalized constriction and inferior nasal field loss.

1.4 Diagnosis

Diagnosis criteria for PTC were reviewed (Binder et al., 2004) (Table 1) and include signs and symptoms attributable to increased ICP, elevated CSF pressure with normal CSF content and normal neuroimaging studies. Other etiologies of intracranial hypertension were excluded. When these criteria are present, neuroimaging is employed to rule out space occupying lesions and sinus vein thrombosis. Lumbar puncture is subsequently performed to measure CSF opening pressure. Generally, an opening pressure of >250mm of water measured in a patient lying in the decubitus position, with outstretched legs and as relaxed as possible, is indicative of increased pressure. A pressure value between 201 and 249mm of water is inconclusive (Corbett & Mehta, 1983); pressure equal to or <200mm of water is considered normal. Often, due to CSF fluctuations, low or inconclusive measurements must be re-evaluated, especially if the clinical picture is indicative of increased ICP.

According to Tibussek et al (2010), a diagnosis of "probable PTC" would be indicated in patients, especially children, with clinical manifestations highly suggestive of PTC, but with a normal CSF opening pressure, presumably due to diurnal fluctuations. Rarely, in these circumstances, is a 24 hour intracranial CSF pressure monitoring, or transducer monitoring for 6 to 24 hours needed to confirm the diagnosis (Spence et al., 1980).

2. Neuroradiological evaluation

A detailed section in this chapter is devoted to diverse imaging modalities in patients with PTC. Imaging plays an important role in excluding intracranial tumors and structural or vascular lesions responsible for intracranial hypertension. CT, although adequate in ruling out hydrocephalus and most mass lesions, conditions such as sinus vein thrombosis, meningeal infiltration, and isodense tumors are undetected by a non-enhanced CT.

An MRI will detect almost all changes and by incorporating MRI venography will further enhance the ability to detect sinus vein thrombosis disguised as PTC (Crassard & Bousser, 2004). In rare cases, imaging of the spinal cord is essential as it excludes rare cases of spinal tumors that cause an increase in intracranial pressure. However, this is typically present with high protein levels in the CSF, therefore making it incompatible with the definition of PTC (Corbett & Mehta, 1983; Friedman & Jacobson, 2004; Ridsdale & Moseley, 1978). Traditionally, slit ventricles were thought to be present in PTC, but a quantitative analysis of ventricular volume noted no differences between patients with PTC and age-matched control patients (Jacobson et al., 1990).

Signs of increased intracranial pressure that may be found on imaging studies include empty sella (70%), flattening of posterior sclera (80%), enhancement of the prelaminar optic nerve (50%), distention of the perioptic subarachnoid space (45%), vertical tortuosity of the orbital optic nerve (40%), and intraocular protrusion of the prelaminar optic nerve (30%) (Brodsky & Vaphiades, 1998).

1.	Symptoms, if present, represent increased intracranial pressure or papilledema.
2.	Signs represent increased intracranial pressure or papilledema.
3.	Documented elevated intracranial pressure during lumbar puncture measured in the lateral decubitus position
4.	Normal cerebrospinal fluid composition.
5.	No evidence of ventriculomegaly, mass, structural, or vascular lesion on magnetic resonance imaging or contrast-enhanced computed tomography and magnetic resonance venography or computerized venography for all others
6.	No other cause (including medication) of intracranial hypertension identified.

Table 1. Clinical criteria for diagnosing idiopathic intracranial hypertension (adapted from Binder et al 2004)

3. Pathogenesis

At present, the pathogenesis of the syndrome is still unknown, however, some explanation must account for elevated intracranial pressure with normal neuroimaging, CSF constituents and neurologic examination (Corbett, 2008). Intracranial pressure is maintained by cerebral arterial pressure which is cerebral autoregulated, resulting in constant intracranial pressure.

CSF is constantly absorbed into the superior sagittal sinus (SSS) at the pacchionian granulation level. This process is carried out by a pressure gradient between the CSF and the venous pressure in the SSS. When there is a rise in the venous pressure, the CSF pressure rises proportionately in order for the CSF to diffuse into the SSS.

According to the Montro-Kellie rule (Greitz et al., 1992; Mokori, 2001), the increase in ICP may be a result of various factors such as an increase in CSF, brain or blood volume. Although many studies have been performed, it is still unclear which factor is responsible for the increase in ICP in cases of PTC.

Different hypotheses have been proposed such as, an increase in cerebral blood volume which was originally proposed by Dandy in 1937. Raichle et al. (1978), using positron emission tomography (PET) found that almost no change occurred in the cerebral blood flow (CBF) in PTC patients, however there were markedly increased cerebral blood or water volumes.

A few years later, Brooks et al (1985) using PET, found no change in cerebral hemodynamics. Recently, Levine demonstrated that vascular compression and dilatation exist in the PTC patient (Levine, 2000).

Bateman et al. (2007) found that the total CBF measured by magnetic resonance (MR) flow quantification and MR venography in the PTC patient, was 46% more elevated then in the control group, which may be secondary to cerebral vascular autoregulation. On the other hand, Lorberboym et al. (2001) reported a reduction in perfusion, noted on single photon emission CT scans in PTC patients a clear correlation between disease severity and CBF reduction. The proposed mechanisms for CBF changes are an increase of the cerebral vascular resistance, impairment of the CBF autoregulation, and a decrease of the tissue vascular density as a result of cerebral edema (Bateman, 2004)).

Bicakci et al (2006) recently studied 16 patients with perfusion and diffusion MRI, finding 6 patients with a statistically reduced CBF, and 2 with a marked increase. All other patients' cerebral blood volume did not significantly increase or decrease compared with the control group. Both vasodilatation and compression occurred in the PTC patient depending on the duration of the disease. The authors claimed that a long standing increase in CSF pressure might result in a decrease in CBF. On the other hand, an increase in CBF may be a result of a failure in autoregulation in the first phases of the disease, as suggested by Bateman's study.

4. Obstruction of venous outflow

The absence of ventricular dilatation in an elevated ICP condition is most likely explained by the presence of venous hypertension. As the pressure in the SSS rises, so does the CSF pressure due to hindered absorption of CSF. Brain parenchimal turgor increases due to an impending resorption of venous blood.

In 1995, King et al's (1995) series of 9 PTC patients with venous hypertension in the SSS and proximal transverse sinuses, cerebral venography and manometry were performed. The authors were able to observe the appearance of the transverse sinuses, ranging from a smooth tapered narrowing to a discrete intraluminal filling defect resembling mural thrombi.

The authors also found a significant drop in venous pressure at the level of the lateral third of the transverse sinus that was not fully explained by the anatomical finding on venography. Furthermore this gradient was eliminated after performing a cervical puncture which reduced the CSF pressure.

Karahalios et al (1996) also described a dural venous outflow obstruction found on cerebral venography and manometry in 5 out of 10 patients. A high pressure gradient was observed while those without obstruction had elevated right atrial pressure as well as elevated venous sinus pressure. The authors concluded that increased venous pressure was common in PTC, secondary to intracranial venous outlet obstruction and without anatomical obstruction.

In the same study, Karahalios proposed other hypotheses, such as obesity related cardiomyopathy with subsequent congestive heart failure, sleep apnea, carbon dioxide retention and increased intra-abdominal pressure. All these conditions benefited from diuretic therapy which reduced CSF production and also reduced the central plasma volume and hence venous pressure.

A recent study by Nodelmann (2009) observed that jugular vein valve insufficiency in patients with PTC supports the hypothesis that increased ICP may be a result of a more general state of venous hypertension, possibly associated with obesity.

Several studies focusing on the appearance of outflow obstruction on MRI and MRV (Farb et al, 2003; Johnston et al., 2002;) produced inconclusive results due to the wide variations of radiological appearances of posterior fossa dural sinuses, which may be confused with a normal anatomical variant (Lee & Brazis, 2000).

Higgins et al (2004) published a study comparing 20 patients with PTC who had undergone MRV and a control group of 40 healthy volunteers, strictly selected. Patients with a history of headaches or other signs or symptoms related to cranial venous involvement were excluded. All subjects were matched for age and sex. A significant difference was observed in the appearance of the lateral sinus between the 2 groups; bilateral lateral sinus flow gaps were seen in 13 out of 20 (65%) PTC patients compared to none in the control group.

A new imaging method proposed by Farb et al. (2003) is auto-triggered elliptic-centric-ordered three-dimensional gadolinium-enhanced MR venography, which may be superior to time of flight MR venography in its flow insensitivity and decreased artifactual signal loss. Using this new technique, bilateral sinovenous stenosis was found in 27 out of 29 (93%) PTC patients compared to only 4 out of 59 (6.5%) in the control group. The authors concluded that the distal transverse sinus is the area of pressure gradient as described in King et al's study (1995).

Farb et al (2003) described two types of dural narrowing a "long smooth tapered narrowing", indicating an extra luminal compressive stenosis, and the "acutely marginated apparent intraluminal filling defect", indicating an enlarged, partially obstructing, intraluminal arachnoid granulation. They concluded that in PTC patients, increased dural venous pressure is measurable; however, whether this is a primary cause, a contributory factor, or a secondary phenomenon is uncertain.

Two opposing hypotheses can be made. The first proposes that dural sinus stenosis should be considered as the primary cause of PTC (fixed stenosis). Kollar et al. (2001) proposed that the transverse sinus is narrowed or obstructed by venous sinus thrombosis, vasculitis, congenital stenosis, enlarged arachnoid granulations or even heterotropic brain.

A recently published paper by De Lucia et al (2006) supports the suggested speculation that PTC is a long term sequela of previous sinus vein thrombosis or of an unidentified thrombus (Nedelmann et al., 2009; Sussman et al., 1997). In their study, 17 PTC patients without radiographic evidence of thrombosis were compared to healthy controls. The results showed a significant predominance of hypercoagulability markers, including protein C deficiency, increased plasma levels of prothrombin fragment 1 and 2, fibrinopeptide A, gene polymorphism for factor V leiden mutation, and high titers of cardiolipin antibodies.

The second hypothesis, in contrast to the fixed stenosis theory, suggests a dynamic one, where venous obstruction is the consequence and not the primary cause of intracranial hypertension. An increased intracranial pressure due to some unknown cause will result in a compression of the vascular compartment and dural sinuses which is in agreement with the Monroe-Kellie doctrine (Corbett, 2004). It is presumed that the predisposition to this phenomenon is due to the anatomy of the distal transverse sinus. Studies have shown that after normalization of the CSF pressure, resolution of the dural sinus narrowing occurs.

5. Endocrinological and metabolic factors

The association between PTC, female gender and obesity suggests an endocrine basis for this disorder. Reports of PTC occurring in corticosteroid deficient states such as Addison's disease, and following the removal of an ACTH secreting pituitary adenoma (Ross & Wilson, 1988), implies abnormalities in the adrenal pituitary axis. Furthermore, corticosteroids effectively treat PTC and corticosteroid withdrawal is associated with PTC (Yasargil et al., 1990). However, Soelberg Sørensen et al. (1986) found no consistent abnormality in pituitary, gonadal, thyroid or adrenal function. Multiple studies have documented the clear association between PTC and polycystic ovaries. In one study conducted by Glueck et al. (2003), 15 women out of 38 PTC patients were found to have

PCOS; 14 were obese, with a body-mass index (BMI) >30 kg/m² and 10 were extremely obese (BMI > or = 40).

6. Excess CSF production

Quincke (1893) was the first to describe excess CSF production. The rate of CSF production can be measured through invasive procedures (Walker, 2001). Donaldson found an increased CSF rate, while other studies failed to demonstrate CSF hypersecretion in PTC patients (Binder et al., 2004; Walker, 2001). A noninvasive technique (MRI) to measure CSF production by recording the flow through the cerebral aqueduct produced highly variable results, which did not support the theory of CSF overproduction in PTC patients (Gideon et al., 1994). In an attempt to rule out this theory, experimental infusion of artificial CSF was injected into the lateral ventricles of dogs which led to ventricular enlargement, not a PTC-like syndrome (Greitz et al., 1992; Walker, 2001).

7. CSF outflow reduction

This theory, supported by most studies, proposes the pathogenesis of CSF outflow obstruction into the venous system, although existing reports are still controversial. Studies have shown that PTC is associated with CSF outflow impairment (Calabrese et al., 1978; Cameron, 1933; Malm et al., 1992; Martins, 1974) and no histological evidence of arachnoid villi granulation dysfunction. Controversy exists as to whether impairment of CSF outflow at the arachnoid granulation level may be pathophysiological. In infancy, agenesis, deficiency, or dyslasia of the arachnoid villi and granulations result in hydrocephalus, not PTC (Gilles & Davidson, 1971).

Studies have demonstrated that in cases of elevated intracranial pressure attributed to high protein concentration in the CSF, (spinal tumor, Guillian-Barre syndrome), some patients develop hydrocephalus while others develop a PTC- like syndrome (Feldmann et al., 1986; Raichle et al., 1978; Ridsdale & Moseley, 1978; Ropper & Marmarou, 1984). It has been suggested that a high concentration of protein in CSF, may lead directly to impairment of CSF outflow.

8. Chronic inflammation

Recent reviews by Binder et al (2004) suggest that increased levels of cytokines and leptins (an adipocyte derivative hormone that circulates in the plasma at levels in proportion to body fat) in the CSF, may contribute to chronic inflammation and pathogenesis of intracranial hypertension in PTC patients.

Hypercoagulable states, devoid of obvious dural sinus thrombosis, have been reported associated with and in some cases used to explain PTC's mechanism. Kesler reported on several individuals found to have antiphospholipid antibodies and hyperfibrinogenemia related to thrombosis (Kesler et al. 2000; Kesler et al., 2010).

9. Drug associated

Numerous published reports and studies have described the correlation between certain drugs and vitamins and the development of increased intracranial pressure. These include antibiotics such as tetracycline or minocycline (Giles & Soble, 1971), fluoroquinolones

(Winrow & Supramaniam, 1990), naladixicacids (Cohen, 1973), sulfamethozaxole (Ch'ien, 1976) and hormonal treatments such as oral contraceptives, growth hormones, progesterone (Hamed et al., 1989; Rogers et al., 1999; Walsh et al., 1965), corticosteroid withdrawal (Neville & Wilson,1970), lithium (Saul et al, 1985) and vitamin A use and its derivatives (Morrice et al., 1960, Spector & Carlisle, 1984; Visani, 1996) in doses exceeding 50,000 UI in adults and over 20,000 UI in children.

10. Systemic conditions

In the literature, various systemic diseases have been found to be associated with PTC, the most common being uremia (Campos & Olitsky, 1995) Toxic conditions, hypervitaminosis A tetracycline therapy, lithium,prolonged steroid therpy, Steroid withdrawal,. Other diseases include anemia (Capriles, et al. 1963), dysthyroidism (Campos & Olitsky, 1995; Huseman & Torkelson, 1984), Addison's disease (Condulis et al., 1997) cerebral sinus thrombosis, and sleep apnea. .

11. Ancillary tests

11.1 Neuroimaging

The rationale for neuroimaging studies in PTC patients is twofold: prior to obtaining the cerebrospinal fluid, a brain imaging study is required to exclude any condition that would put the patient at risk of herniation, such as a tumor and to assure no secondary cause of increased ICP. The recommended study type has been modified together with the advance in neuroimaging technology. A CT scan is generally adequate as to ensure that the patient is not at risk when undergoing a lumbar puncture. The resolution is insufficient to exclude posterior fossa abnormalities, isodense lesions gliomatosis cerebri or venous sinus thrombosis. As either neuroimaging is acceptable, MRI of the brain with gadolinium is preferred over CT scanning with contrast.

11.2 MRI

Brain MRI is typically normal in the PTC patient, with a ventricular size normal for the patient's age. An asymptomatic empty sella is a well known neuroimaging finding in patients with increased intracranial pressure and may be present in over 50% of cases (Silbergleit et al., 1989). The empty sella (Figure 2) is attributed to longstanding effects of pulsatile CSF under high pressure, leading to downward herniation of an arachnocele through a defect in the diaphragma sella (George, 1989). The incidence of empty sella ranged from 10% when plain radiographs of the skull were analyzed (Sorenson et al., 1989) to 94% when third-generation CT scans were analyzed (Gibby et al., 1993).

Over the past few decades, other radiographic evidence of increased ICP in PTC patients has been detected using various neuroimaging techniques. Flattening of the posterior sclera is the most sensitive sign of elevated intracranial pressure, and was observed in 80% of patients with pseudotumor cerebri in Brodsky's study (Brodsky & Vaphiades, 1988). The flattening indicated transmission of elevated perioptic CSF pressure to the compressible posterior sclera. Jacobson (1995) found similar findings of bilateral posterior scleral flattening and distension of the perioptic subarachnoid space on MR imaging (Figure 3)in a patient with elevated intracranial pressure and unilateral papilledema. Furthermore, he emphasized that the constellation of acquired hyperopia and choroidal folds may indicate the presence of pseudotumor cerebri in rare patients whose distal optic nerves are structurally resistant to developing papilledema.

A study by Jinkins et al (1996) found intraocular protrusion of the swollen optic disc in 10 out of 15 patients with pseudotumor cerebri while examining the prelaminar optic nerves via MRI. The optic disc appeared hypointense to vitreous on T2-weighted images.

Upon administration of intravenous gadolinium, enhancement on T1 and T2 was produced in areas where the blood-brain barrier was absent or disrupted. Intraocular enhancement of the swollen disc was found in 50% of MR images of patients with PTC resulting from diffuse prelaminar capillary leakage secondary to severe venous congestion. Distension of the perioptic subarachnoid space was present in 45% of patients with pseudotumor cerebri. A finding of intraocular protrusion of the prelaminar optic nerve can be visualized well on CT scanning (Lam et al., 1997; Jinkins et al., 1996), however, on MRI, no signal differential between the swollen optic disc and the vitreous cavity was observed (Connolly et al., 1992; Foley & Posner, 1975; 1989; Gass et al., 1996; Gideon et al., 1995; Mashima et al., 1996; Silbergleit et al.).

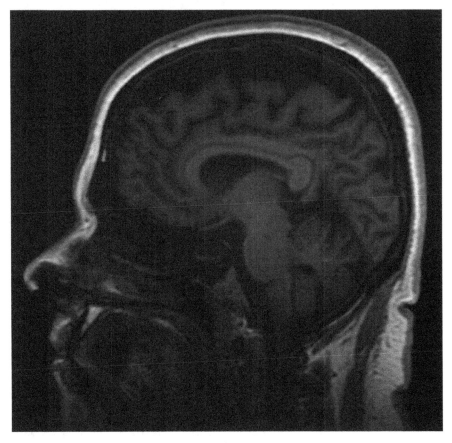

Fig. 2. MRI image demonstrating an empty sella in a 26 year old PTC patient

Brodsky (1998) observed vertical tortuosity of the optic nerves in 8 out of 20 (40%) patients with pseudotumor cerebri compared to only one control subject. Since some tortuosity may exist in normal subjects, the ability of axial MR imaging to display relatively minor degrees of horizontal tortuosity, makes it a relatively nonspecific finding. Furthermore, vertical tortuosity of the orbital optic nerve is often accompanied by a "smear sign" on T1-weighted images where the midportion of the optic nerve is displaced from the field of view, causing it to appear obscured by a "smear" of orbital fat. The optic nerve tortuosity or kinking in patients with elevated intracranial pressure is attributable to the distal fixation of the optic nerves by the globes tethered to the orbits by their rectus muscles and check ligaments.

Every patient suspected of PTC must routinely undergo an MRV or CTV examination. Both exams are equally reliable in identifying sinus vein thrombosis and therefore the decision of which examination to perform is entirely up to the expertise of the neurologist at the medical center.

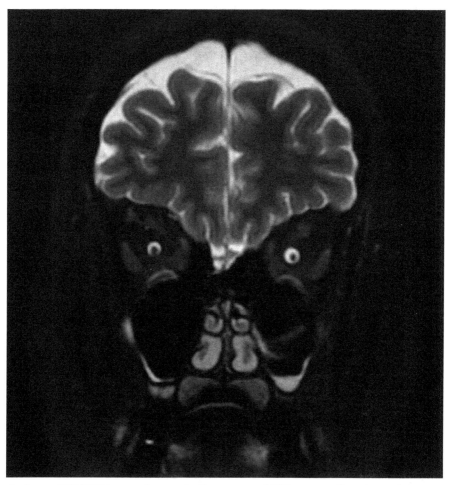

Fig. 3. Coronal T2 MRI image, demonstrating excess of CSF surrounding the optic nerves

11.3 MRV

PTC is consistently associated with venous outflow disturbances. Sinus venous stenosis are found on MR venography in the large majority of PTC patients and may have various conformations, ranging from functional smooth narrowing of sinus segments associated or not associated with definite flow gaps, to segmental hypoplasia or aplasia of one or more central venous collectors. Stenosis is currently believed to be a consequence of primary altered cerebrospinal fluid (CSF) pressure since it may normalize after CSF subtraction with lumbar puncture or shunting procedures (De Simone et al., 2010).

At present, the pathophysiologic mechanism of the elevated intracranial pressure in PTC remains unknown. Evidence suggests that perturbed venous efflux from the head may play a role in the etiology of the disease. Many studies suggest that elevated intracranial venous pressure, an underlying component of PTC, is the result of intracranial venous hypertension due to raised central venous pressure or disturbances of transverse sinuses (TSs) outflow (Brodsky et al., 1998; Friedman & Jacobson, 2002; Gass et al., 1996; Jacobson et al., 1990).

Occasionally, the clinical picture of PTC is the only clue to the presence of cerebral venous thrombosis, which may be a potentially devastating condition. Thus, every patient diagnosed with PTC must undergo an MRV or CTV to rule out this condition.

MRV is a noninvasive technique effective in visualizing cerebral venous sinuses (Mattle et al., 1991). Different MRV sequences offer the capability of investigating cerebral sinovenous outflow from multiple orientations such as two-dimensional time-offlight (2D-TOF) and three-dimensional phase-contrast (3D-PC) techniques. However, all these techniques have limitations and pitfalls (Ayanzen et al., 2000; Pipe, 2001).

A prospective study by Farb et al. (2003) suggested an auto-triggered elliptic-centric-ordered three-dimensional gadolinium enhanced MR venography (ATECO MRV) to evaluate the cerebral venous outflow of patients with PTC in combination with a novel scoring system. They found substantial bilateral sinovenous stenoses in 27 out of 29 (93%) patients with PTC compared to only 4 out of 59 in the controls and concluded that using ATECO MRV and a novel grading system for quantifying sinovenous stenoses, the authors could identify PTC patients with a sensitivity and specificity of 93%.

Higgins et al. (Higgins et al., 2004) described a distinctive pattern in the signal phase of contrast MRV in PTC patients. They found "signal gaps" in both lateral sinuses of PTC patients, unobserved in their control group. These "signal gaps" may indicate that flow velocities over that specific segment are outside the range prescribed in their study.

This finding does not necessarily mean that a thrombus is present nor does it inevitably indicate that abnormal arachnoid granulations might have caused a local alteration of blood flow. However, it does raise the possibility of stenosis or occlusion.

Higgins et al. (2002) reported the first patient with refractory PTC and transverse sinus stenosis treated with a stent. Direct cerebral venography and manometry confirmed the presence of stenoses with raised pressure, proximal to the obstructions. Dilation of one of the sinuses with a stent reduced the pressure gradient with dramatic symptomatic improvement.

Current evidence (Higgins et al., 2003; Metellus et al.; Ogungbo et al., 2003; 2005; Rajpal et al., 2005) suggests that selected patients with PTC may benefit from a transverse sinus (TS) stent. Restoring the patency of stenotic TSs with a stent in patients with refractory IIH resulted in a resolution or significant improvement in headache and papilledema.

11.4 CT and CTV

Neuroimaging utilizing CT offers rapid image acquisition, wide availability and excellent spatial resolution. The speed and ability of a CT to detect acute blood or bone abnormality makes this technique very valuable in traumatic cases.

Due to the rise in availability of MRI and MRV during the past few decades, and their known advantages over CT scans, the use of a CT as a neuroimaging tool in diagnosing PTC patients has lessened over the years. Current studies in the literature are focusing mainly on MRI and MRV findings in neuroimaging rather the CT.

Almost 25 years ago, Jinkins (1987) first reported on the reversal of the optic nerve head in a variety of conditions associated with increased intracranial pressure, including pseudotumor cerebri. Enlarged optic nerve sheaths have also been observed in patients with pseudotumor cerebri. Weisberg (1985) found that 2/28 patients had enlarged optic nerves, although no measurements were provided and no control values were available. Six out of 28 patients were described as having a "small-sized ventricular system." These examinations were performed on a second-generation CT scanner, without controls and in a non-blinded manner.

Almost two decades ago, Gibby et al. (1993) published a paper on CT findings in their PTC patients. The purpose of their study was to evaluate and compare orbital and cerebral CT findings in PTC patients with those of age and sex matched controls. Ventricular size in both groups was evaluated. Their findings matched Huckman et al's (1976) who found no differences between ventricular sizes of patients with pseudotumor cerebri and those of a control population.

Empty sellae have been associated with many conditions causing increased intracranial pressure. Gibby et al. in 1993 observed empty sellae in 5% of 788 autopsies (Kesler et al., 2001). In the PTC group, 16 (94%) out of 17 patients had at least partial empty sella. The degree of empty sellae was significantly greater than in the controls. The high prevalence noted in patients with pseudotumor cerebri is compatible with their chronic elevated intracranial pressure, which averaged 370 mm H2O. CT angiography uses a high speed spiral scanner, providing excellent vessel resolution with a 3-dimensional capability, comparable to an MRA. The technique requires iodinated dye and ionizing radiation and takes approximately 15 minutes. Sensitivities in detecting aneurysms >3mm or stenosis >70% are approximately 95%. Some centers prefer the use of a CTA over an MRA in identifying cerebral aneurysms, including those causing ocular motor cranial nerve palsies.

11.5 Visual field perimetry

Visual field testing by either automated Humphrey static or manual Goldmann perimetry reveals enlargement of the physiological blind spot in virtually all patients with PTC. Other common visual field defects include inferonasal loss and generalized constriction of the fields. Central defects, arcuate and altitudinal defects may occur but are highly unlikely. However, if found, a search is warranted for another cause, unless a large serous retinal detachment from a high-grade optic edema, spreading to the macula area, is found.

Almost all PTC patients suffer from some type of visual field loss over time. In prospective (Wall & George, 1987; Wall & George, 1991) studies of patients with PTC, visual field loss in at least 1 eye (other than an enlargement of the blind spot due to the edematous optic nerve) was found in 96% of patients using a Goldmann perimetry, a disease specific strategy and in 92% with automated perimetry. Approximately one third of this visual field loss was mild and was usually not noticed by the patient (Wall & George, 1991).

Wall et al's study (1991) showed that with treatment, about 50% of patients experience a significant visual field improvement. They further demonstrated that the only subgroup of patients who had a worsening of their visual fields were those with a recent weight gain. This was the only factor significantly associated with a decline in vision.

11.6 Ultrasound of optic nerve

Ultrasound has been used to identify intracranial hypertension by measuring the optic nerve sheath diameter. The modality is extremely safe and does not have any contraindications for use, except for ocular globe injuries (Munk et al., 1991). In most modern medical facilities, multipurpose ultrasound units with high-frequency transducers (>7.5 MHz) provide high lateral and axial precision (Berges et al., 2006).

Hayreh (1964) in an experimental study of monkeys and humans showed that the subarachnoid spaces surrounding the optic nerve is in continuity with the intracranial cavity, and therefore changes in cerebrospinal fluid pressure may be transmitted along the optic nerve sheath (Hayreh, 1964). The retrobulbar enlarged optic nerve sheath can therefore inflate as a consequence of raised pressure in the cerebrospinal fluid.

It has been confirmed that the optic nerve sheath diameter (ONSD) increases in patients with intracranial hypertension (Blaivas et al., 2005; Geeraerts et al., 2007; Girisgin et al., 2007; Karakitsos et al., 2006; Malayeri et al., 2005; Munk et al., 1991; Salgarello et al., 1996; Stone, 2009). ONSD alterations are correlated with head CT scan results in brain injured adults (Karakitsos et al., 2006) as well as with the invasive and noninvasive measurements of the ICP (Soldatos et al., 2008).

During US evaluation, it is important to perform a 30° test to evaluate excess of fluids within the arachnoid sheaths of the optic nerve. The patient is asked to turn approximately 30° toward the probe placed temporally on the globe. The measurements in abduction are compared with the measurements at the primary position. If fluid excess is present, the diameter at 30° will be smaller than that found in the primary position.

11.7 Optical coherence tomography (OCT)

OCT is a non-invasive imaging technique yielding high-resolution, cross-sectional images of the retina. More importantly, it is a valuable modality used to identify the status of the retinal nerve fiber layer as well as to measure macular thickness. The technique is principally based on measuring the time required for light to reflect from the tissue to an external detector (i.e. "echo time delay"). Duration of time and intensity of the backscattered light corresponds directly to the depth and density of the tissue being imaged. OCT produces in vivo cross-sections which can be serially acquired (in thin sections) in order to obtain tomographic images (Schuman et al., 2004).

The principles underlying OCT are similar to those of ultrasound imaging, except that light is utilized instead of sound. The axial resolution of OCT images is at least 1-2 orders of magnitude greater than those of ultrasound. OCT images of the retina provide a spatial resolution as low as 3-5 microns (Huang et al., 1991; Schuman et al., 2004).

Currently, two main types of OCT are utilized in practice: the time-domain, employing low-coherence interferometry for imaging tissue structures, and the spectral-domain OCT. Spectral-domain imaging provides faster and more spatially detailed images than the time-domain method. In addition, spectral domain OCT allows for imaging at a speed of 18,000 to approximately 40,000 A-scans per second, fast enough to eliminate artifacts from eye movements. It also provides a greater resolution of the retina with subsequent better visualization of the laminar structure and clarification of details at the cellular level within the nuclear layers (Choi et al., 2008). Several reports have also described particularly good reproducibility of RNFL and optic disc measurements with the newer spectral-domain technique (Gonzalez-Garcia, et al., 2009; Leung et al., 2009; Menke et al., 2008).

Computer-aided image processing algorithms have been developed to estimate NFL thickness from circumpapillary OCT images acquired in cylindrical sections surrounding the optic disc. A circumpapillary scan pattern of a typically ¾ mm diameter is used, because it effectively intercepts all nerve fibers originating from the optic disc, thus enabling a quantitative measurement of the circumferential variations in NFL thickness around the optic disc as well as visualization of the nerve fiber bundles.

Studies have demonstrated the effectiveness of time-domain OCT in providing a quantitative measure of the severity of disease, response to treatment and follow up monitoring of patients with PTC (Ophir et al., 2005; Rebolleda & Munoz-Negrete, 2009). RNFL thickness decreased correspondingly, with the improvement recorded at the patients' clinical evaluation. The study outcomes provided a basis for using OCT to predict which patients would ultimately fare better in terms of visual functional status (Rebolleda & Munoz-Negrete, 2009).

Precise measurements obtained with OCT allow the physician to more accurately evaluate the treatment effect than the subjective interpretation of the funduscopic appearance of the optic nerve heads. Recently, studies have emphasized the importance of viewing the macula in these patients. Hoye et al. (2001) evaluated the detection and monitoring of sub-retinal fluids extending from the optic nerve head to the macula in patients with papilledema. The authors found that the fluids accounted for the reduced visual acuity in 7 out of 55 patients, and when the volume of sub-retinal fluids decreased, an improvement in the visual acuity function was noted.

Future OCT assessment of papilledema will be evaluating the total optic nerve head disc volume and maximal optic nerve head height, as these measures potentially correlate with the response to medication and ultimate visual outcome. At present, clinical evaluation of the optic nerve head volume, better reflects the overall degree of optic nerve head edema rather than the thickness of the RNFL alone, since volume measurement incorporates the volume of both the total optic nerve height and the sub-retinal hypo reflective space. (Johnson et al., 2009).

11.8 Fluorescein angiography

Fluorescein angiography was initially developed as a tool for studying retinal vascular flow characteristics. Extensive use of fluorescein angiography and technique refinement has allowed the clinician and researcher to better understand the pathophysiologic and histopathologic changes of fundus disease in vivo. Fluorescein angiography may aid the clinician in accurately diagnosing papilledema by the appreciation of leakage or late hyperfluorescence surrounding the optic disc. Blocked hypofluorescence may be noted at the optic nerve head during papilledema as a result of bleeding, which is present at the level of the neurosensory retina, blocking the fluorescence from the underlying choroid (Rabb et al., 1978).

12. Management

There are nonsurgical and surgical approaches to PTC, decisions based on symptomatology and visual function status. If a headache is controlled by common analgesics and no optic nerve dysfunction is observed, therapy may not be required. Asymptomatic patients with preserved vision and minimal papilledema warrant only frequent follow-ups as well as monitoring disc swelling and visual function, including visual fields (Nonne, 1904).

12.1 Medical (nonsurgical) approach

Acetazolamide, a carbonic anhydrase inhibitor that decreases CSF production by the choroid plexus, is generally accepted as first-line medication, although its efficacy has not been proven in prospective trials. Based on our experience, a starting regimen of acetazolamide 500 mg, orally two or three times per day, is preferred. The dose can be increased to a total of 3 grams per day, if necessary. Major side effects include diuresis, loss of appetite, abnormal taste (metallic taste with carbonated beverages) paresthesias of the lips, fingers and toes, malaise, renal colic and metabolic acidosis (Corbett et al., 1982). Most of these side effects resolve with potassium and magnesium-rich dietary supplements such as bananas and oranges. Severe adverse effects experienced with acetazolamide treatment include acute tubular necrosis, hepatic dysfunction, and aplastic anemia.

Teratogenic effects in animals such as limb malformations and cortical dysgenesis have been reported (Quincke, 1893). Although sacrococcygeal teratoma in neonates (Tibussek et al., 2010) have been documented in the past, there is little clinical or experimental evidence to support any adverse effect of the drug on pregnancy outcome in humans (Spence et al., 1980). If acetazolamide fails, topiramate, an anti-epileptic drug, may be used. Its therapeutic effects are due to its carbonic anhydrase inhibitory properties. The drug is particularly useful as a prophylaxis for headaches, appetite suppression and weight loss (Nonne, 1904). The dose should be built up slowly over weeks (25 mg/week) in order to reduce the risk of cognitive side effects. It is of utmost importance to regularly check the intraocular pressure (IOP) of patients undergoing this treatment, as elevation of IOP is a known side effect of topamax.

Short-term oral corticosteroids may be considered as a treatment option in patients presenting with severe headaches, marked papilledema, and very high intracranial pressure. High doses of intravenous corticosteroid treatment may occasionally be administered when there is rapidly progressive vision loss or while the patient awaits surgery (Mathews et al., 2003).

Treatment medication is usually given over a long period of time. ICP-lowering agents may be tapered and eventually discontinued when the patient's visual status and optic nerve appearance have improved and stabilized. Patients should be periodically monitored post treatment, since recurrences are common. If symptoms reoccur, reinstitution of medications is usually indicated (Friedman & Jacobson, 2004).

Weight loss is a crucial part of the treatment program, as even moderately obese patients may significantly benefit from a sensible diet and exercise program (Mathews et al., 2003). Medications known as associated risk factors for pseudotumor syndromes, such as vitamin A, vitamin A derivatives, and tetracycline should be discontinued if possible.

12.2 Lumbar puncture

In the past, repeated lumbar punctures were an acceptable treatment modality due to improvement of symptoms after the procedure. Nowadays, this type of treatment approach is less acceptable. Currently, lumbar puncture may be indicated in pregnant women or when the clinical picture points to rapidly declining vision, thus temporarily lowering the CSF pressure while planning a more aggressive treatment (Friedman & Jacobson, 2004). In the past serial lumbar punctures (e.g., twice weekly) have been proposed as an alternative to surgery for patients with papilledema, when the disease cannot be controlled medically. Complications of the procedure such as infection, tonsillar herniation, radiculopathy, and arachnoiditis are rare.

12.3 Surgical approach
The most frequent and accepted indication for surgery is a progressive loss of vision despite maximal medical therapy. Surgery should be carried out as soon as a visual field defect worsens or remains unimproved despite maximal treatment. Medical treatment fails in approximately 18% to 22% of patients with PTC (Burgett et al., 1997; Corbett & Thompson, 1989; Lorberboym et al., 2001; Lueck & McIlwaine, 2002; Pearson et al., 1991). According to Friedman et al (2004), ophthalmological indications for surgical intervention are severe or rapid visual loss at onset ("malignant IIH"), severe papilledema causing macular edema or exudates without improvement while undergoing medical treatment. Even if there is no consensus among the specialists (Friedman & Jacobson, 2004), surgery should be considered in the management of intractable headaches (Binder et al., 2004; Mathews et al., 2003). Surgical treatment options include optic nerve sheath fenestration (ONSF) and CSF diversion procedures. A CSF shunt reduces intracranial hypertension, whereas ONSF focuses on protecting the vulnerable optic nerve head.

12.4 Optic nerve sheath decompression (ONSD)
The mechanism by which ONSD works has not been clarified, but several theories have been suggested. Keltner (1988) suggests that it may provide a filtering effect, with a subsequent decrease in the local CSF pressure, improvement of the peripapillary circulation (Keltner, 1988), or produce a generalized decrease in ICP. According to another hypothesis, the scarring of the arachnoid by the procedure itself may protect the nerve head from elevated CSF pressure (Friedman & Jacobson, 2004). Technically, ONSD is performed by uncovering the optic nerve sheath through a lateral orbitotomy or through a medial approach via a transconjunctival incision. Multiple linear incisions are made or a window is cut into the anterior dural that covers the optic nerve sheath, creating a CSF drainage outlet (Mathews et al., 2003).
The overall complication rate of ONSD ranges from 4.8% to 45% (151,165,166,167,168), the most common being extraocular motility problems due to lateral rectus palsy which is usually transient, and papillary abnormalities. Other complications may include long-term and transient blindness due to ischemic injury to the optic nerve, orbital hemorrhage, visual field defects and globe perforation (Friedman & Jacobson, 2004). In the majority of patients, post-ONSD vision stabilizes or improves in the long-term, but as many as 32% of operated eyes may experience deterioration following initially successful surgery (McHenry & Spoor, 1993). A reoperation can be performed, but based on clinical experience, a shunting procedure is recommended in these cases.

12.5 Lumbar peritoneal shunt (L-P shunt)
Although an L-P shunt is considered an effective procedure, failure and low pressure-related headaches are common. Shunts may be efficiently placed in the lumbar cistern,

cisterna magna, or the ventricles. The lumboperitoneal (L-P) technique has traditionally been the method of choice in PTC.
A review of the literature Binder et al (2004) found that the efficacy of L-P shunting is maintained as long as the shunt remains patent. The failure rate for LP shunts range from 38% to 64% (Burgett et al., 1997; Gupta et al., 2007; Johnston et al., 1988). Major causes include catheter obstruction, over-shunting (low pressure headaches), catheter migration, and lumbar radiculopathy.

12.6 Ventriculoperitoneal (V-P) shunts
A V-P shunt is difficult to perform due to relatively small or normal ventricle size. However, this technique is becoming increasingly popular in treating PTC (Binder et al., 2004; Maher et al., 2001; Tulipan et al., 1998).
In the long-term, V-P shunts offer advantages compared to the L-P shunt method, especially with regard to shunt revision (Kang, 2000; Maher et al., 2001). The procedure does not present the risk of inducing a Chiari I malformation, and may be less likely to over-drain.
A wider range of shunts are available for the V-P route. Usually, PTC patients benefit from relatively high-pressure valves (possibly with an antisiphon system to limit over-drainage), which are able to retain sufficient intracranial CSF to compensate the changing intracranial volume conditions and limit the collapse of the ventricular system around the shunt catheter. Flow-regulated valves have also been proposed (Garton, 2004).

12.7 Subtemporal decompression
The first neurosurgical technique to treat PTC patients, by a subtemporal decompression, was performed in 1937 (Dandy, 1937). Dandy performed a unilateral subtemporal craniectomy with excellent initial results in alleviating headaches and preventing visual loss. The long-term efficacy of the procedure was uncertain, since a high rate of morbidity and complications were reported, including seizures, infections, focal brain damage, cosmetic disfigurement, intracranial hematomas, and further visual deterioration (Binder et al., 2004). After introducing stenting procedures for treating IIH, this procedure became obsolete; nonetheless, subtemporal decompression is still an option, when other surgical methods have failed.

12.8 Endovascular stenting
It is highly controversial whether venous sinus narrowing is the cause or the result of elevated intracranial pressure. Based on the frequent findings in MRI venography of narrowed transverse sinuses, endovascular stenting of the venous sinuses has been recently advocated by some authors (Higgins et al., 2002; Higgins et al., 2003; Metellus et al., 2005; Metellus et al., 2007; Donnet et al., 2008; Paquet et al., 2008).
Higgins et al (2002) was the first to report on a 30 year old patient with refractory PTC, papilledema and bilateral TS stenosis found on an MR venogram, that was successfully treated with dilation of 1 of the sinuses with a stent, thus reducing the pressure gradient with dramatic symptomatic improvement.
As of today, only about 40 patients with PTC, treated with sinovenous stent placement, have been reported in the literature. Most were women aged 15-65, symptomatic with PTC for 2 weeks to 15 years. After stent placement, 33 out of the 40 (82.5%), reported a significant improvement in their headaches. Papilledema improved or resolved in 30 out of 33 (91%)

patients who presented with active papilledema. Although the promising initial results of long term efficiency of the procedure still needs to be proven, further investigation is still warranted to prove the procedure as a useful treatment technique.

12.9 Pregnancy and PTC

Current reports suggest that pregnant patients with PTC can be safely managed similarly to nonpregnant patients with PTC. No increase in the rate of spontaneous abortion or fetal wastage has been reported. A therapeutic abortion to limit the progression of the disease is not indicated. (Tang et al., 2004).

Acetazolamide had previously been considered as the preferred therapy after 20 weeks of gestation, since sacrococcygeal teratoma was reported with earlier use (Digre et al., 1984). A recent report of 12 women treated with acetazolamide for PTC during pregnancy, showed no adverse pregnancy outcomes in terms of fetal loss or congenital malformation. Acetazolamide at high doses may produce birth defects in animals, but there is little clinical or experimental evidence to support any adverse effect on pregnancy outcome in humans. If the clinical situation mandates acetazolamide use in PTC, the drug can be offered after appropriate informed consent (Lee et al., 20050). Management of labor and indications for cesarean delivery for a parturient with PTC are controversial. Regular labor may be allowed with a cesarean delivery reserved for obstetric indications.

13. Natural history and visual prognosis

The natural history of PTC is unknown. In some cases, it is a self-limited condition, while in others ICP may remain elevated for many years even if systemic and visual symptoms resolve. In some patients, the process may last from months to years. Individuals with mild to moderate visual loss tend to recover vision following medical therapy. Papilledema usually resolves after a few weeks or months, but many patients are left with some residual disc elevation, especially nasally. Severe visual impairment may be a serious and permanent complication of PTC. PTC produces significant visual impairment in approximately 25% of patients. The risk of visual loss in the pediatric PTC population is similar to that of adults (Corbett & Thompson, 1989). Recurrent symptoms have been reported in 8 to 37% of patients, years after being diagnosed (Corbett & Thompson, 1989). Visual deterioration in PTC patients is usually gradual, but in cases of fulminant papilledema, blindness may appear rather quickly. In Corbett et al's (1989) follow up study of 5 - 41 years after the initial diagnosis of 57 patients, revealed severe visual impairment in 14 patients (24.6%). In Kesler et al's experience (2004), recurrence was frequently associated with weight gain. The long-term prognosis and visual outcome of 54 patients with IIH was observed over a period of 6.2 years. The results showed that recurrences occurred in almost 40% of the cases. None of these exacerbations occurred during the first 10 months, and none occurred while the patients continued treatment.

14. References

Ahlskog, J.E., & O'Neill, B.P. (1982). Pseudotumor cerebri. *Annals of Internal Medicine*, Vol. 97, No. 2 (August 1982), pp. 249-256

Ayanzen, R.H., Bird, C.R., Keller, P.J., McCully, F.J., Theobald, M.R., & Heiserman, J.E. (2000). Cerebral MR venography: normal anatomy and potential diagnostic pitfalls. *American Journal of Neuroradiology* Vol. 21, No. 1, (January 2000), pp. 74-78

Balcer, L.J., Liu, G.T., Forman, S., Pun, K., Volpe, N.J., Galetta, S.L., & Maguire, M.G. (1999). Idiopathic intracranial hypertension: relation of age and obesity in children. *Neurology* Vol. 52, No. 4, (March 1999), pp. 870-872

Bateman, G.A., Smith, R.L., & Siddique, S.H. (2007). Idiopathic hydrocephalus in children and idiopathic intracranial hypertension in adults: two manifestations of the same pathophysiological process? *Journal of Neurosurgery*, Vol. 107, No. 6 Suppl, pp. 439-444.

Bateman, G.A. (2004). Idiopathic intracranial hypertension: priapism of the brain? *Medical Hypotheses*, Vol. 63, No. 3, (March 2004), pp, 549-552.

Berges, O., Koskas, P., Lafitte, F., & Piekarski, J.D. (2006). Sonography of the eye and orbit with a multipurpose ultrasound unit. *Journal of Radiology*, Vol. 87, No. 4 Pt 1, pp. 345-353.

Bicakci, K., Bicakci, S., & Aksungur, E. (2006). Perfusion and diffusion magnetic resonance imaging in idiopathic intracranial hypertension. *Acta Neurologica Scandinavica*, Vol. 114, No. 3, (September 2006), pp. 193-197.

Binder, D.K., Horton, H.C., Lawton, M.T., & McDermott, M.W. (2004). Idiopathic intracranial hypertension. *Neurosurgery* Vol. 54, No. 3, (March 2004), pp. 538-552.

Blaivas, M., Theodoro, D., & Sierzenski, PR. (2003). Elevated intracranial pressure detected by bedside emergency ultrasonography of optic nerve sheath. *Academic Emergency Medicine*, Vol. 10, No. 4, (April 2003), pp. 376-381.

Brodsky, M.C., & Vaphiades, M. (1998). Magnetic resonance imaging in pseudotumor cerebri. *Ophthalmology* Vol. 105, No. 5, (September 1998), pp. 1686-1693.

Brooks, D.J., Beaney, R.P., Leenders, K.L., Marshall, J., Thomas, D.J., & Jones, T. (1985). Regional cerebral oxygen utilization, blood flow, and blood volume in benign intracranial hypertension studied by positron emission tomography. *Neurology* Vol. 35, No. 7, (July 1985), pp. 1030-1034.

Burgett, R.A., Purvin, V.A., & Kawasaki, A. (1997). Lumboperitoneal shunting for pseudotumor cerebri. *Neurology* Vol. 49, No. 3, (September 1997), pp. 734-739.

Busch, W. (1951). Die Monphologie den Sella Turcica und ihre Heziehungen zur Hypophyse. *Virchows Archiv A: Pathological Anatomy Histopathology*, Vol. 320, No. 5, (September 1951), pp. 437-458.

Campos, S.P., & Olitsky, S. (1995). Idiopathic intracranial hypertension after l-thyroxine therapy for acquired primary hypothyroidism. *Clinical Pediatrics*, Vol. 34, No. 6, (June 1995), pp. 334-337.

Calabrese, V.P., Selhorst, J.B., & Harbison, J.W. (1978). CSF infusion test in pseudotumor cerebri. *Transactions of the American Neurological Association*, Vol. 103, pp. 146-150.

Cameron, A.J. (1933). Marked papilloedema in pulmonary emphysema. *British Journal of Ophthalmology*, Vol. 17, No. 3, (March 1933), pp. 167-169.

Capriles, L.F. (1963). Intracranial hypertension and iron-deficiency anemia. *Archives of Neurology,*Vol. 9, pp. 147-153.

Chang, D., Nagamoto, G., & Smith, W.E. (1992). Benign intracranial hypertension and chronic renal failure. *Cleveland Clinic Journal of Medicine,*Vol. 59, No. 4, (July-August 1992), pp. 419-422.

Ch'ien, L.T. (1976). Intracranial hypertension and sulfamethoxazole. *New England Journal of Medicine*, Vol. 283, No. 1, (July 1970), pp. 47.

Choi, S.S., Zawadzki, R.J., Keltner, J.L., & Werner, J.S. (2008). Changes in cellular structures revealed by ultra-high resolution retinal imaging in optic neuropathies. *Investigative Ophthalmology & Visual Science*, Vol. 49, No. 5, (May 2008), pp. 2103-2119.

Cinciripini, G.S., Donahue, S., & Borchert, M.S. (1999). Idiopathic intracranial hypertension in prepubertal pediatric patients: characteristics, treatment, and outcome. *American Journal of Ophthalmology*, Vol. 127, No. 2, (February 1999), pp. 178-182.

Corbett, J.J. (2008). The first Jacobson Lecture. Familial idiopathic intracranial hypertension. *Journal of Neuroophthalmology*, Vol. 28, No. 4, (December 2008), pp. 337-347.

Corbett, J.J., & Mehta, M.P. (1983). Cerebrospinal fluid pressure in normal obese subjects and patients with pseudotumor cerebri. *Neurology* Vol. 33, No. 10, (October 1983), pp. 1386-1388.

Cohen, D.N. (1973). Intracranial hypertension and papilledema associated with nalidixic acid. *American Journal of Ophthalmology*, Vol. 76, No. 5, (November 1973), pp. 680-682.

Condulis, N., Germain, G., Charest, N., Levy, S., & Carpenter, T.O. (1997). Pseudotumor cerebri: a presenting manifestation of Addison's disease. *Clinical Pediatrics*, Vol. 36, No. 12, (December 1997), pp. 711-713.

Connolly, M.B., Farrell, K., Hill, A., & Flodmark, O. (1992). Magnetic resonance imaging in pseudotumor cerebri. *Development Medicine and Child Neurology*, Vol. 34, No. 12, (December 1992), pp. 1091-1094.

Corbett, J.J. (2004) Increased intracranial pressure: idiopathic and otherwise. *Journal of Neuro-Ophthalmology*, Vol. 24, No. 2, (June 2004), pp. 103-105.

Corbett, J.J., Savino, P.J., Thompson, H.S., et al. (1982).Visual loss in pseudotumor cerebri. Follow-up of 57 patients from five to 41 years and a profile of 14 patients with permanent severe visual loss. *Archives of Neurology*, Vol. 39, No. 8, (August 1982), pp. 461-474.

Crassard, I., & Bousser, M.G. (2004). Cerebral venous thrombosis. State of the art. *Journal of Neuro-Ophthalmology*, Vol. 24, No. 10, (October 1989), pp. 156-163.

Dandy, W.E. (1937). Intracranial pressure without brain tumor: diagnosis and treatment. *Annals of Surgery*, Vol. 106, No. 4, (October 1937), pp. 492-513.

De Lucia, D., Napolitano, M., Di Micco, P., *et al.* (2006). Benign intracranial hypertension associated to blood coagulation derangements. *Thrombosis Journal* Vol. 24, No. 4, (December 2006), pp. 21.

De Simone, R., Ranieri, A., & Bonavita, V. (2010). Advancement in idiopathic intracranial hypertension pathogenesis: focus on sinus venous stenosis. *Neurological Sciences*, Vol. 31, Supplement 1, (June 2010), pp. S33-S39.

Digre, K.B., Varner. M.W., & Corbett, J.J. (1984). Pseudotumor cerebri and pregnancy. *Neurology*, Vol. 34, No. 6, (June 1984), pp. 721-729.

Donnet, A., Metellus, P., Levrier, O., et al. (2008). Endovascular treatment of idiopathic intracranial hypertension: clinical and radiologic outcome of 10 consecutive patients. *Neurology*, Vol. 70, No.8, (February 2008), pp. 641-647.

Durcan, F.J., Corbett, J.J., & Wall, M. (1988). The incidence of pseudotumor cerebri: population studies in Iowa and Louisiana. *Archives of Neurology*, Vol. 45, No. 8, (August 1988), pp. 875-877.

Farb, R.I., Vanek, I., Scott, J.N., Procopis, P. & Antony, J. (2003). Idiopathic intracranial hypertension: the presence and morphology of sinovenous stenosis. *Neurology,* Vol. 60, No. 9, (May 2003), pp. 1418-1424.

Farb, R.I.,Vanek, I., Scott, J.N. *et al.* (2003). Idiopathic intracranial hypertension: The prevalence and morphology of sinovenous stenosis. *Neurology* Vol. 60, No. 9, (May 2003), pp. 1418-1424.

Feldmann, E., Bromfield, E., Navia, B., Pasternak, G.W., & Posner, J.B. (1986). Hydrocephalic dementia and spinal cord tumor. *Archives of Neurology,* Vol. 43, No. 7, (July 2006), pp. 714-718.

Foley, K.M. & Posner, J.B. (1975). Does pseudotumor cerebri cause the empty sella syndrome? *Neurology,* Vol. 25, No. 6, (June 1975), pp. 565-569.

Foley, J. (1955). Benign forms of intracranial hypertension. Toxic and otitic hydrocephalus. *Brain,* Vol. 78, No. 1, pp. 1-41.

Friedman, D.I., & Jacobson, D.M. (2002). Diagnostic criteria for idiopathic intracranial hypertension. *Neurology,* Vol. 59, No. 10, (November 2002), pp.1492-1495.

Friedman, D.I. & Jacobson, D.M. (2004). Idiopathic intracranial hypertension. State of art. *Journal of Neuro-Ophthalmology,* Vol. 24, No. 2, (June 2004), pp. 138-145.

Garton, H.J.L. (2004). Cerebrospinal fluid diversion procedures. *Journal of Neuro-Ophthalmology,* Vol. 24, No. 2, (June 2004), pp. 146-155.

Gass, A., Barker, G.J., Riordan-Eva, P., *et al.* (1996). MRI of the optic nerve in benign intracranial hypertension. *Neuroradiology* Vol. 38, No. 8, (November 1996), pp. 769 - 773.

Geeraerts, T., Launey, Y., Martin, L., *et al.* (2007). Ultrasonography of the optic nerve sheath may be useful for detecting raised intracranial pressure after severe brain injury. *Intensive Care Medicine,* Vol. 33, No. 10, (October 2007), pp. 1704-1711.

George, A.E. (1989). Idiopathic intracranial hypertension: pathogenesis and the role of MR imaging. *Radiology,* Vol. 170 (1 Pt 1), pp. 21-22.

Gideon, P., Sfrensen, P.S., Thomsen, C. *et al.* (1995). Increased brain water self- diffusion in patients with idiopathic intracranial hypertension. *American Journal of Neuroradiology,* Vol. 16, No. 2, (February 1995), pp. 381-387.

Gideon, P., Sorensen, P.S., Thomsen, C., *et al* (1994) Assessment of CSF dynamics and venous flow in the superior sagittal sinus by MRI in idiopathic intracranial hypertension: a preliminary study. *Neuroradiology,* Vol. 36, No. 5, (July 1994), pp. 350-354.

Gibby, W.A., Cohen, M.S., Goldberg, H.I., & Sergott, R.C. (1993). Pseudotumor cerebri: CT findings and correlation with vision loss. *American Journal of Roentgenology,* Vol. 160, No. 1, (January 1993), pp. 143-146.

Giles, C., & Soble, A. (1971). Intracranial hypertension and tetracycline therapy. *American Journal of Ophthalmology,* Vol. 72, No. 2, (November 1971), pp. 981-982.

Gilles, F.H., & Davidson, R.I. (1971). Communicating hydrocephalus associated with deficient dysplastic parasagittal arachnoidal granulations. *Journal of Neurosurgery,* Vol. 35, No. 4, (October 1971), pp. 421-426.

Girisgin, A.S., Kalkan, E., Kocak, S., *et al.* (2007). The role of optic nerve ultrasonography in the diagnosis of elevated intracranial pressure. *Emergency Medicine Journal,* Vol. 24, No. 4, (April 2007), pp. 251-254.

Glueck, C.J., Iyengar, S., Goldenberg, N., Smith, L.S., & Wang, P. (2003). Idiopathic intracranial hypertension: associations with coagulation disorders and polycystic-ovary syndrome. *Journal of Laboratory and Clinical Medicine*, Vol. 142, No. 1, (July 2003), pp. 35-45.

Gonzalez-Garcia, A.O., Vizzeri, G., Bowd, C., *et al.* (2009). Reproducibility of RTVue retinal nerve fiber layer thickness and optic disc measurements and agreement with stratus optical coherence tomography measurements. *American Journal of Ophthalmology*, Vol. 147, No. 6, (June 2009), pp. 1067-1074.

Greitz, D., Wirestam, R., Franck, A., *et al.* (1992). Pulsatile brain movement and associated hydrodynamics studied by magnetic resonance phase imaging. The Monro-Kellie doctrine revisited. *Neuroradiology*, Vol. 34, No. 5, pp. 370-380.

Gupta, A.K., Gupta, A., Kumar, S., & Lal, V. (2007). Endoscopic endonasal management of pseudotumor cerebri: is it effective? *Laryngoscope*, Vol. 117, No. 7, (July 2007), pp. 1138-1142.

Hamed, L.M., Glaser, J.S., Schatz, N.J., & Perez, T.H. (1989). Pseudotumor cerebri induced by danazol. *American Journal of Ophthalmology*, Vol. 107, No. 2, (February 1989), pp. 105-110.

Hayreh, S.S. (1964). Pathogenesis of oedema of the optic disk (papilloedema), a preliminary report. *British Journal of Ophthalmology*. Vol. 48, (October 1964), pp. 522-543.

Hayreh, S.S. (1977). Optic disc edema in raised intracranial pressure. VI. Associated visual disturbances and their pathogenesis. *Archives of Ophthalmology*, Vol. 95, No. 9, (September 1977), pp. 1566-1579.

Higgins, J.N., Owler, B.K., Cousins, C., *et al.* (2002). Venous sinus stenting for refractory benign intracranial hypertension. *Lancet*, Vol. 359, No. 9302, (January 2002), pp. 228-230.

Higgins, J.N.P., Cousins, C., Owler, B.K., *et al.* (2003). Idiopathic intracranial hypertension: 12 cases treated by venous sinus stenting. *Journal of Neurology, Neurosurgery & Psychiatry*, Vol. 74, No. 12, (December 2003), pp. 1662-1666.

Higgins, J.N.P., Gillard, J.H., Owler, B.K., Harkness, K., & Pickard, J.D. (2004). MR venography in idiopathic intracranial hypertension: unappreciated and misunderstood. *Journal of Neurology, Neurosurgery & Psychiatry*, Vol. 75, No. 4, (April 2004), pp. 621-625.

Holt, G.R., & Holt, J.E. (1983). Incidence of eye injuries in facial fractures: an analysis of 727 cases. *Otolaryngology- Head and Neck Surgery*. Vol. 91, No. 3, (June 1983), pp. 276-279.

Hoye, V.J., III, Berrocal, A.M., Hedges, T.R., III, & Maro-Quireza, M.L. (2001). Optical coherence tomography demonstrates subretinal macular edema from papilledema. *Archives of Ophthalmology*, Vol. 119, No. 9, (September 2001), pp. 1287-1290.

Huang, D., Swanson, E.A., Lin, C.P., *et al.* (1991). Optical coherence tomography. *Science*, Vol. 254, No. 5035, (November 1991), pp. 1178-1181.

Huckman, M.S., Fox, J.S., Ramsey, R.G., *et al.* (1976). Computed tomography in the diagnosis of pseudotumor cerebri. *Radiology*, Vol. 119, No. 3, (June 1976), pp. 593-597.

Huseman, C.A., & Torkelson, R.D. (1984). Pseudotumor cerebri following treatment of hypothalamic and primary hypothyroidism. *American Journal of Diseases of Children*, Vol. 138, No. 10, (October 1984), pp. 927-931.

Jacobson, D.M. (1995). Intracranial hypertension and the syndrome of acquired hyperopia with choroidal folds. *Journal of Neuroophthalmology*, Vol. 15, No. 3, (September 1995), pp. 178-185.

Jacobson, D.M., Karanjia, P.N., Olson, K.A., & Warner, J.J. (1990). Computed tomography ventricular size has no predictive value in diagnosing pseudotumor cerebri. *Neurology*, Vol. 40, No. 9, (September 1990), pp. 1454-1455.

Jinkins, J.R. (1987). "Papilledema": neuroradiologic evaluation of optic disk protrusion with dynamic orbital CT. *American Journal of Radiology*, Vol. 149, No. 4, (October 1987), pp. 793-802.

Jinkins, J.R., Athale, S., Xiong, L., *et al.* (1996). MR of optic papilla protrusion in patients with high intracranial pressure. *American Journal of Neuroradiology*, Vol. 17, No. 4, (April 1996), pp. 665-668.

Johnson, L.N., Diehl, M.L., Hamm, C.W., Sommerville, D.N., & Petroski, G.F. (2009). Differentiating optic disc edema from optic nerve head drusen on optical coherence tomography. *Archives of Ophthalmology*, Vol. 127, No. 1, (January 2009), pp. 45-49.

Johnston, I., Besser, M., & Morgan, M. (1988). Cerebrospinal fluid diversion in the treatment of benign intracranial hypertension. *Journal of Neurosurgery*, Vol. 69, No. 2, (August 1988), pp. 195-202.

Johnston, I., Kollar, C., Dunkley, S., Assaad, N., & Parker, G. (2002). Cranial venous outflow obstruction in the pseudotumour syndrome: incidence, nature and relevance. *Journal of Clinical Neuroscience*, Vol. 9, No. 3, (May 2002), pp. 273-278.

Kang, S. (2000). Efficacy of lumbo-peritoneal versus ventriculoperitoneal shunting for management of chronic hydrocephalus following aneurismal subarachnoid hemorrhage. *Acta Neurochirurgia* (Wien), Vol. 142, No. 1, pp. 45-49.

Karahalios, D.G., Rekate, H.L., Khayata, M.H., & Apostolides, P.J. (1996). Elevated intracranial venous pressure as a universal mechanism in pseudotumor cerebri of varying etiologies. *Neurology*, Vol. 46, No. 1, (January 1996), pp. 198-202.

Karakitsos, D., Soldatos, T., Gouliamos, A., Armaganidis, A., *et al.* (2006). Transorbital sonographic monitoring of optic nerve diameter in patients with severe brain injury. *Transplantation Proceedings*, Vol. 38, No. 10, (December 2006), pp. 3700-3706.

Kelman, S.E., Heaps, R., Wolf, A., & Elman, M.J. (1992). Optic nerve decompression surgery improves visual function in patients with pseudotumor cerebri. *Neurosurgery*, Vol. 30, No. 3, (March 1992), pp. 391-395.

Keltner, J.L. (1988). Optic nerve sheath decompression. How does it work? Has its time come? *Archives of Ophthalmology*, Vol. 106, No. 10, (October 1988), pp. 1365-1369.

Kesler, A., Ellis, M.H., Reshef, T., Kott, E., & Gadoth, N. (2000). Idiopathic intracranial hypertension and anticardiolipin antibodies. *Journal of Neurology Neurosurgery & Psychiatry*, Vol. 68, No. 3 (March 2000), pp. 379-380.

Kesler, A., Goldhammer, Y., & Gadoth, N. (2001). Do men with pseudomotor cerebri share the same characteristics as women? A retrospective review of 141 cases. *Journal of Neuroophthalmology*, Vol. 21, No.1, (March 2001), pp. 15-7.

Kesler, A., Hadayer, A., Goldhammer, Y., Almog, Y. & Korczyn, A.D. (2004). Idiopathic intracranial hypertension: risk of recurrences. *Neurology*, Vol. 63, No. 9, (November 2004), pp. 1737-1739.

Kesler, A., Kliper, E., Assayag, E.B., *et al.* (2010). Thrombophilic factors in idiopathic intracranial hypertension: a report of 51 patients and a meta-analysis. *Blood Coagulation & Fibrinolysis*, Vol. 21. No. 4, (June 2010), pp. 328-33.

Killer, H.E., Laeng, H.R., & Groscurth, P. (1999). Lymphatic capillaries in the meninges of the human optic nerve. Journal of Neuro-Ophthalmology, Vol. 19, No. 4, (December 1999), pp. 222-228.

King, J.O., Mitchell, P.J,, Thomson, K.R., & Tress, B.M. (1995). Cerebral venography and manometry in idiopathic intracranial hypertension. *Neurology*, Vol. 45, No. 12, (December 1995), pp. 2224-2228.

Kollar, C., Parker, G., & Johnston, I. (2001). Endovascular treatment of cranial venous sinus obstruction resulting in pseudotumor syndrome. Report of three cases. *Journal of Neurosurgery*, Vol. 94, No. 4, (April 2001), pp. 646-651.

Lam, B.L., Glasier, C.M., & Feuer, W.J. (1997). Subarachnoid fluid of the optic nerve in normal adults. Ophthalmology, Vol. 104, No. 10, (October 1997), pp. 1629-1633.

Lee, A.G., & Brazis, P.W. (2000), Magnetic resonance venography in idiopathic pseudotumor cerebri. *Journal of Neuroophthalmology*, Vol. 20, No. 1, (March 2000), pp. 12-13.

Lee, A.G., Pless, M., Falardeau, J., *et al.* (2005). The use of acetazolamide in idiopathic intracranial hypertension during pregnancy. *American Journal of Ophthalmology*, Vol. 139, No. 5 (May 2005), pp. 855-915.

Lessell, S. (1992). Pediatric pseudotumor cerebri (idiopathic intracranial hypertension). *Survey of Ophthalmology*, Vol. 37, No. 3, (November 1992), pp. 155-166.

Leung, C.K., Cheung, C.Y., Weinreb, R.N., *et al.* (2009). Retinal nerve fiber layer imaging with spectral-domain optical coherence tomography: a variability and diagnostic performance study. *Ophthalmology*, Vol. 116, No. 7, (July 2009), pp. 1257-1263.

Levine, D.N. (2000). Ventricular size in pseudotumor cerebri and the theory of impaired CSF absorption. *Journal of the Neurological Sciences*, Vol. 177, No. 2, (August 2000), pp. 85-94.

Lorberboym,M., Lampl, Y., Kesler, A., Sadeh, M., & Gadot, N. (2001). Benign intracranial hypertension: correlation of cerebral blood flow with disease severity. *Clinical Neurology and Neurosurgery*, Vol. 103, No.1, (April 2001), pp. 33-36.

Lueck, C., & McIlwaine, G. (2002). Interventions for idiopathic intracranial hypertension. *Cochrane Database System Review*, Vol 3, pp. CD003434.

Maher, C.O., Garrity, J.A., & Meyer, F.B. (2001). Refractory idiopathic intracranial hypertension treated with stereotactically planned ventriculoperitoneal shunt placement. *Neurosurgery Focus*, Vol. 10, No. 2, (February 2001), pp. 1-4.

Malayeri, A.A., Bavarian, S., & Mehdizadeh, M. (2005). Sonographic evaluation of optic nerve diameter in children with raised intracranial pressure. *Journal of Ultrasound Medicine*, Vol. 24, No. 2, (February 2005), pp. 143-147.

Malm, J., Kristensen, B., Markgren, P., & Ekstedt, J. (1992). CSF hydrodynamics in idiopathic intracranial hypertension: a longterm study. *Neurology*, Vol. 42, No. 4, (April 1992), pp. 851-858.

Mashima Y, Oshitari K, Imamura Y, et al.(1996) High-resolution magnetic resonance imaging of the intraorbital optic nerve and subarachnoid space in patients with papilledema and optic atrophy. *Arch Ophthalmol* Vol. 114, No. 10, (October 1996), pp. 1197–203.

Mathew, N.T., Ravishankar, K., & Sanin, L.C. (1996). Coexistence of migraine and idiopathic intracranial hypertension without papilledema. *Neurology*, Vol. 46, No. 5, (May 1996), pp. 1226-1230.

Mathews, M.K., Sergott, R.C. & Savino, P.J. (2003). Pseudotumor cerebri. *Current Opinion in Ophthalmology*, Vol. 14, No. 6, (December 2003), pp. 364-370.

Mattle, H.P.,Wentz ,K.U., Edelman, R., *et al.* (1991). Cerebral venography with MR. *Radiology*, Vol. 178, No. 2, (February 1991), pp. 453-458.

Martins, A.N. (1973). Resistance to drainage of cerebrospinal fluid: clinical measurement and significance. *Journal of Neurology Neurosurgery & Psychiatry*, Vol.36, No. 2, (April 1973), pp. 313-318.

Maxner, C.E., Freeman, M.I. & Corbett, J.J. (1987). Asymmetric papilledema and visual loss in pseudotumor cerebri. *Canadian Journal Neurological Sciences*, Vol. 4, No. 4, (November 1987), pp. 593-596.

McHenry, J.G., & Spoor, T.C. (1993). Optic nerve sheath fenestration for treatment of progressive ischemic optic neuropathy. *Archives of Ophthalmology*, Vol. 111, No. 12, (December 1993), pp. 1601-1602.

Menke, M.N., Knecht, P., Sturm,V., Dabov, S., & Funk, J. (2008). Reproducibility of nerve fiber layer thickness measurements using 3D fourier-domain OCT. *Investigative Ophthalmology & Visual Science*, Vol. 49, No. 12, (December 2008), pp. 5386-5391.

Metellus, P., Levrier, O., Fuentes, S., *et al.* (2005). Endovascular treatment of benign intracranial hypertension by stent placement in
the transverse sinus: therapeutic and pathophysiological considerations illustrated by a case report [in French]. *Neurochirurgie*, Vol. 51, No. 2, (May 2005), pp. 113-120.

Mokri, B. (2001). The Monro-Kellie hypothesis: applications in CSF volume depletion. *Neurology*, Vol. 56, No. 12, (June 2001), pp. 1746-1748.

Morrice, G., Havener, W.H., & Kapetanxky, F. (1960). Vitamin A intoxication as a cause of pseudotumor cerebri. *Journal of the American Medical Association*, Vol. 173, (August 1960), pp. 1802-1805.

Munk, P.L., Vellet, A.D., Levin, M., Lin, D.T., & Collyer, R.T. (1991). Sonography of the eye. *American Journal of Roentgenology*, Vol. 157, No. 5, (November 1991), pp. 1079-1086.

Nedelmann, M., Kaps, M., & Mueller-Forell, W. (2009). Venous obstruction and jugular valve insufficiency in idiopathic intracranial hypertension. *Journal of Neurology*, Vol. 256, No. 6, (June 2009), pp. 964-969.

Neville, B.G.R., & Wilson, J. (1970). Benign intracranial hypertension following corticosteroid withdrawal in childhood. *British Medical Journal*, Vol. 3, No. 5722, (September 1970), pp. 554-556.

Nonne, M. (1904). Ueber Falle vom Symptomkomplex "tumor cerebri" mit Ausgang in Heilung (pseudotumor cerebri*). Dtsch Z Nervenheil*, Vol. 27, pp. 169-216.

Ogungbo, B., Roy, D., Gholkar, A., *et al.* (2003). Endovascular stenting of the transverse sinus in a patient presenting with benign intracranial hypertension. *British Journal of Neurosurgery*, Vol. 17, No. 6, (December 2003), pp. 565-568.

Ophir, A., Karatas, M., Ramirez, J.A., & Inzelberg, R. (2005). OCT and chronic papilledema. *Ophthalmology*, Vol. 112, No. 12, (December 2005), pp. 2238.

Paquet, C., Poupardin, M., Boissonnot, M., *et al.(2008).* Efficacy of unilateral stenting in idiopathic intracranial hypertension with stenosis: a case report. *European Neurology*, Vol. 60, No. 1, (May 2008), pp. 47-48.

Pearson, P.A., Baker, R.S., Khorram, D., & Smith, T.J. (1991). Evaluation of optic nerve sheath fenestration in pseudotumor cerebri using automated perimetry. *Ophthalmology*, Vol. 98, No. 1, (January 1991), pp. 99-105.

Pipe, J.G. (2001). Limits of time-of-flight magnetic resonance angiography. *Topics in Magnetic Resonance*, Vol. 12, No. 13, (June 2001), pp. 163-174.

Plotnik, J.L., & Kosmorsky, G.S. (1993). Operative complications of optic nerve sheath decompression. *Ophthalmology*, Vol. 100, No. 5, (May 1993), pp. 683-690.

Quincke, H. (1893). Meningitis serosa. *Samml Klin Vortr, Leipzig*, Vol. 67: Inn Med 23:655.

Quincke H (1897) Ueber meningitis serosa und verwande Zustande. *Dtsch Z Nervenheil*, Vol. 9, pp. 140-168.

Rabb, F., Burton, T.C., Schatz, H., & Yannuzzi, L.A. (1978) Fluorescein angiography of the fundus: A schematic approach to interpretation. *Survey of Ophthalmology*, Vol. 22, No. 6, (May 1978), pp. 387-403.

Radhakrishnan, K., Ahlskog, J.E., Cross, S.A., *et al.* (1993). Idiopathic intracranial hypertension (pseudotumor cerebri). Descriptive epidemiology in Rochester, Minn, 1976 to 1990. *Archives of Neurology*, Vol. 50, No. 1, (January 1993), pp. 78-80.

Radhakrishnan, K., Ahlskog, J.E., Garrity, J.A., & Kurland, L.T. (1994). Idiopathic intracranial hypertension. *Mayo Clinic Proceedings*, Vol. 69, No. 2, (February 1994), pp. 169-180.

Raichle, M.E., Grubb, R.L., Jr, Phelps, M.E., Gado, M.H. & Caronna, J.J. (1978). Cerebral hemodynamics and metabolism in pseudotumor cerebri. *Annals of Neurology*, Vol. 4, No. 2, (August 1978), pp. 104-111.

Rajpal, S., Niemann, D.B., & Turk, A.S. (2005). Transverse venous sinus stent placement as treatment for benign intracranial hypertension in a young male: case report and review of the literature. *Journal of Neurosurgery*, Vol. 102, No. 3(suppl), (April 2005), pp. 342-346.

Rangwala, L.M., & Liu, G.T. (2007). Pediatric idiopathic intracranial hypertension. *Survey of Ophthalmology*, Vol. 52, No. 6, (November 2007), pp. 597-617.

Rebolleda, G., & Munoz-Negrete, F.J. (2009). Follow-up of mild papilledema in idiopathic intracranial hypertension with optical coherence tomography. *Investigative Ophthalmology & Visual Science*, Vol. 50, No. 11, (November 2009), pp. 5197-5200.

Reid, A.C., Teasdale, G.M., Matheson, M.S., & Teasdale, E.M. (1981). Serial ventricular volume measurements: further insights into the aetiology and pathogenesis of benign intracranial hypertension. *Journal of Neurology Neurosurgery & Psychiatry*, Vol. 44, No. 7, (July 1981), pp. 636-40.

Ridsdale, L., & Moseley, I. (1978). Thoracolumbar intraspinal tumours presenting features of raised intracranial pressure. *Journal of Neurology Neurosurgery & Psychiatry*, Vol. 41, No. 8, (August 1978), pp. 737-745.

Rogers, A.H., Rogers, G.L., Bremer, D.L., & McGregor, M.L. (1999). Pseudotumor cerebri in children receiving recombinant human growth hormone. *Ophthalmology*, Vol. 106, No. 6, (June 1999), pp. 1186-1190.

Ropper, A.H., & Marmarou, A. (1984). Mechanism of pseudotumor in Guillain-Barré syndrome. *Archives of Neurology*, Vol. 41, No. 3, (March 1984), pp. 259-261,

Ross, D.A & Wilson, C.B. (1988). Results of transsphenoidal microsurgery for growth Hormone secreting pituitary adenoma in a series of 214 patients. *Journal of Neurosurgery*, Vol. 68, No. 6, (June 1988), pp. 854-867.

Rothman, M.I., & Zoarski, G.H. (2003). The orbit. In: *Textbook of Radiology and Imaging* Vol. 2. 7th ed, Sutton, D. pp. 1573-1595, Churchill Livingstone, London.

Salgarello T., Tamburrelli, C., Falsini, B., Giudiceandrea, A., & Colotto, A. (1996). Optic nerve diameters and perimetric thresholds in idiopathic intracranial hypertension. *British Journal of Ophthalmology*, Vol. 80, No 6, (June 1996), pp. 509-514.

Saul, R.F., Hamburger, H.A., & Selhorst, J.B. (1985). Pseudotumor cerebri secondary to lithium carbonate. *Journal of the American Medical Association*, Vol. 253, No. 19, (May 1985), pp. 2869-2870.

Schuman, J.S., Puliafito, C.A., & Fujimoto, J.G. (2004). *Optical coherence tomography of ocular diseases*. Slack Incorporated, Thorofare, NJ.

Silbergleit, R., Junck, L., Gebarski, S.S., & Hatfield, M.K. (1989). Idiopathic intracranial hypertension (pseudotumor cerebri): MR imaging. *Radiology*, Vol. 170, No. 1, (January 1989), pp. 207-209.

Soelberg Sørensen, P., Gjerris, F., & Svenstrup, B. (1986). Endocrine studies in patients with pseudotumor cerebri. Estrogen levels in blood and cerebrospinal fluid. *Archives of Neurology*, Vol. 43, No. 9, (September 1986), pp. 902-906.

Soldatos, T., Karakitsos, D., Chatzimichail, K., *et al.* (2008). Optic nerve sonography in the diagnosis evaluation of adult brain injury. *Critical Care*, Vol. 12, No. 3, (May 2008), pp. R67

Sorensen, P.S., Thomsen, C., & Gjerris, F. et al. (1989). Increased brain water content in pseudotumor cerebri measured by magnetic resonance imaging of brain water self diffusion. *Neurology Research*, Vol. 11, No. 3, (September 1989), pp. 160-4.

Spector, R.H., & Carlisle, J. (1984). Pseudotumor cerebri caused by a synthetic vitamin A preparation. *Neurology*, Vol. 34, No. 11, (November 1984), pp. 1509-1511.

Spence, J.D., Amacher, A.L & Willis, N.R. (1980). Benign intracranial hypertension without papilledema: role of 24-hour cerebrospinal fluid pressure monitoring in diagnosis and management. *Neurosurgery* Vol.7, No. 4, (October 1980), pp. 326-336.

Spoor, T.C., & McHenry, J.G. (1993). Long-term effectiveness of optic nerve sheath decompression for pseudotumor cerebri. *Archives of Ophthalmology*, Vol. 111, No. 5, (May 1993), pp. 632-635.

Stone, M.B. (2009). Ultrasound diagnosis of papilledema and increased intracranial pressure in pseudotumor cerebri. *American Journal of Emergency Medicine*, Vol. 27, No. 3, (March 2009), pp. e1-376

Sussman, J., Leach, M., Greaves, M., Malia, R., & Davies-Jones, GA. (1997). Potentially prothrombotic abnormalities of coagulation in benign intracranial hypertension. *Journal of Neurology Neurosurgery & Psychiatry*, Vol. 62, No. 3, (March 197), pp. 229-233.

Tang, R.A., Dorotheo, E.U., Schiffman, J.S., & Bahrani, H.M. (2004). Medical and surgical management of idiopathic intracranial hypertension in pregnancy. *Current Neurology and Neuroscience Reports*, Vol. 4, No. 5, (September 2004), pp. 398-409.

Tibussek, D., Schneider, D.T., Vandemeulebroecke, N., *et al.* (2010). Clinical spectrum of the pseudotumor cerebri complex in children. *Child's Nervous System*, Vol. 26, No. 3, (March 2010), pp. 313-321.

Tulipan, N., Lavin, P.J., & Copeland M.(1998). Stereotactic ventriculoperitoneal shunt for idiopathic intracranial hypertension: technical note. *Neurosurgery* Vol. 43, No. 1, (July 1998), pp. 175-176.

Visani, G., Manfroi, S., Tosi, P., & Martinelli, G. (1996). All-trans-retinoic acid and pseudotumor cerebri. *Leukemia & Lymphoma*. Vol. 23, No. 5-6, (November 1996), pp. 437-442.

Walker, R.W.H. (2001). Idiopathic intracranial hypertension: any light on the mechanism of the raised pressure? *Journal of Neurology Neurosurgery & Psychiatry*, Vol. 71, No. 1, (July 2001), pp. 1-5.

Wall, M., & George, D. (1987). Visual loss in pseudotumor cerebri. Incidence and defects related to visual field strategy. *Archives of Neurology*, Vol. 44, No. 2, (February 1987), pp. 170-175.

Wall, M., & George, D. (1991). Idiopathic intracranial hypertension. A prospective study of 50 patients. *Brain*. Vol. 114, No. 1A, (January 1991), pp. 155-180.

Wall, M., & White, W.N. II. (1998). Asymmetric papilledema in idiopathic intracranial hypertension: prospective interocular comparison of sensory visual function. *Investigative Ophthalmology & Visual Science*, Vol. 39, No. 1, (January 1998), pp. 134-142.

Walsh, F.B., Clark, D.B., Thompson, R.S., & Nicholson, D.H. (1965). Oral contraceptives and neuro-ophthalmologic interest. *Archives of Ophthalmology*, Vol. 74, No. 5, (November 1965), pp. 628-640.

Wang, S.J., Silberstein, S.D., Patterson, S., & Young, W.B. (1998). Idiopathic intracranial hypertension without papilledema: a case-control study in a headache center. *Neurology* Vol. 51, No. 1, (July 1998), pp.245-249.

Weisberg, L.A. (1985). Computed tomography in benign intracranial hypertension. *Neurology*, Vol. 35, No. 7, (July 1985), pp.1075-8.

Wessel, K., Thron, A., Linden, D., *et al.* (1987). Pseudotumor cerebri: clinical and neuroradiological findings. *European Archives of Psychiatry & Neurological Sciences*, Vol. 237, No. 1, pp. 54-60.

Winner, P., & Bello, L. (1996). Idiopathic intracranial hypertension in a young child without visual symptoms or signs. *Headache*, Vol. 36, No. 9, (October 1996), pp. 574-576.

Winrow, A.P., & Supramaniam, G. (1990). Benign intracranial hypertension after ciprofloxacin administration. *Archives Disease of Childhood*, Vol. 65, No. 10, (October 1990), pp.1165-1166.

Worsham, F. Jr, Beckman, E.N., & Mitchell, E.H. (1978). Sacrococcygeal teratoma in a neonate. Association with maternal use of acetazolamide. *Journal of the American Medical Association*, Vol. 240, No. 3, (July 1978), pp. 251-2.

Yaşargil, M.G., Curcic, M., Kis, M., *et al.* (1990). Total removal of craniopharyngiomas. Approaches and long-term results in 144 patients. *Journal of Neurosurgery*, Vol. 73, No. 1, (July 1990), pp. 3-11.

Neuroimaging in Fragile X-Associated Tremor/Ataxia Syndrome (FXTAS)

Laia Rodriguez-Revenga[1,2], Beatriz Gómez-Ansón[3,4],
Esther Granell Moreno[3], Javier Pagonabarraga[4,5] and Montserrat Mila[1,2]
[1]Biochemistry and Molecular Genetics Department, Hospital Clínic, IDIBAPS Barcelona
[2]CIBER de Enfermedades Raras (CIBERER), Barcelona
[3]Neuroradiology Unit, Radiology Department, Hospital Sant Pau, Barcelona
[4]CIBER de Enfermedades Neurodegenerativas (CIBERNED), Barcelona
[5]Neurology Service, Hospital Sant Pau, Barcelona
Spain

1. Introduction

Fragile X syndrome (FXS, OMIM #300624) is the most common form of inherited mental retardation. The real incidence of the syndrome is not known, but epidemiological studies indicate that it is responsible for mental retardation in 1 in 4,000-6,000 males and in 1 in 7,000-10,000 females of European descendent (for review Hagerman, 2002). In a study performed in Catalonia it gave an incidence of 1:2,466 male and 1:8,333 females (Rife *et al.*, 2003). It is also important to highlight the high incidence of premutation carriers, 1 in 1,233 males and 1 in 411 females (Rife *et al.*, 2003). FXS is inherited as X-linked dominant trait, with a reduced penetrance (80% for males and 30% for females).

In 1991 the responsible gene was identified by positional cloning and named the fragile X mental retardation-1 gene (*FMR1*) (Oberle *et al.*, 1991; Verkerk *et al.*, 1991; Yu *et al.*, 1991). The *FMR1* gene is located in the long arm of the X chromosome at Xq27.3, it expands 17 exons, and 40 kb of genomic DNA. It transcribes an mRNA of 3.9 kb, and the translated protein is called fragile X mental retardation protein (FMRP). The lack of this protein, which plays an important role in synaptogenesis and synaptic plasticity (Basell & Warren, 2008), is the cause of the FXS.

FXS is almost exclusively caused by a dynamic mutation, a CGG repeat expansion in the 5′ untranslated region of the *FMR1* gene (Oberle *et al.*, 1991; Verkerk *et al.*, 1991; Yu *et al.*, 1991). In a normal situation the number of CGG repeats is polymorphic with alleles between 6 to about 54, with the most common allele presenting 30 CGG repeats. In this situation the CpG island, which is located in the promoter of the gene acting as a switch depending on its methylation status, is unmethylated. Thus the gene is active, *FMR1* is transcribed and translated. Repeats at this size remain stable upon transmission. A second class of alleles that overlaps with the upper range of the wild-type is those with ~40-55 CGGs. This range, known as the gray zone, no expands to full mutation but it is transmitted slightly unstable to subsequent generations with the possibility of creating a premutated allele. In the premutation, alleles range from 55 to about 200 CGG repeats. At this situation, the *FMR1* gene is also transcribed as the CpG island is unmethylated. Therefore, premutated carriers have normal or lightly reduced synthesis of FMRP and they are asymptomatic for FXS. However, they have risk of having affected descendence since the number of CGG is unstable, and in each cellular division it can increase, and can be transmitted with a higher number of repeats to the next generation. Finally, when the CGG number is beyond 200 repeats (known as full mutation), the CpG island is methylated, and as consequence, the gene is transcriptionally silenced, and no protein is translated. These individuals are always affected if they are males and in about 30% of females.

In this chapter we review the clinical, molecular and neuroradiological aspects of FXTAS syndrome, a late-onset neuropsychiatric degenerative disorder that occurs predominantly in male carriers of the *FMR1* premutation. Based on our experience we describe in detail the different aspects that characterize the syndrome as well as the new findings.

2. Fragile X syndrome premutation and FXTAS identification

The possibility of clinical involvement in carriers of premutation expansions (55 to 200 CGG repeats) of *FMR1* gene was initially discounted, since carrier mothers of FXS children have a normal cognitive functioning (Bennetto *et al.*, 2001; Reiss *et al.*, 1993). Even though, and contrary to expectation, there are reported several subgroups of male and female premutation carriers displaying features consistent with the typical clinical spectrum of FXS. For instance, Riddle and co-workers (1998) and Hagerman (2002) described a group of premutation carriers with prominent ears and joint laxity; or with learning disabilities, attention deficit/hyperactivity disorder (ADHD), or difficulty with math (Riddle *et al.*, 1998, reviewed in Hagerman & Hagerman 2004). In addition, some carriers have emotional problems, including anxiety, obsessional thinking, schizotypy, and/or depression (Hagerman *et al.*, 2002; Rodriguez-Revenga *et al.*, 2008a). Such findings were observed to be more likely to occur in carriers with a lowered FMRP levels and particularly in those carrier females with larger CGG expansions (>100 repeats) (Johnston *et al.*, 2001).

There are, however, two forms of clinical involvement among carriers of premutation alleles that are not consistent with the clinical spectrum of the FXS. These two disorders are the primary ovarian insuffiency (FXPOI) and the fragile X-associated tremor/ataxia syndrome (FXTAS). FXPOI, which refers to the cessation of menses before age 40, is seen in ~20% of female who carry permutation alleles. Therefore, the genetic counseling for premutated women has to include a fertility advice since delaying the reproduction may not be a good option.

FXTAS, the second form of clinical involvement described among permutation carriers, was identified in 2001 by Hagerman and co-workers as a late-onset neurodegenerative disorder (Hagerman *et al.*, 2001). It took more than 10 years after the *FMR1* gene identification to recognize FXTAS as a *FMR1* permutation associated phenotype. One explanation for this is that the movement disorder experienced by older carriers, who were thought to be clinically normal, was not associated with the FXS (a childhood disorder) affecting children. Mothers of FXS children, being seen in clinics, were often expressing concerns about their fathers (*FMR1* premutation carriers) who were experiencing problems with hand tremor and unsteady gait. When Hagerman and co-workers evaluated these male carriers they found that they all have a common neurological profile, consisting of intention tremor and gait ataxia (reviewed in Hagerman & Hagerman 2004). Therefore, FXTAS was firstly identified among older male carriers of premutation alleles, including progressive action tremor and ataxia with associated radiological findings (Hagerman & Hagerman 2004). However, to date FXTAS has also been described among premutated women although it has been suggested that it occurs less frequently and that the phenotype is milder with older age at onset (Hagerman *et al.*, 2001; Jacquemont *et al.*, 2004a). An explanation for this difference is the presence of a second normal allele and a random X-inactivation of the premutated one; however, there may be additional sex-specific effects that reduce penetrance among females (Hagerman & Hagerman, 2004).

Not all *FMR1* premutation carriers develop FXTAS and it remains unknown which carriers will do so and when. It has been estimated that at least one-third of all male carriers will develop a FXTAS syndrome, although the penetrance increases with age, exceeding 50% for men aged 70-90 years. Moreover, there is significant variability in the progression of neurological dysfunction (Hagerman & Hagerman 2004; Jacquemont *et al.*, 2004a, 2004b). In an attempt to provide an estimation of FXTAS penetrance among premutation carriers in Spanish FXS families, we evaluated 398 families among which 151 were composed of at least three generations. Our results showed that signs of FXTAS were detected in 16.5% of female premutation carriers and in 45.5% of premutated males older than 50 years. Overall, the mean age and the mean of CGG repeat number for the FXTAS men group was of 72.05 ± 6.85 and 85 ± 21.5 (mean ± SD), respectively. Similarly it was of 75.8 years old ± 10.2 and 82 CGG repeats ± 18 (mean ± SD) for the FXTAS women group (Rodriguez-Revenga *et al.*, 2009).

The description and characterization of FXTAS syndrome is of great interest to the population, because the prevalence of *FMR1* premutation in the general population is relatively high. Several studies have been performed in order to determine the real role of FXTAS in undiagnosed adult patients with movement disorders. The results obtained in European populations ranges from 0% to 4% (Brussino *et al.*,2005; Macpherson *et al.*, 2003; Van Esch *et al.*, 2005; Zuhlke *et al.*, 2004). Our studies show an estimated FXTAS prevalence of 2% among patients presenting with ataxia or movement disorders of unknown etiology (Rodriguez-Revenga *et al.*, 2007, 2008b). Although large studies are necessary to better define FXTAS prevalence in this kind of population, on the basis of premutation male frequency in general population, the prevalence of FXTAS has been estimated in ~1/3,000 males aged over 50 years of age (~1/10,000 males of all ages) (Hagerman & Hagerman, 2004).

3. Clinical and cognitive overview

FXTAS syndrome is a neurodegenerative disease that eventually appears in adult subjects who carry a CGG repeat length between 55 and 200 trinucleotides in the *FMR1* gene of chromosome X (Jacquemont *et al.*, 2007). These subjects are categorized as *FMR1* premutation carriers. As stated above, it was originally described in grandparents of children with FXS. Different specialized centres in diagnosing and attending children with FXS observed that their grandparents and uncles were more likely to develop, from 50 years onwards, a stereotyped clinical picture characterized by unsteadiness while walking and action tremor in both hands (Hagerman *et al.*, 2001).

Neurological examination of children's relatives disclosed the presence of predominant intention tremor in hands and wide-base cerebellar ataxia. Both symptoms used to follow a progressive course, and were often accompanied by progressive cognitive and behavioral disturbances (Hagerman *et al.*, 2001).

Clinical descriptions published in the past 10 years have demonstrated that *FMR1* premutation carriers are very prone to develop cerebellar dysfunction from the age of 50 years. Seveirty of symptoms usually impairs gait and associates mild to moderate dysmetria, repeated falls, intention tremor, and speech difficulties. The combination of cerebellar dysfunction, cognitive impairment and the appearance of characteristic radiologic features in the brain MRI has been claimed to constitute a nosological entity that has been named Fragile X-associated Tremor/Ataxia syndrome (FXTAS).

In the only study about the natural history of patients with FXTAS, this syndrome has been observed to represent a disabling condition impacting on motor daily activities, thinking, and social skills after 15 years of evolution (Jacquemont *et al.*, 2003).

Mean age of onset of FXTAS is 60 years. Mild intention tremor, affecting both hands, symmetrically, is usually the first symptom. Within the first 5 years, tremor becomes more apparent and some balance and speech problems develop. At this stage, balance problems are mild and are only noticed by patients as a feeling of unsteadiness while walking for long periods of time or when turning. Between 5 and 15 years from disease onset balance problems progress in severity and are usually the main complain, provoking repeated falling and limiting the ability to drive, walking autonomously in the streets, or using public transportation. At this stage, moreover, is when the first cognitive and behavioural disturbances appear. After 15 years, autonomous walk is greatly impaired, and patients need the help of a walker or the supervision of another person. Finally, dysphagia and severe ataxia are associated with immobility and recurrent urinary and respiratory infections (Leehey *et al.*, 2007).

The penetrance of FXTAS is not well established. Penetrance increases with age, and it has been reported to range from 15% at 50 years of age to 75% at age 80 (Jacquemont *et al.*, 2004b).

Being a relatively newly described condition, the clinical spectrum of the disease has expanded in the past years. As in other diseases, such as Parkinson's disease, FXTAS was initially conceived as a predominant motor disease. New data have evidenced that many clinically relevant cognitive and behavioural disturbances may also develop in FXTAS patients. Also, while FXTAS was originally described in males, the number of women developing FXTAS symptoms has increased exponentially in the past five years. Women have been reported to develop the same motor, cognitive and behavioural problems than males, although women are more likely to develop a milder form of the disease (Coffey *et al.*, 2008). Nevertheless, cognitive dysfunction severe enough to accomplish criteria for dementia has been reported in FXTAS women with inactivation of the healthy X-chromosome (Rodriguez-Revenga *et al.*, 2010).

Cognitive impairment in FXTAS is characterized by recent episodic memory problems, difficulties in sustained attention, and other executive problems such as organizing new material and inhibiting automatic responses. In males, initially mild cognitive problems can accomplish criteria for dementia after 5 to 10 years of evolution (Grisby *et al.*, 2007). Extension of the neurodegenerative process to prefrontal and temporal structures seems to account for the progression of cognitive defects in FXTAS patients (Seritan *et al.*, 2008). While balance problems and tremor seem to be the consequence of the progressive degeneration of middle cerebellar peduncles and associated cerebellar structures, both cognitive and behavioural problems in FXTAS are associated with diffuse cortical and white-matter subcortical degeneration (Hashimoto *et al.*, 2011).

The dysexecutive problems of FXTAS patients affect different prefrontal dominions. Cognitive tasks dependent on the dorsolateral prefrontal cortex are affected since the early stages of the disease. Problems in working memory, set-shifting and mental flexibility have been described in patients with mild ataxia and tremor (Grisby *et al.*, 2007). Later in the disease, cognitive alterations more dependent on the medial prefrontal cortex, such as difficulties in inhibiting automatic responses, arise. Response inhibition in go-no go tasks, inability to perform Luria's promotor series, and signs of environmental dependency were seen not only to limit the ability of FXTAS' patients to cope with cognitive strategies in the daily life, but also accounted for the behavioral disorders of the disease (Moore *et al.*, 2004a). Memory problems develop due to both prefrontal and medial temporal dysfunction. Numerous eosinophylic inclusions have been observed bilaterally in the hippocampus and the entorrhinal cortex. Progressive deterioration and atrophy of medial temporal lobe structures explains the progressive nature of temporal disorientation and both verbal and visual recent episodic memory. (Grisby *et al.*, 2008). In comparison with Alzheimer's disease, FXTAS patients show a higher impairment in dysexecutive tasks and less memory impairment, and in comparison with Parkinson's disease, visuospatial skills seem to be more preserved. In addition, compared to both Parkinson's disease and dementia with Lewy bodies, FXTAS patients are less likely to manifest visual hallucinations and psychosis (Grisby *et al.*, 2008).

Neuropsychiatric disturbances in FXTAS are characterized by a change in premorbid personality. Patients with FXTAS, as in frontotemporal dementia, may develop irritability, psychomotor agitation, a tendency to selfishness, blunted emotions, apathy, and sometimes even social and personal disinhibition. Similarities with frontotemporal dementia correlate with the evidence of predominant medial prefrontal and anteromedial temporal atrophy in neuroimaging studies (Bacalman *et al.*, 2006).

In summary, fronto-temporal cognitive and behavioral disturbances seem to characterize FXTAS patients. Frontal cognitive symptoms are present in early stages and progress through disease evolution, medial prefrontal behavioral disturbances appear in the middle stages and progress also in severity, and finally, from medium to late FXTAS stages, temporal cognitive symptoms impair even more global cognitive function and lead to dementia. A better delineation of each one of these components would help to refine the progression of cognitive and behavioural symptoms in different FXTAS subgroups (age, gender, etc...).

Other neurological disturbances described in FXTAS patients are the development of rigid-akinetic parkinsonism with predominant axial involvement (35%), unilateral resting tremor (10%), peripheral neuropathy (30%), dysautonomia (40-50%; urinary urgency, erectile dysfunction, orthostatic hypotension), nistagmus (10%), and hyporreflexia (10%).

In some patients, postural and intention tremor may present in isolation, making the diagnosis of essential tremor very likely. Reported cases stress the importance of considering the diagnosis of FXTAS in patients diagnosed of essential tremor who develop ataxia or with a family history of mental retardation (Leehey *et al.*, 2003). Other patients present with isolated and progressive adult-onset ataxia. Currently, genetic testing for FXTAS must be considered in any patient with ataxia developing after the age of 50. The screening of FXTAS in a prospective series of patients with multiple system atrophy showed that 4% of patients with an initial diagnosis of multiple system atrophy of the cerebellar type were actually *FMR1* premutation carriers (Kamm *et al.*, 2005). Taking into account the consequences of a diagnosis of FXTAS on genetic counselling, FXTAS should be categorized as a new kind of spinocerebellar ataxia (Milà *et al.*, 2009).

4. Molecular genetics overview

FXTAS is an allelic disorder to the FXS, and therefore should be considered as a distinct neurodegenerative disorder. In fact, the molecular mechanism leading to FXTAS is distinct from the *FMR1* silencing mechanism and/or a deficit in FMRP operating in FXS. In premutated patients the *FMR1* gene is rarely silenced and FMRP levels are generally normal or only slightly lowered (Hagerman & Hagerman, 2004) (Fig.1a). The only known molecular abnormality among premutation carriers is the presence of markedly elevated levels (~2-8 fold) of *FMR1* mRNA (Fig.1b).

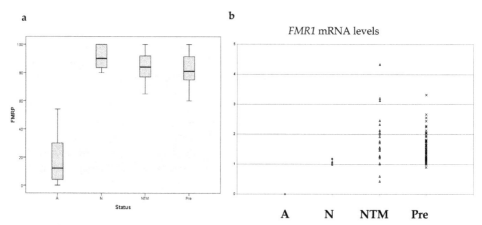

Fig. 1. a) Schematic representation of FMRP levels detected in A: FXS affected individuals, N: individuals with a normal CGG repeat number; NTM: *FMR1* premutation male carriers and Pre: *FMR1* premutation female carriers. B) Schematic representation of *FMR1* mRNA levels detected in A: FXS affected individuals, N: individuals with a normal CGG repeat number; NTM: *FMR1* premutation male carriers and Pre: *FMR1* premutation female carriers.

The increased transcriptional activity of the *FMR1* gene seems to be positively correlated with the size of the CGG repeat. That is, CGG repeats in the upper range (100-200 CGG) result in average 5-8 fold elevation, whereas CGGs in the lower range (50-100 CGG) result in an average 2-fold elevation (Kenson *et al.*, 2001; Oostra & Willemsen, 2003; Tassone *et al.*, 2000a, 2000b). Although the precise mechanism for this overexpression is unknown, several possible mechanisms have been postulated. A feedback mechanism suggests that the cell attempts to compensate for reduced levels of FMRP by increasing the amount of available FMR1 transcript (reviewed in Galloway & Nelson, 2009; Tassone & Hagerman, 2003). Alternatively, it is likely that the increasing length of the CGG repeat near the *FMR1* promoter proportionally opens the chromatin, allowing more ready access to transcription factors (Tan *el al.*, 2009). The presence of these elevated levels of abnormal (expanded CGG repeat) *FMR1* mRNA led to propose an RNA "toxic gain-of-function" model for FXTAS, in which the mRNA itself, with the abnormal CGG repeat tract, is causative of the neurological disorder (Greco et al., 2002: Hagerman & Hagerman, 2004; Hagerman et al., 2001: Jacquemont et al., 2003). Although several evidences support the RNA-based mechanism, the precise form of how the CGG-repeat RNA is responisble for FXTAS pathogenesis is not yet resolved (Garcia-Arocena & Hagerman, 2010) The same RNA "toxic gain-of-function" mechanism has been proposed for myotonic dystrophy (DM1 and DM2), in which either the expanded repeat tract of CUG in DM1 or CCUG in DM2 sequestered CUG-binding proteins that disrupts mRNA processing of other genes or transport of other mRNAs (Mankodi & Thornton, 2002). In fact, this model has been demonstrated for DM1 by placing an expanded CTG tract in 3' UTR region of the DMPK mRNA in a transgenic mouse (Mankodi et al., 2000). A part from this finding, FXTAS and myotonic dystrophy have another important similarity that supports the RNA gain-of-function mechanism. Both disorders show nuclear inclusions produced as a result of the binding proteins sequestered by the respectively mRNA, with a cytotoxic effect that lead to cell death. In a study performed by Greco and co-worker (2002) eosinophilic intranucelear inclusions in neurons and astrocytes throughout the cortex and in deep cerebellar nuclei of FXTAS post-mortem samples were reported. Furthermore, in a subsequent study, there is described a highly significant association between CGG length and both the number of inclusions and the age of death, which correlates with the progressive character of the disease (Greco et al., 2006). The intranuclear inclusions associated with FXTAS have characteristic features different than those found in tauopathies (e.g., Pick disease), synucleinopathies (e.g., Lewy body dementias and Parkinson disease) or polyglutamine disorders (SCAs). It is important to note that, unlike the polyglutamine disorders, there is no known structurally abnormal protein with FXTAS (reviewed in Galloway & Nelson, 2009; Iwahashi et al., 2006). Taken together, these facts define FXTAS as a new class of inclusion disorder.

In order to test the RNA gain-of-function hypothesis for FXTAS, a "knock-in" mouse model has been generated in which the endogenous mouse CGG repeat was replaced by a human CGG tract carrying 98 CGGs (Bontekoe et al., 2001; reviewed in Oostra & Willemsen, 2009). Further studies of the brain of these expanded-repeat mice (at 20-72 weeks) evidenced elevated Fmr1 mRNA levels and ubiquitin-positive intranuclear inclusions (Willemsen et al., 2003). An increase was also observed in both the number and the size of the inclusions in specific brain region during the course of life (Oostra & Willemsen, 2003). The presence of inclusions in this mouse, that has normal levels of FMRP, provides evidences against a protein-deficiency model for FXTAS, and supports a direct role of the Fmr1 gene, by either CGG expansion per se or by elevated Fmr1 mRNA levels, in the pathology.

There are several other animal and cell-based studies that provide evidence of direct RNA toxicity (Galloway & Nelson, 2010; reviewed in Garcia-Arocena & Hagerman, 2010). Most of these studies have demostrated a sequestartion of several candidates CGG-repeat binding proteins from their normal function. Remarkably, they have also demonstrated at least partial rescue of the wild-type phenotype by overexpressing the sequestered protein. The number of candidate proteins for sequestration has been lately increased and surprisingly, it has also been shown that inclusions are dynamic structures that expanded over time, resulting in giant inclusions (Sellier et al., 2010). Continuous enlargements of CGG RNA aggregates suggest that these repeats may constantly recruit proteins, implying a founding RNA-protein interaction event that would subsequently trap other proteins through indirect RNA-protein or protein-protein interactions (Sellier et al., 2010). The protein components of FXTAS inclusions fell into eight major functional categories, including: histone family; intermediate filament; microtubule; myelin-associated proteins; RNA-binding proteins;

stress-related proteins; chaperones and ubiquitin-proteasome-related proteins (reviewed Galloway & Nelson, 2010).

Interestingly, an antisense transcript, *ASFMR1*, has recently been identified to overlap the CGG repeat region of the *FMR1* gene (Ladd *et al.*, 2007). Similar to *FMR1*, the *ASFMR1* transcript is silenced in full mutation individuals and overexpressed in permutation carriers. However, whether *ASFMR1* contributes to the pathogenesis of either FXTAS or FXS remains to be determined (Tan *et al.*, 2009).

5. Neuroimaging findings – Conventional MRI strenghts and limitations

FXTAS was originally described in men, older than 50 years of age, having a typical clinical picture of progressive intention tremor, and cerebellar ataxia (Hagerman *et al* 2001). Magnetic resonance imaging (MRI) of the brain was obtained in these patients searching for specific features, and the finding of hyperintensities in the cerebellar white matter and middle cerebellar peduncles on T2-weighted images was reported as a characteristic feature and called the "MCP sign" (Fig. 2a), as it was seen in nearly all FXTAS-premutated carriers, and not in controls (Brunberg *et al.*, 2002). Other typical MR features described originally in patients with FXTAS included cerebellar, pontine, and cerebral atrophy, as well as white matter hyperintensities (Fig. 2 b-d) (Brunberg *et al.*, 2002).

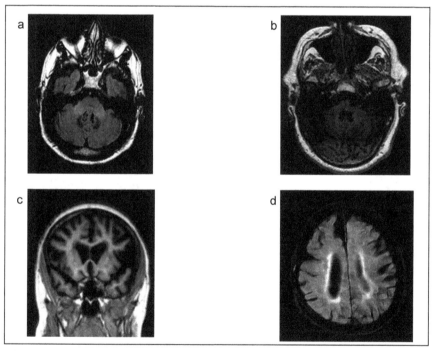

Fig. 2. MR images showing characteristic findings in FXTAS. 1a. Axial FLAIR- MCP sign (middle cerebellar peduncle hyperintensities); 1b. Axial T1- Cerebellar and pontine atrophy; 1c. Coronal T1- Cerebral atrophy; 1d. Axial FLAIR- Hyperintensities in the cerebral white matter.

Thus, characteristic findings described on conventional MRI in patients with FXTAS, were classified into two categories -major and minor criteria-, and proposed, together with clinical findings, as diagnostic criteria for FXTAS (Jacquemont *et al.*, 2003). Major criteria included the MCP sign, as well as white matter and brainstem hyperintensities. Cerebellar and brain atrophy were proposed as minor criteria (Jacquemont *et al.*, 2003) (Table 1).

Examination and Degree	Observation
Radiological:	
Major	MRI white matter lesions in MCPs and or brain stem
Minor	MRI white matter lesions in cerebral white matter
Minor	Moderate-to-severe generalized atrophy
Clinical:	
Major	Intention tremor
Major	Gait ataxia
Minor	Parkinsonism
Minor	Moderate-to-severe short-term memory deficiency
Minor	Executive function deficit

Inclusion criterion: CGG repeat number between 55 and 200.
Note. Data described by Jacquemont *et al*. 2003.

Table 1. Clinical Criteria for FXTAS. The diagnostic categories described by Jaquemont et al. 2003 are as follows:
Definite (1 major radiological sign plus 1 major clinical symptom)
Probable (1 major radiological sign plus 1 minor clinical symptom or two major clinical symptoms)
Possible (1 minor radiological sign plus 1 major clinical symptom)

Early neuropathological, postmortem studies of the brain of patients with FXTAS revealed intranuclear inclusions in neurons and astrocytes throughout the cortex and in deep cerebellar nuclei, but not in Purkinje cells of the cerebellum (Greco *et al.*, 2002). Further evidence has shown that there is significant cerebral and cerebellar white matter disease, associated astrocytic pathology in the cerebral white matter, and intranuclear inclusions in both brain and spinal cord (Greco *et al.*, 2006). Additionally, there seems to be an association between the number of CGG repeats and the number of intranuclear inclusions in neurons and astrocytes, so that CGG repeat has been suggested as a predictor for clinical and neuropathological involvement (Greco *et al.*, 2006). Unfortunately, there is no histopathological evidence from brains of premutated, non-FXTAS subjects, who died because of an unrelated condition, being either asymptomatic neurologically, or little symptomatic. This evidence would certainly add in the understanding of the pathogenetic processes underlying glial and neuronal damage, and eventual neurological dysfunction. Brain banks and collaborative actions may represent a good opportunity in this regard.
Penetrance of FXTAS among premutation carriers has been studied, and reported to be relevant, mainly in men (Jacquemont *et al.*, 2004). As premutation carriers are relatively common in the general population, it has been proposed that older men with ataxia and intention tremor should be screened for the *FMR1* mutation (Jacquemont 2004). Using the previously described criteria for FXTAS (Jacquemont *et al.*, 2003), a study among adult Spanish patients with ataxia, revealed an estimated FXTAS prevalence varying between

1.15% for males, and 3% for females (Rodriguez-Revenga *et al.*, 2007). Similarly, a frequency of 1.6% of patients with FXTAS has been reported among adult patients with movement disorders who tested negative for the Huntington gene (Rodriguez-Revenga *et al.*, 2008b). The importance of neuroradiological findings that could be used as an additional screening tool for FXTAS is demonstrated by these studies.

In this regard, the MCP sign, which was originally proposed to be a characteristic and specific feature for FXTAS, that could be used for screening purposes, has been also reported in patients with other forms of adult-onset cerebellar ataxia, thus lacking specificity for FXTAS (Okamoto *et al.*, 2003). Patients with atypical parkinsonism, and particularly those having a clinical picture including dysautonomia, and ataxia -a condition currently known as the cerebellar form of Multiple System Atrophy (MSA)-, may show the MCP sign on MRI, so that middle cerebellar peduncles hyperintensities in a patient with parkinsonism should be regarded as a non-specific finding, which can be seen in FXTAS, but also in MSA (Kamm et al., 2005). Additionally, the sensitivity of the MCP sign may be less than previously thought, as the frequency of the MCP sign among women with FXTAS seems to be less (Hagerman *et al.*, 2004), and its presence among premutated men with subtle neurological, psychiatric, or cognitive dysfunction remains unknown.

As more evidence among *FMR1* premutation carriers developing neurological features, and particularly parkinsonism, is being gained, the spectrum and variability of MRI features becomes broader. Also, the severity of disease, which may relate to CGG repeat number, or other unknown factors, may influence the presence and magnitude of MRI findings. In this context, a correlation between CGG repeat length and reductions in IQ and cerebellar volume, and increased ventricular volume and whole-brain white matter hyperintensities, have been reported in *FMR1* premutation carriers (Cohen *et al.*, 2006). It may well then be the case, that patients with a longer duration of neurological disturbances, or a greater severity, are those showing the so-known "typical MRI findings" of FXTAS. In this regard, more evidence is needed among younger premutated patients. Additionally, premutated women and women with FXTAS seem to have a different phenotype (Berry *et al.*, 2004; Hagerman *et al.*, 2004; Hessl *et al.*, 2005), so that the frequency and relevance of MRI findings in women may be different from that in men. In this regard, less pronounced reductions in cerebellar volume and a lower incidence of the MCP sign has been reported in women with FXTAS compared to men (Adams *et al.*, 2007). Also, an absence of significant associations between reduced cerebellar volumes and increased FXTAS severity, and increased length of the CGG repeat expansion was reported in women, differently from men having FXTAS (Adams *et al.*, 2007).

Conventional MRI, as including T1- and T2- weighted MR images, suffers from several limitations as a tool to investigate patients with a neurodevelopmental disorder that develop a neurodegenerative process later in life, as happens in the *FMR1* premutation/FXTAS condition. Today, with the advent of high field strength MRI, and stronger gradients, there are more specific sequences such as susceptibility- or gradient-echo-weighted MR-images, which can provide more specific assessment of mechanisms underlying neuronal degeneration, such as iron deposition. Iron deposition is seen with normal aging in specific brain structures. Up to date, increased and/or iron deposition in certain brain structures has not been demonstrated among FXTAS patients, to the best of our knowledge, but this may only be a question of time or of the cohorts being studied.

Also, recently FLAIR imaging has somehow substituted T2-weighted imaging for the assessment of white matter and brainstem T2- signal changes. Findings on FLAIR images may not be exactly the same as seen on T2-weighted images, and thus, more evidence is needed with these more recent techniques. Finally, Arterial Spin Labeling, a non-invasive MRI method that allows detection of specific perfusion patterns of involvement linked to brain metabolism, is currently being applied to several neurodegenerative brain conditions, and may also be useful in the context of *FMR1* premutation/FXTAS.

6. Advances in neuroimaging in FXTAS and future needs

The advancing field of Neuroradiology, and particularly of MRI, has provided insight in neurodegenerative conditions. Typical MRI findings have been described, that allow prompt and more precise characterization of many conditions, such as FXTAS. Additionally, MRI has provided non-invasive markers of disease, which may be potentially useful in early and differential diagnosis, in prognosis, and eventually in therapeutic response. This is the case for triplet expansion, genetic conditions, such as Huntington´s disease (HD), which offers some similarities to FXTAS. Originally, conventional MRI was used and typical MRI findings were described in HD, but recently, more sophisticated imaging methods, such as MR-Spectroscopy, have been applied not only to patients with HD, but also to asymptomatic carriers, searching for markers for early diagnosis and conversion to disease. In this regard, metabolic (Gomez-Anson *et al.*, 2007) and structural (Gomez-Anson *et al.*, 2009) MR-alterations in the prefrontal regions of asymptomatic HD carriers have been recently described, linked to neuropsychological dysfunction, and proposed as early markers for disease, related to underlying pathology. Knowledge in field of *FMR1* premutation carriers, who will eventually develop FXTAS, may follow a similar course. Although until now, mainly conventional MRI features have been described, there is growing evidence from more sophisticated MR techniques, which has and will continue adding knowledge in the field.

Advances in Neuroimaging in *FMR1* premutation/FXTAS may, perhaps, come from two distinct contributions. Firstly, more recent developments in MR are being applied to these patients. This is particularly the case of functional MR techniques, which not only provide information about structural brain changes in these patients, but also of brain functioning. As an example, MR-Spectroscopy (MRS) is a technique which allows studying non-invasively brain metabolism in vivo. Metabolic information can be linked to cellular pools, thus to histopathological changes, and to neuropsychological and clinical features. There is very little evidence about MRS in FXTAS. However, MRS changes indicating neuronal loss/dysfunction have been described in the pons of patients with FXTAS having the typical MCP sign on conventional imaging (Ginestroni *et al.*, 2007). More recent evidence has shown altered metabolism on MRS in the middle cerebellar peduncles of patients with *FMR1* premutation, which may be more marked in FXTAS (Gomez-Anson *et al.*, abstract 2007). These findings indicate a potential usefulness of MRS, adding in differential diagnosis of patients with ataxias, and being able, perhaps, to identify those patients that will develop FXTAS. However, more longitudinal evidence and larger cohorts of carriers and patients from multicentric studies are needed in this regard. Functional MRI may also prove to be useful in the field of, as it has been recently demonstrated that there is altered prefrontal cortex activity underlying executive and memory deficits in permutated carriers and patients (Hashimoto *et al.*, 2011).

Secondly, contributions from more sophisticated postprocessing tools will certainly add during the near future in the field. In this context, assessment and quantification of volume changes in the brain is now feasible non-invasively using MRI and volumetric techniques. One of these techniques, the Voxel Based Morphometry method (VBM) allows determination of focal changes of grey and white matter density in the brain on MRI (Ashburner *et al.*, 2000). However, the evidence of volumetric studies in FXTAS and premutation carriers is scarce (Gomez-Anson *et al.*, 2007; Hashimoto *et al.*, 2011; Moore *et al.*, 2004b). Automated postprocessing tools are also being currently applied to study regional changes of volume in the brain, which may be specific to a condition, and related to certain cognitive tasks. This is the case of the hippocampus and memory impairment, which are relevant in Alzheimer´s disease, for example (Sanchez-Benavides *et al.*, 2010). Evidence of the application of these tools to research in the FXTAS condition is still lacking.

The potential usefulness of neuroimaging in providing insight in FXTAS becomes more evident as cognitive decline in FXTAS is resulting in an important field of research. As the phenotypic spectrum has expanded among *FMR1* premutated carriers, and FXTAS patients, psychiatric and cognitive disturbances are increasingly being recognized as relevant features

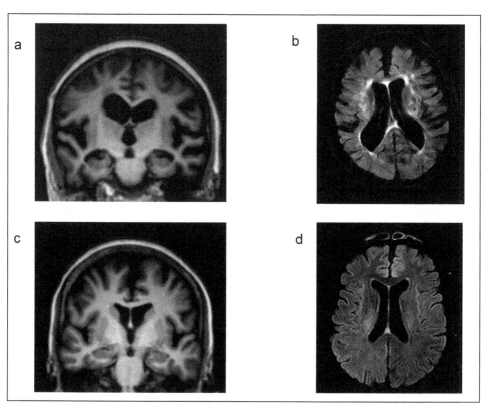

Fig. 3. Magnetic resonance imaging findings of two female patients with dementia and FXTAS. A) Coronal T1-weighted, 3D MPRAGE MR image of patient 1 shows asymmetrical frontal, and bilateral, symmetrical, medial temporal atrophy. B) Axial 3D FLAIR of patient 1 shows marked hyperintensities in the cerebral white matter. C) Coronal T1-weighted, 3D MPRAGE MR image of patient 2 shows moderate cerebral atrophy involving the frontal lobes, while the medial temporal lobes appeared normal.; K) Axial 3D FLAIR of patient 2 shows no marked HI in the white matter.

(Sevin *et al.*, 2009). Cognitive decline in FXTAS usually occurs in men, after a long duration of extrapyramidal disturbances, but it may also occur in women. Typically in men, a clinical picture similar distinct from Alzheimer´s disease (Seritan *et al.*, 2008), and more similar to patients with fronto-temporal lobar degeneration occurs (FTLD) (Burgeois *et al.*, 2009).

Although there is little evidence from MRI in these patients, particularly in women (Al Hinti *et al.*, 2007; Karmon *et al.*, 2008), more recently, two cases of mother-to-daughter transmission were reported (Rodriguez-Revenga *et al.*, 2010). In these two female patients with FXTAS and dementia, a radiological pattern of brain atrophy resembling that of patients with FTLD, was described. However, radiological heterogeneity may be large in this condition, as shown by the fact that prominent white matter hyperintensities were only seen in one case, as had been previously described (Al Hinti *et al.*, 2007; Karmon *et al.*, 2008), the second case lacking these, as well as hippocampal atrophy (Fig. 3).

There is very recent evidence about the use of VBM for studying the brain changes of *FMR1* premutated carriers, with and without FXTAS, and their correlation to neuropsychology (Hashimoto *et al.*, 2011). In this study, patients with FXTAS demonstrated a distinct pattern of grey matter volume loss, involving multiple cortical and subcortical regions. This included different parts of the cerebellum, as well as of the medial surface of the brain, including the dorsomedial prefrontal cortex, anterior cingulate and precuneus. Additional volume loss was seen in the lateral prefrontal cortex, orbitofrontal cortex, amygdala, and insula. More interestingly, there were significant correlations between grey matter loss in different brain regions, behavioral scales, and CGG repeats (Hashimoto *et al.*, 2011).

7. Conclusion

FXTAS is a relatively new disorders that is currently regarded as a late-onset neurodegenerative disorder; however, the underlying pathogenic process may begin very early in life. It is essential to fathom the molecular mechanism of FXTAS and to increase our knowledge of disease pathology in order to understand of FXTAS disease progression. Although the RNA gain-of-function hypothesis for FXTAS is well accepted, further analysis of the pathogenic effect of the expanded CGG-repeat *FMR1* mRNA are still required. A better understanding of the molecular basis of FXTAS should shed light on therapeutic approaches that will combat neurodegeneration and improve cognitive and motor performance. Furthermore, it can also help unraveling common mechanisms in other neurodegenerative diseaser which will bring hope to treatments more effective and specific to the underlying dysfunction.

MRI findings in FXTAS patients classically include middle cerebellar and white matter hyperintensities, as well as cerebellar, pontine and brain atrophy. Neuroimaging, and particularly MR techniques, offer an excellent opportunity to gain insight into the FXTAS condition. In vivo biomarkers may be identified non-invasively, which may be potentially useful in improving recognition, and early characterization of patients with FXTAS, so that treatment strategies can be developed and applied.

As the prevalence of premutated alleles is relatively high in general population, FXTAS may represent one of the more common monogenic causes of tremor, ataxia, and dementia. For this reason, it is probably that many carriers with FXTAS are being seen by a clinical specialist without awareness of the underlying genetic basis for the symptoms. The early diagnosis of those patients not only benefits themselves but also the rest of the family that should be advised for the FXS.

8. Acknowledgments

This work has received financial support from grant PI09/0413 and FISS PI/770 both financed by "Instituto Carlos III". We would like to acknowledge GIRMOGEN and the Catalan Association of Fragile X syndrome as well as all FXS families that collaborate with us. The CIBER de Enfermedades Raras is an initiative of the ISCIII

9. References

Adams, JS., Adams, PE., Nguyen, D., Brunberg, JA., Tassone, F., Zhang, W., Koldewyn, K., Rivera, SM., Grigsby, J., Zhang, L., DeCarli, C., Hagerman, PJ., & Hagerman, RJ. (2007). *Neurology* 28,69 ,851-859.

Al-Hinti, JT., Nagan, N., & Harik, SI. (2007). *Alzheimer Disease & Associated Disorders* 21,262-264.

Ashburner, J., & Friston, KJ. (2000). *Neuroimage* 11,805-821.

Bacalman, S., Farzin, F., Bourgeois, JA., Cogswell, J., Goodlin-Jones, BL., Gane, LW., Grigsby, J., Leehey, MA., Tassone, F., & Hagerman, RJ. (2006). *Journal of Clinical Psychiatry* 67,87-94.

Bassell, GJ., & Warren, ST. (2008). *Neuron* 60,201-214.

Bennetto, L; Pennington, BF; Porter, D; Taylor, AK; Hagerman, RJ. (2001). *Neuropsychology* 15,290-299.

Berry-Kravis, E., Potanos, K., Weinberg, D., Zhou, L., & Goetz, CG. (2004). *Annals of Neurology* 57,144–147.

Bontekoe, CJ; Bakker, CE; Nieuwenhuizen, IM; van der Linde, H; Lans, H; de Lange, D; Hirst, MC; & Oostra, BA. (2001). *Human Molecular Genetics* 10,1693-1639.

Bourgeois, JA., Coffey, SM., Rivera, SM., Hessl, D., Gane, LW., Tassone, F., Greco, C., Finucane, B., Nelson, L., Berry-Kravis, E., Grigsby, J., Hagerman, PJ., & Hagerman, RJ. (2009). *Journal of Clinical Psychiatry* 70,852-862.

Brunberg J., Jacquemont S., Hagerman RJ., Berry-Kravis, E., Grigsby, J., Leehey, M., Tassone, F., Brown, T., Greco, C., & Hagerman. PJ. (2002). *American Journal of Neuroradiology*.23,1757-1766.

Brussino, A., Gellera, C., Saluto, A., Mariotti, C., Arduino, C., Castellotti, B., Camerlingo, M., de Angelis, V., Orsi, L., Tosca, P., Migone, N., Taroni, F., & Brusco, A. (2005) *Neurology* 64,145-147.

Coffey, SM., Cook, K., Tartaglia, N., Tassone, F., Nguyen, DV., Pan, R., Bronsky, HE., Yuhas, J., Borodyanskaya, M,, Grigsby, J., Doerflinger, M., Hagerman, PJ., & Hagerman, RJ. (2008) *American Journal of Medical Genetics Part A* 146,1009-1016.

Cohen, S., Masyn, K., Adams, J., Hessl, D., Rivera, S., Tassone, F., Brunberg, J., DeCarli, C., Zhang, L., Cogswell, J., Loesch, D., Leehey, M., Grigsby, J., Hagerman, PJ., & Hagerman, R. (2006). *Neurology* 67,1426–1431.

Galloway, JN., & Nelson, DL. (2009) *Future Neurology* 4,785.

Garcia-Arocena, D., & Hagerman PJ. (2010). *Human Molecular Genetics* 19,R83-R89.

Ginestroni, A., Guerrini, L., Della Nave, R., Tessa, C., Cellini, E., Dotti, MT., Brunori, P., De Stefano, N., Piacentini, S., & Mascalchi, M. (2007). *AJNR - American Journal of Neuroradiology.* 28,486-488.

Gómez-Ansón, B., Alegret, M., Muñoz, E., Sainz, A., Monte, GC., & Tolosa, E. (2007). *Neurology* 68,906-910.

Gómez Ansón, B., Monte, GC., Rotger, R., Rodriguez-Revenga, L., Mila, M., & Capurro, S. (2007). MR characterization of premutated carriers of the fragile X syndrome: a VBM and 1H-MRS study. *Proceedings of* Congress of European Society of Neuroradiology (ESNR), Genova, September 2007.

Gómez-Ansón, B., Alegret, M., Munoz, E., Monte, GC., Alayrach, E., Sanchez, A., Boada, M., & Tolosa, E. (2009). *Parkinsonism & Related Disorders* 15,213-219.

Greco, CM., Hagerman, RJ., Tassone, F., Chudley, AE., Del Bigio, MR., Jacquemont, S., Leehey, M., & Hagerman, PJ. (2002). *Brain* 125,1760-1771.

Greco, CM., Berman, RF., Martin, RM., Tassone, F., Schwartz, PH., Chang, A., Trapp, BD., Iwahashi, C., Brunberg, J., Grigsby, J., Hessl, D., Becker, EJ., Papazian, J., Leehey, MA., Hagerman, RJ., & Hagerman, PJ. (2006). *Brain* 129:243-255.

Grigsby, J., Brega, AG., Leehey, MA., Goodrich, GK., Jacquemont, S., Loesch, DZ., Cogswell, JB., Epstein, J., Wilson, R., Jardini, T., Gould, E., Bennett, RE., Hessl, D., Cohen, S., Cook, K., Tassone, F., Hagerman, PJ., & Hagerman, RJ. (2007). *Movement Disorders* 22,645-650.

Grigsby, J., Brega, AG., Engle, K., Leehey, MA., Hagerman, RJ., Tassone, F., Hessl, D., Hagerman, PJ., Cogswell, JB., Bennett, RE., Cook, K., Hall, DA., Bounds, LS., Paulich, MJ., & Reynolds, A. (2008). *Neuropsychology* 22,48-60.

Hagerman, RJ., Leehey, M., Heinrichs, W., Tassone, F., Wilson, R., Hills, J., Grigsby, J., Gage, B., & Hagerman, PJ. (2001). *Neurology* 57,127-130.

Hagerman, RJ. (2002). Physical and behavioral phenotype, In: *Fragile X Syndrome: Diagnosis, treatment and research* Hagerman RJ & Hagerman PJ (3rd edition). The Johns Hopkins University Press, Baltimore, MD.

Hagerman, PJ., & Hagerman, RJ. (2004). *The American Journal of Human Genetics* 74,805-816.

Hashimoto, RI., Backer, KC., Tassone, F., Hagerman, RJ., & Rivera, SM. (2011). *Movement Disorder* 11.

Hessl, D., Tassone, F., Loesch, DZ., Berry-Kravis, E., Leehey, MA., Gane, LW., Barbato, I., Rice, C., Gould, E., Hall, DA., Grigsby, J., Wegelin, JA., Harris, S., Lewin, F., Weinberg, D., Hagerman, PJ., & Hagerman, RJ. (2005). *American Journal of Medical Genetics Part A* 139,115–121.

Iwahashi, CK., Yasui, DH., An, HJ., Greco, CM., Tassone, F., Nannen, K., Babineau, B., Lebrilla, CB., Hagerman, RJ., & Hagerman, PJ. (2006). *Brain* 129,256-271.

Jacquemont, S., Hagerman, RJ., Leehey, M., Grigsby, J., Zhang, L., Brunberg, JA., Greco, C., Des Portes, V., Jardini, T., Levine, R., Berry-Kravis, E., Brown, WT., Schaeffer, S., Kissel J., Tassone, F., & Hagerman, PJ. (2003). *The American Journal of Human Genetics* 72,869-878.

Jacquemont, S., Hagerman, RJ., Leehey, MA., Hall, DA., Levine, RA., Brunberg, JA., Zhang, L., Jardini, T., Gane, LW., Harris, SW., Herman, K., Grigsby, J., Greco, CM., Berry-Kravis, E., Tassone, F., & Hagerman, PJ. (2004a). *JAMA, the Journal of the American Medical Association* 291,460-469.

Jacquemont, S., Farzin, F., Hall, D., Leehey, M., Tassone, F., Gane, L., Zhang, L., Grigsby, J., Jardini, T., Lewin, F., Berry-Kravis, E., Hagerman, PJ., & Hagerman, RJ. (2004b). *American Journal Of Mental Retardation* 109,154-164.

Jacquemont, S., Hagerman, R., Hagerman, PJ., Leehey, MA. (2007). *The Lancet Neurology* 6,45-55.

Johnston, C., Eliez, S., Dyer-Friedman, J., Hessl, D., Glaser, B., Blasey, C., Taylor, A., & Reiss, A. (2001). *American Journal of Medical Genetics* 103,314-319.

Kamm, C., Healy, DG., Quinn, NP., Wüllner, U., Moller, JC., Schols, L., Geser, F., Burk, K., Børglum, AD., Pellecchia, MT., Tolosa, E., del Sorbo, F., Nilsson, C., Bandmann, O., Sharma, M., Mayer, P., Gasteiger, M., Haworth, A., Ozawa, T., Lees, AJ., Short, J., Giunti, P., Holinski-Feder, E., Illig, T., Wichmann, HE., Wenning, GK., Wood, NW., Gasser, T., & European Multiple System Atrophy Study Group. (2005). *Brain* 128,1855-1860.

Karmon, Y., & Gadoth, N. (2008). *Journal of Neurology, Neurosurgery & Psychiatry* 79,738-739.

Kenneson, A., Zhang, F., Hagedorn, CH., & Warren, ST. (2001). *Human Molecular Genetics* 10,1449-1454.

Ladd, PD., Smith, LE., Rabaia, NA., Moore, JM., Georges, SA., Hansen, RS., Hagerman, RJ., Tassone, F., Tapscott, SJ., & Filippova, GN. (2007). *Human Molecular Genetics* 16,3174-3187.

Leehey, MA., Munhoz, RP., Lang, AE., Brunberg, JA., Grigsby, J., Greco, C., Jacquemont, S., Tassone, F., Lozano, AM., Hagerman, PJ., & Hagerman, RJ. (2003). *Archives of Neurology* 60,117-121.

Leehey, MA., Berry-Kravis, E., Min, SJ., Hall, DA., Rice, CD., Zhang, L., Grigsby, J., Greco, CM., Reynolds, A., Lara, R., Cogswell, J., Jacquemont, S., Hessl, DR., Tassone, F., Hagerman, R., & Hagerman PJ. (2007). *Movement Disorders* 22,203-206.

Macpherson, J., Waghorn, A., Hammans, S., & Jacobs, P. (2003). *Human Genetics* 112,619-620.

Mankodi, A., Logigian, E., Callahan, L., McClain, C., White, R., Henderson, D., Krym, M., & Thornton, CA. (2000). *Science* 289,1769-1773.

Mankodi, A., & Thornton, CA. (2002). *Current Opinion in Neurology* 15,545-552.

Milà, M., Madrigal, I., Kulisevsky, J., Pagonabarraga, J., Gómez, B., Sánchez, A., & Rodríguez-Revenga, L. (2009). *Medicina Clínica* 133, 252-4.

Moore, CJ., Daly, EM., Schmitz, N., Tassone, F., Tysoe, C., Hagerman, RJ., Hagerman, PJ., Morris, RG., Murphy, KC., & Murphy, DG. (2004a). *Neuropsychologia* 42,1934-1947.

Moore, CJ., Daly, EM., Tassone, F., Tysoe, C,. Schmitz, N., Ng, V., Chitnis, X., McGuire, P., Suckling, J., Davies, KE., Hagerman, RJ., Hagerman, PJ., Murphy, KC., & Murphy, DG. (2004b). *Brain* 127,2672-2681.

Oberle, I., Rousseau, F., Heitz, D., Kretz, C., Devys, D., Hanauer, A., Boue, J., Bertheas, MF., & Mandel, JL. (1991). *Science* 252,1097-1102.

Okamoto, J., Tokiguchi, S., Furusawa, T., Ishikawa, K., Quardery, AF., Shinbo, S., & Sasai S. (2003). *AJNR Am American Journal of Neuroradiology* 24,1946-1954.

Oostra, BA., & Willemsen, R. (2003). *Human Molecular Genetics* 12,R249-R257.

Oostra BA., & Willemsen R. (2009). *Biochimica et Biophysica Acta* 1790,467-477.

Reiss, AL., Freund, L., Abrams, MT., Boehm, C., & Kazazian, H. (1993). *The American Journal of Human Genetics* 52,884-894.

Riddle, JE., Cheema, A., Sobesky, WE., Gardner, SC., Taylor, AK., Pennington, BF., & Hagerman, RJ. (1998). *American Journal Of Mental Retardation* 102,590-601.

Rife, M., Badenas, C., Mallolas, J., Jimenez, L., Cervera, R., Maya, A., Glover, G., Rivera, F., & Mila, M. (2003). *Genetic Testing* 7,339-343.

Rodriguez-Revenga, L., Gómez-Anson, B., Muñoz, E., Jiménez, D., Santos, M., Tintoré, M., Martín, G., Brieva, L., & Milà, M. (2007). *Molecular Neurobiology* 35,324-328.

Rodriguez-Revenga, L., Madrigal, I., Alegret, M., Santos, M., & Milà, M. (2008a). *Psychiatric Genetics* 18,153-155.

Rodriguez-Revenga, L., Santos, MM., Sánchez, A., Pujol, M., Gómez-Anson, B., Badenas, C., Jiménez, D., Madrigal, I., & Milà, M. (2008b). *Genetic Testing* 12,135-138.

Rodriguez-Revenga, L., Madrigal, I., Pagonabarraga, J., Xunclà, M., Badenas, C., Kulisevsky, J., Gomez, B., & Milà, M. (2009). *European Journal of Human Genetics* 17,1359-1362.

Rodriguez-Revenga, L., Pagonabarraga, J., Gómez-Anson, B., López-Mourelo, O., Xunclà. M., & Milà, M. (2010). *Neurology* 75,1370-1376.

Sánchez-Benavides, G., Gómez-Ansón, B., Sainz, A., Vives, Y., Delfino, M., & Peña-Casanova, J. (2010). *Psychiatry Research* 181,219-225.

Sellier, C., Rau, F., Liu, Y., Tassone, F., Hukema, RK., Gattoni, R., Schneider, A., Richard, S., Willemsen, R., Elliott, DJ., Hagerman, PJ., & Charlet-Berguerand, N. (2010). *The EMBO Journal* 29,1248-1261.

Seritan, AL., Nguyen, DV., Farias, ST., Hinton, L., Grigsby, J., Bourgeois, JA., & Hagerman, RJ. (2008). *American Journal of Medical Genetics Part B: Neuropsychiatric Genetics* 147,1138-1144.

Sevin, M., Kutalik, Z., Bergman, S, Vercelletto, M., Renou, P., Lamy, E., Vingerhoets,FJ., Di Virgilio, G., Boisseau, P., Bezieau, S., Pasquier, L., Rival, JM., Beckmann, JS., Damier, P., & Jacquemont. S. (2009). *Journal of Medical Genetics* 46,818-824.

Tan, H., Li, H., & Jin, P. (2009). *Neuroscience Letters* 466,103-108.

Tassone, F., Hagerman, RJ., Taylor, AK., Gane, LW., Godfrey, TE., & Hagerman, PJ. (2000a). *The American Journal of Human Genetics* 66,6-15.

Tassone, F., Hagerman, RJ., Taylor, AK., Mills, JB., Harris, SW., Gane, LW., & Hagerman, PJ. (2000b). *American Journal of Medical Genetics* 91,144-1152.

Tassone, F., & Hagerman, PJ. (2003). *Cytogenetic and Genome Research* 100,124-128.

Van Esch, H., Matthijs, G., & Fryns, JP. (2005). *Annals of Neurology* 57,932-933.

Verkerk, AJ., Pieretti, M., Sutcliffe, JS., Fu, YH., Kuhl, DP., Pizzuti, A., Reiner, O., Richards, S., Victoria, MF., Zhang, FP., et al. (1991). *Cell* 65,905-914.

Willemsen, R., Hoogeveen-Westerveld, M., Reis, S., Holstege, J., Severijnen, LA., Nieuwenhuizen, IM., Schrier, M., van Unen, L., Tassone, F., Hoogeveen, AT., Hagerman, PJ., Mientjes, EJ., & Oostra, BA. (2003). *Human Molecular Genetics* 12,949-959.

Yu, S., Pritchard, M., Kremer, E., Lynch, M., Nancarrow, J., Baker, E., Holman, K., Mulley, JC., Warren, ST., Schlessinger, D; *et al.* (1991). *Science* 252,1179-1181.

Zuhlke, Ch., Budnik, A., Gehlken, U., Dalski, A., Purmann, S., Naumann, M., Schmidt, M., Burk, K., & Schwinger, E. (2004). *Journal of Neurology* 251:1418-1419.

Dopamine Transporter Imaging for Distinguishing Between Idiopathic Parkinson's Disease and Secondary Parkinsonism

Chin-Chang Huang[1], Tzu-Chen Yen[2] and Chin-Song Lu[3]
*[1]Department of Neurology, Chang Gung Memorial Hospital
and Chang Gung University College of Medicine, Taipei
[2]Department of Nuclear Medicine, Chang Gung Memorial
Hospital and Chang Gung University
[3]Department of Neurology, Chang Gung Memorial Hospital
and Chang Gung University
Taiwan*

1. Introduction

Idiopathic Parkinson's disease (IPD), first described by James Parkinson in 1817, is a sporadic neurodegenerative disorder. The main clinical features include masked face, resting tremor, bradykinesia, rigidity, festinating gait, and loss of postural reflexes. The clinical features are most insidious and usually asymmetric at onset. The asymmetry may persist even in a late stage and progress slowly. The pathological findings are characterized by loss of pigmented dopamine neurons in the substantia nigra, particularly the pars compacta and locus ceruleus, and the presence of Lewy bodies. The cause of IPD remains unknown.

Parkinsonism (PM) is not a single disease but a common clinical presentation. The clinical syndrome is characterized by tremors, bradykinesia, rigidity, and postural instability. Exposure to toxins such as 1-methyl-4-phenyl-1,2,3,6-tetrahydropyridine (MPTP), which was sold as "synthetic heroin," manganese (Mn), carbon disulfide (CS_2), carbon monoxide (CO), methanol, cyanide, and other organic solvents may cause brain damage, leading to features similar to PM. Many neurodegenerative disorders may present with PM, including progressive supranuclear palsy (PSP), multiple system atrophy (MSA), spinocerebellar atrophy (SCA), and corticobasal sundrome (CBS). Several genetic diseases, including dopa-responsive dystonia (DRD), Wilson's disease (WD), and Huntington's disease (HD), may cause degeneration in the basal ganglia or affect the dopaminergic pathway. Furthermore, some dementia syndromes may be associated with PM, including vascular parkinsonism (multiple infarct parkinsonism), dementia with Lewy bodies (DLB), and frontotemporal dementia, and parkinsonism linked to chromosome 17 (FTD-17).

The main treatment of IPD includes the use of dopamine, dopamine agonists, monoamine oxidase inhibitors, and catechol-*o*-methyltransferase inhibitors. The above medications are usually effective in IPD patients, whereas their effects are usually limited in patients with secondary parkinsonism. Although definite diagnosis of IPD is based on typical pathological findings, early diagnosis is very important as it leads to early treatment.

IPD and PM are distinguished on the basis of the onset of symptoms, symmetry of clinical features, characteristics of tremors, rigidity, bradykinesia, and other associated symptoms, such as cognitive impairment, limitation of eye ball movement, ataxia, and autonomic dysfunction. In addition, information concerning family history, smoking and alcohol exposure, diabetes with hypertension, and exposure to toxic substances are also essential for diagnosis. Despite differences in the clinical features of IPD and PM, definite diagnosis may be difficult; therefore, reliable imaging is helpful for early and accurate diagnosis.

2. Dopamine transporter (DAT) scan

Dopamine transport is one of the primary mechanisms that can modulate the dopaminergic tone via an active transport system that involves the re-uptake of dopamine. Cocaine analogues including (1r) 2β-carbomethoxy-3β-(4-iodophenyl) tropane (β-CIT), and ^{123}I-FP-CIT have been developed as single photon emission computed tomography (SPECT) imaging agents. Both agents can bind at the DAT site of dopamine neuron terminals in normal human subjects and IPD patients. In addition, ^{99m}Tc-TRODAT-1 is a promising ^{99m}Tc-labelled radiotracer for imaging DAT in the human brain. Since a cyclotron and well-trained radiochemists are required for clinical usage of ^{123}I-β-CIT and ^{123}I-FP-CIT SPECT, they are more difficult to use in clinical settings. ^{99m}Tc-TRODAT-1 is much easier to prepare and can be made in many nuclear medicine departments. Previous studies have shown that ^{99m}Tc-TRODAT-1 is very reliable in detecting dopamine neurons in the striatum; therefore, it is an important tool for understanding the role of DAT in various neurological diseases.

3. DAT scan in IPD

Similar to ^{123}I-β-CIT and ^{123}I-FP-CIT, ^{99m}Tc-TRODAT-1 activity in the basal ganglia can demonstrate a stable target/non-target ratio, and at a reduced level in IPD patients than in healthy volunteers. Serial ^{99m}Tc-TRODAT-1 SPECT images taken 2, 3, and 4 h after injection of 925 MBq ^{99m}Tc-TRODAT into healthy volunteers show a consistent increase of the uptake with time. Furthermore, the relative concentration of ^{99m}Tc-TRODAT-1 in the basal ganglia regions decreases significantly with age in healthy volunteers. The rate of decline is significantly faster in young individuals than in the elderly. The effect seems to occur during young adulthood, particularly in individuals younger than 40 years. The putamen/occipital and caudate/occipital ratios show a statistically significant difference between IPD patients and healthy volunteers.

4. Secondary parkinsonism

4.1 Toxin-induced PM
4.1.1 1-Methyl-4-phenyl-1,2,3,6-tetrahydropyridine (MPTP)
MPTP is a byproduct of a meperidine analogue, 1-methyl-4-proprion-oxypeperidine (MPPP), which is a synthetic heroin. Injection of the contaminated synthetic drug may cause the victims to develop acute severe parkinsonian features such as bradykinesia and severe rigidity in about 7 days. Since its discovery, MPTP has been used in animal models of

parkinsonism, which is responsive to dopamine and dopamine agonist treatment. Although dementia and autonomic dysfunction, typical dyskinesia, prominent wearing off phenomena, and psychiatric impairments in MPTP victims occur more rapidly than in subjects with IPD, the clinical features of these individuals are indistinguishable from those of IPD patients. The MPTP toxin may damage the dopamine neurons in the substantia nigra via 1-methyl-4-phenyl-pyridinium (MPP+), a metabolite of MPTP, that may inhibit the production of ATP and stimulate the formation of superoxide radicals. The neurotoxic effect of MPTP is permanent, even though the patients have an excellent response to levodopa treatment. 6F-Dopa positron emission tomography (PET) of the brain showed that a subclinical exposure to MPTP might result in a reduction of fluorodopa uptake in the striatum. In some experimental studies that used brain SPECT, ^{99m}Tc-TRODAT-1 binding was significantly lower in the MPTP-treated monkeys than in the control monkeys.

4.1.2 Manganese (Mn) intoxication

Chronic exposure to manganese may induce parkinsonism similar to IPD. However, the clinical features of manganism, including lower body parkinsonism, frequent gait disturbance (particularly cock gait), increased dystonia, and reduced action tremor, also differ from IPD. In addition, in Mn-induced PM, a reduced response to anti-parkinsonian drugs, gait-freezing during turns, and difficulty in walking backwards were also noted. Although relative symmetry was noted, clinical asymmetry was also reported. Unlike patients with multiple system atrophy, patients with manganism did not show postural hypotension, sexual dysfunction, and sphincter disturbance.

Brain magnetic resonance imaging (MRI) is a promising technique to demonstrate the presence of manganese in the brain. T1-weighted MR images showed an increased intensity in the globus pallidus area of welders, smelters, patients undergoing parenteral nutrition, and in patients with hepatic failure. However, the increase in signal intensity in T1-weighted MR images only indicates an exposure to manganese in recent months but does not indicate manganism.

Previous PET scans with 6-FD had shown a normal nigrostriatal dopaminergic uptake in the caudate or putamen in manganism patients. In addition, brain PET scans with raclopride showed a mild decrease (less than 20%) of caudate dopamine D2 receptors. However, the minimal decrease of D2 receptor density could not account for the prominent clinical features in manganese intoxication patients.

Both 6-FD PET and DAT are sensitive detectors for dopamine neurons. In a previous study, DAT density with ^{123}I-β-CIT SPECT was decreased in PM patients with manganese exposure. However, these findings seemed to be more consistent with IPD than with Mn-induced parkinsonism. The brain ^{99m}Tc-TRODAT-1 SPECT showed no significant changes in the putamen and the putamen/caudate ratio of manganism patients and normal controls. However, a statistically significant decrease was noted in the uptake of ^{99m}Tc-TRODAT-1 in the putamen area of IPD patients than in the manganism patients. Figure 1 shows the DAT findings in a manganism patient, an IPD patient, and a normal control. The data indicate that presynaptic dopaminergic terminals are not the main targets of chronic manganese intoxication. Pathologic changes in monkeys after manganese chloride injection included prominent gliosis in the globus pallidus and in the substantia nigra pars reticularis that differs from the target lesion-substantia nigra pars compacta in IPD.

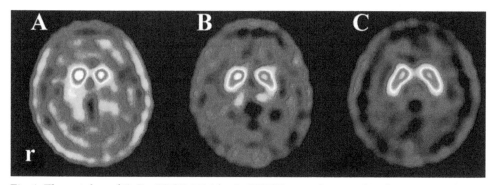

Fig. 1. The uptakes of ^{99m}Tc -TRODAT-1 brain SPECT were decreased in the corpus striatum particularly in the left side in a PD patient (A), and nearly normal in a patient with chronic manganism (B) and a normal control (C). r=right.

4.1.3 Carbon disulfide (CS$_2$) intoxication

CS$_2$ is a colorless liquid organic solvent frequently used in the production of viscose rayon fibers and cellophane films. Acute exposure to CS$_2$ may cause psychosis, delirium, seizures,

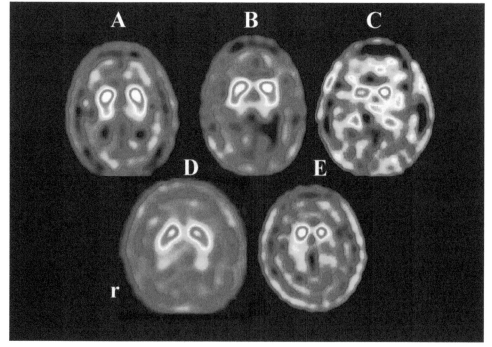

Fig. 2. Normal DAT bindings with ^{99m}Tc -TRODAT-1 brain SPECT were noted in 2 patients with CS$_2$ intoxication (A), and (B) but a decreased DAT binding in another patient who had IPD with CS$_2$ exposure (C), as compared with those of a normal control (D) and a PD patient (E). r=right.

and even death. Chronic exposure to CS_2 manifests as a diffuse encephalopathy including parkinsonism, intention tremor, emotional lability, and neurobehavioral disorders as well as polyneuropathy. Brain MRI may reveal diffuse hyperintense lesions in T2-weighted images in the subcortical white matter, basal ganglia, and brainstem. A brain CT perfusion study showed a decrease of regional cerebral flow and prolonged regional mean transit time in the subcortical white matter and the basal ganglia. The diffuse white matter lesions are better explained by vascular insufficiency than demyelination. In CS_2 intoxicated patients with parkinsonism, brain ^{99m}Tc-TRODAT-1 SPECT showed a normal uptake of the dopamine transporter, indicating a normal presynaptic dopaminergic pathway (Figure 2). Therefore, CS_2 intoxication-induced parkinsonism is probably due to post-synaptic lesions in the basal ganglia rather than the presynaptic dopaminergic pathway.

4.1.4 Carbon monoxide (CO) intoxication

Acute CO intoxication may induce hypoxic changes in the brain with variable degree of consciousness disturbance from confusion, delirium, and stupor to deep coma. Most patients recover after appropriate oxygen therapy; however, sequelae such as dystonia and cognitive impairment may persist. Approximately 0.2–40% of survivors developed delayed encephalopathy within 2 months. The common manifestations include cognitive changes, sphincter disturbance, akinetic mutism, and parkinsonian features. Brain MRI studies showed hyperintense lesions in the basal ganglia, particularly in the globus pallidus and subcortical white matter. A steady improvement was found after 1–2 years of supportive therapy; however, residual parkinsonism may develop in some patients. Moreover, a poor response to levodopa is noted. Brain ^{99m}Tc-TRODAT-1 may show a normal uptake in the basal ganglia, indicating that the presynaptic pathway of the nigrostriatral system is normal.

4.1.5 Others: Methanol and cyanide

Acute intoxication with methanol may cause metabolic acidosis and severe anionic gaps, leading to blindness and parkinsonism including masked face, rigidity, bradykinesia, gait disturbance, and dystonia. Brain MRI may show damage in the bilateral putaminal areas. Acute cyanide intoxication may also cause parkinsonism such as hypomimia, rigidity, and gait disturbance within a few days, and subsequent dystonia and dementia. The response to levodopa therapy is usually disappointing. Table 1 summarizes the clinical features and DAT findings in toxin-induced PM.

4.2 Other neurodegenerative parkinsonian syndromes
4.2.1 Progressive supranuclear palsy (PSP)

PSP, first described in the early 1900s, is a devastating neurodegenerative disease. In 1963, Steele, Richardson, and Olszewski reported a series of patients with pathologically confirmed heterogeneous system degeneration. The syndrome is characterized by parkinsonism, axial rigidity, frequent falls, vertical gaze palsy, pseudobulbar palsy, and dementia. In addition, atypical features include asymmetrical parkinsonism, dystonia, tremor, apraxia, and pure akinesia. The pathological changes include neuronal loss, neurofibrillary tangles, and gliosis in the basal ganglia, brainstem, and cerebral cortex. The response to levodopa treatment for parkinsonian symptoms is usually poor. The most common subtypes of PSP syndrome include Richardson's syndrome (RS) and progressive supranuclear palsy-parkinsonism (PSP-P). The clinical features of RS are similar to the classic type of PSP, whereas PSP-P has features similar to IPD, such as asymmetric onset of symptoms, tremor, and initial response to levodopa.

	MPTP	Mn	CS$_2$	CO	Methanol
Clinical features					
Parkinsonism	+	+	+	+	+
Rigidity	+	+	+	+	+
Tremor	+	Less	-	-	-
Bradykinesia	+	+	+	+	+
Loss of postural reflex	+	+	+	+	+
Mental disorders	+	+	+	+	+
Cerebellar sign	-	Less	+	-	-
Polyneuropathy	-	-	+	-	-
Autonomic dysfunction	+	+	+	-	-
Neuroimaging					
Brain CT/MRI	N/N	N/+ (T1 high)	+/+ (Vascular changes)	+/+ (GP)	+/+ (Putamen lesion)
DAT uptake in striatum (^{99m}Tc-TRODAT-1 SPECT)	Decrease (in monkey)	N	N	N	NA
Prognosis	Permanent	Deterioration	Poor	Partial recovery	Blindness
Response to Levodopa	Good	No	No	No	Poor
Source of exposure	Synthetic heroin	Smelter, miner, welder	Viscose rayon worker	Accidental, suicidal attempts	Accidental

+: presence; -: absence; GP: globus pallidus; N: normal; NA: not available
MPTP: 1-methyl-4-phenyl-1, 2, 3, 6-tetrahydropyridine; Mn: manganese; CS$_2$: carbon disulfide; CO: carbon monoxide.

Table 1. Toxins induced secondary parkinsonism

Dopamine transporter (DAT) scans with ^{123}I-β-CIT showed a reduction of DAT activities in the caudate and putamen areas, particularly the caudate areas in PSP patients. However, the dopamine D2 receptor images with IBZM were variable. The inconsistent findings are probably because of the grouping of both RS and PSP-P types. In our previous studies with

^{99m}Tc-TRODAT-1 scans, the mean striatal uptake was reduced in the RS group than in the PSP-P group, even though uptake did not reach statistical significance. The putamen/caudate ratios were significantly different between IPD and PSP patients. However, there was no difference between RS and PSP-P patients. In the IBZM scan, the uptake was significantly reduced in the RS group, but mildly increased in the PSP-P group. The data indicate that DAT imaging is helpful to distinguish PSP-P from IPD patients in the early stages. DAT activities showed a greater decrease in the RS group than in the PSP-P group. In addition, activities of the D2 receptor were reduced in the RS group but not in the PSP-P group.

4.2.2 Multiple system atrophy (MSA)

Multiple system atrophy (MSA) was originally described as 3 distinct disorders: olivopontocerebellar atrophy (OPCA), Shy–Drager syndrome (SDS), and striatonigral degeneration (SND). MSA is a sporadic progressive neurodegenerative disease characterized by variable degrees of parkinsonism, cerebellar ataxia, and autonomic dysfunction. According to the motor dysfunction, MSA can be divided into 2 subtypes: parkinsonian type (MSA-P) and cerebellar type (MSA-C). The pathologic changes reveal a variable involvement of neuronal loss in the corpus striatum, globus pallidus, substantia nigra, locus ceruleus, Edinger–Westphal nucleus, olivary nuclei, cerebellar peduncles, cerebellar Purkinje cells, intermediolateral column, and Onuf's nucleus of the spinal cord. The diagnosis of MSA is still based on clinical criteria. The clinical distinction between MSA-P and IPD is sometimes difficult, particularly in the early stages, because both have a good response to levodopa.

In IPD patients, a severe reduction of DAT uptake in the putamen and relative sparing of the caudate nucleus is noted. However, a variable uptake of 6-^{18}F-fluorodopa was noted in MSA patients. ^{99m}Tc-TRODAT-1-brain SPECT revealed a more symmetrical reduction of the striatal binding in MSA-P and MSA-C patients; this was in contrast with the greater asymmetric reduction seen in IPD patients. In addition, the reduction of P/O and S/O ratios is greater for the MSA-P patients than for the MSA-C patients. P/C ratios showed that MSA-P and IPD patients have a similar pattern of nigral involvement but that MSA-C patients had a different pattern.

4.2.3 Spinocerebellar degeneration (SCA)

Hereditary ataxias are a clinically and genetically heterogeneous group of disorders transmitted most frequently as autosomal dominant or autosomal recessive traits. Three common phenotypes including SCA1, SCA2 and SCA3 (Machado–Joseph disease, MJD) are characterized by variable degrees of cerebellar signs, pyramidal dysfunction, anterior horn cell involvement, and/or peripheral neuropathy but some patients may develop parkinsonian symptoms, which may also respond to levodopa treatment.

4.2.3.1 SCA1

The early pictures include cerebellar syndrome and upper motor neuron signs. Later, ophthalmoplegia, slow saccades, and a sensory predominant polyneuropathy, amyotrophy, chorea, and dystonia may develop. Dysarthria, dysphagia, and cognitive impairment are also noted. The gene mutation is an unstable CAG expansion in the *ataxin 1* gene on chromosome 6p. Brain ^{99m}Tc-TRODAT-1 SPECT imaging revealed a decrease of dopamine transport in the striatum.

4.2.3.2 SCA2

SCA2 has a wider phenotypical spectrum than SCA1. The presence of slow saccades and peripheral neuropathy early in the disease may lead to the diagnosis of SCA2. In addition, dystonia, levodopa-responsive parkinsonism, and cognitive decline are also noted. The mutation is a CAG expansion in the *ataxin 2* gene on chromosome 12 with alleles ranging from 32–64 (normal, 15–31). ^{99m}Tc-TRODAT-1 SPECT of the brain showed a significantly asymmetric reduction of the striatal dopamine transporter in these patients; this was similar to the finding in IPD patients. The presynaptic impairment of nigrostriatal function is probably the reason for levodopa responsiveness.

4.2.3.3 SCA3

This is the most prevalent type of spinocerebellar ataxia. The clinical manifestations include cerebellar and brainstem signs such as facial and tongue fasciculations or myokymia, with facial atrophy, and dysphonia. Non-cerebellar eye signs such as slow saccades, impairment in conjugate eyeball movement, ophthalmoparesis, ptosis, eyelid retraction, and blepharospasm have also been reported. Dystonia is commonly seen. In addition, the parkinsonian features may respond to dopamine therapy. The mutation is an unstable CAG expansion in the *ataxia 3* gene on chromosome 14 with 53–86 CAG repeats (normal limit < 47). ^{99m}Tc-TRODAT-1 scan of the brain revealed a significant decrease in the uptake of tracers in MJD patients than in healthy controls. The decreased uptakes of ^{99m}Tc-TRODAT-1 indicated a defect in the nigrostriatal dopaminergic pathway in symptomatic MJD patients with and without extrapyramidal signs. However, the severity of the DAT abnormality did not correlate well with the length of the CAG repeat, age at disease onset, or disease duration.

4.2.4 Corticobasal syndrome (CBS)

Corticobasal syndrome was first described in 1967 in 3 patients who had asymmetric motor symptoms with an involvement of frontoparietal atrophy and neuronal loss at autopsy. CBS is an adult onset and slowly progressive degeneration with asymmetric akinetic-rigid syndrome. A limited response to levodopa treatment is noted in such patients. Some other extrapyramidal symptoms include tremor, dystonia, cortical dysfunction, cortical sensory impairment, apraxia, and alien hand phenomenon. Brain MRI may show focal cortical atrophy, particularly in the parietal lobe. Brain ^{18}F-FDG PET reveals a frequently asymmetric hypometabolism in both the cerebral hemispheres. Brain ^{99m}Tc-TRODAT SPECT reveals an asymmetric involvement in the corpus striatum with equal involvement in both caudate and putamen regions.

The clinical and DAT findings in the above-described neurodegenerative diseases are shown in Table 2.

4.3 Gene-related parkinsonism/dystonia degenerative diseases
4.3.1 Dopa-responsive dystonia (DRD)

Dopa-responsive dystonia, also known as Segawa's disease, is characterized by foot dystonia since childhood, diurnal fluctuation, and a dramatic and sustained response to low-dosage levodopa. Some patients with DRD may also show adult-onset parkinsonism similar to IPD. Pathologic degeneration of dopaminergic nigral cells is found in IPD, whereas synthesis defects in dopamine neurons without cell loss are noted in DRD.

	PSP		MSA		SCA			CBS
	RS	PSP-P	MSA-P	MSA-C	SCA1	SCA2	SCA3	
Clinical features								
Parkinsonism	+(sym)	+(asym)	+	+	+	+	+	+ (asym)
Rigidity	+(axial)	+(axial)	+	+	+	+	+	+ (asym)
Tremor	-	+	+	+	+(action)	+(action)	+(action)	+
Bradykinesia	+	+	+	+	+	+	+	-
Loss of postural reflex	+	+	+	+	+	+	+	-
Akinetic- rigid syndrome	+	-	+	-	-	-	-	+
Dystonia	+(facial)	+(facial)	-	-	+	+	+	+
Retrocollis	+	+	-(anticollis)		-	-	-	-
Cognitive dysfunction	+	+	+	-	+	-	-	+
Alien hand	-	-	-	-	-	-	-	+
Cortical sensory impairment	-	-	-	-	-	-	-	+
Cerebellar sign	-	-	+	+	+	+	+	-
Ataxia	-	-	-	+	+	+	+	-
Slow saccade	-	-	-	+	+	+	+	-
Peripheral neuropathy	-	-	-	-	+	+	-	-
Autonomic dysfunction	+	+	+	+	-	?	?	?
EOM limitation	+ (VGP)	+ (VGP)	-	-	+	-	+	-
Ptosis	-	-	-	-	-	-	+	-
Fasciculation	-	-	-	-	-	-	+	-
Face	-	-	-	-	-	-	+	-
Tongue	-	-	-	-	-	-	+	-
Dysarthria	+	+	+	+	+	+	+	-
Dysphagia	+	+	+	+	+	+	+	-
Apraxia	-	-	-	-	-	-	-	+
Response to Levodopa	Poor	Initial good	Initial good	Partial	Partial	Initial good	Partial	+ (limited)
Neuroimaging								
CT/MRI	+/+	+/+	+/+	+/+	+/+	+/+	+/+	+/+
DAT uptake	D	D	D (sym)	D (sym)	D	D (asym)	D	D (asym)
IBZM uptake	D	Increase (mild)	Possible D	Possible D	NA	NA	NA	D
6 FD-PET uptake	NA	NA	D	D	NA	NA	NA	D (asym)

+: presence; -: absence; D: decrease; I: increase; sym: symmetrical; asym: asymmetrical; VGP: vertical gaze palsy; NA: not available

Table 2. Clinical features and DAT data in neurodegenerative diseases

Molecular genetic studies revealed a mutation in GTP cyclohydrolase 1 (*GCH1*) in autosomal-dominant inherited DRD and mutations in tyrosine hydroxylase (*TH*) in autosomal-recessive inherited DRD. In DRD patients, ^{18}F-Dopa PET reveals normal uptakes in the corpus striatum; these findings may distinguish DRD from IPD, which reveals a decreased uptake even in the early stage of IPD patients. Dopamine transporter images with ^{99m}Tc-TRODAT-1 SPECT also show a normal uptake in DRD, indicating that presynaptic nigrostriatal dopaminergic terminals are normal (Figure 3).

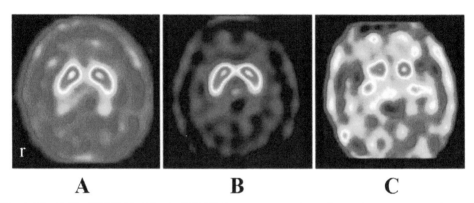

A   B   C

Fig. 3. The [99m]Tc -TRODAT-1 brain SPECT shows a normal uptake in the putamen and caudate in a patient with DRD (B) compared with those in a normal control (A) and a PD patient (C). A reduction of the uptake in the corpus striatum, particularly in the right side was observed in the PD patient. r=right.

4.3.2 Wilson's disease (WD)
Wilson's disease, hepatolenticular degeneration, is an autosomal recessive disorder characterized by a decreased serum concentration of ceruloplasmin, low serum copper concentration, and excessive deposition of copper in the liver, brain, and other organs.

The most common neurological manifestations include akinetic-rigid syndrome, dystonia, and cerebellar ataxia with action tremor. Pathologically, the most severely affected lesions include the basal ganglia involving the putamen, caudate, and globus pallidus. A brain CT scan may show low-density lesions with cystic degeneration in the basal ganglia, particularly the putamen and globus pallidus, as well as cortical atrophy and ventricular enlargement. Brain MRI reveals increased signal intensities in T2-weighted images of the lenticular nuclei, thalamus, and brainstem including the pons, midbrain, and even the substantia nigra. Occasionally, double panda signs were found in the brainstem. A poor therapeutic response to levodopa is noted in WD patients. However, brain 6F-DOPA PET studies have shown an involvement of the nigrostriatal presynaptic dopaminergic pathway. In addition, SPECT with ^{123}I-iodobenzamide (^{123}I-IBZM) and PET images with ^{18}F-methylspiperone have showed a reduction of postsynaptic striatal D2 receptor, reflecting striatal neuronal damage. Some DAT studies with ^{123}I-β-CIT SPECT disclosed a severe or differential loss of the DAT in the striatum of WD patients, indicating a presynaptic defect in the terminals of the nigrostriatal dopaminergic neurons. However, in some WD patients with akinetic-rigid syndrome, a normal presynaptic dopaminergic pathway may occur; brain MRI also reveals the involvement of substantia nigra in these patients. (Figure 4).

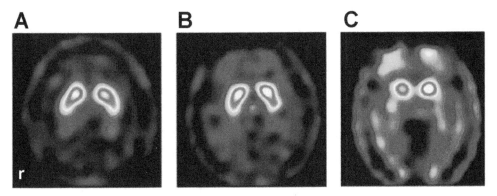

Fig. 4. Demonstration of ^{99m}Tc-TRODAT-1 uptake in an age-matched normal control (A), a WD patient (B) and a PD patient (C). Normal uptake of ^{99m}Tc-TRODAT-1 in the putamen and caudate nucleus was noted in a normal control and a WD patient (A and B). In PD patient, there was an asymmetrically decreased ^{99m}Tc-TRODAT-1 uptake, predominantly in the putamen (C). r=right.

4.3.3 Huntington's disease (HD, Westphal type)

Huntington's disease, the most common cause of hereditary chorea, is an autosomal dominant disorder caused by an expansion of an unstable trinucleotide repeat in chromosome 4. The most striking feature is the appearance of chorea movements that seem purposeless and abrupt. However, some patients may present with the so-called akinetic-rigid variant form (Westphal variant). This form of the disease is rapidly progressive with a fatal outcome in less than 10 years after the onset of symptoms. Brain CT/MRI show enlarged ventricles with atrophy of the caudate nucleus. MRI of patients with the a kinetic-rigid form of the disease may reveal T2 hyperintense lesions in the striatum. FDG-PET may show hypometabolism in the caudate and putamen regions.

The clinical features and neuroimages of DRD, WD, and HD with Westphal variant are summarized in Table 3.

4.4 Dementia syndromes with parkinsonism
4.4.1 Vascular parkinsonism (VP) or multiple infarct parkinsonism

Vascular parkinsonism is characterized by clinical symptoms of gait disturbance with freezing, lower body parkinsonism, and loss of postural reflexes. Tremor is rarely seen. The onset is usually insidious and the course is progressive. Brain MRI usually reveals hyperintense T2-weighted signals in the basal ganglia and/or white matter; these findings are compatible with those of multiple infarctions. Hypertension is a common risk factor for the disorder. A poor or insufficient response to anti-parkinsonian drugs is also noted in these patients. Early diagnosis of VP is important because the prognosis and response to treatment in these patients are different from those of patients with IPD. However, VP may have a wide spectrum of clinical features, which make the differential diagnosis of these diseases difficult. A study using DAT with ^{99m}Tc-TRODAT-1 showed that specific binding in the putamen and caudate areas was slightly lower in VP patients than in healthy individuals; however, a significant decrease in the uptake of ^{99m}Tc-TRODAT-1 in the striatum was noted in IPD patients. A significant striatal asymmetry was observed in IPD patients but not in VP patients.

	DRD	WD	HD (Westphal)
Clinical features			
Diurnal fluctuation	+	-	-
Chorea	-	-	+
Dystonia	+	+	+
Parkinsonism	+	+	+
Cerebellar sign	-	+	-
Cognitive impairment	-	+	+
Liver dysfunction	-	+	-
Autonomic dysfunction	-	+	-
Response to levodopa	Excellent	Partial	No
Neuroimaging			
CT/MRI	N/N	Abn/Abn	Abn/Abn (caudate atrophy)
DAT-SPECT	N	Abn	NA
FDG-PET	N	Abn	Abn
6 FD-PET	N	Abn	NA

+: presence; -: absence; N: normal; Abn: abnormal; NA: not available

Table 3. Clinical features and DAT findings in gene- related PM/dystonia degenerative diseases

4.4.2 Dementia with Lewy bodies (DLB)

DLB is the second most common cause of neurodegenerative dementia after Alzheimer's disease (AD). The diagnostic criteria of DLB were established by the consensus conference for DLB in 2005. In the early stage of DLB, deficits in attention, executive function, and visuospatial ability are very prominent. The core clinical features include fluctuation of cognition, visual hallucination, and spontaneous parkinsonism. Recent suggestive features include REM sleep behavioral disorder, severe neuroleptic sensitivity, and low dopamine transporter uptake in the basal ganglia on SPECT or PET imaging. Supportive features of DLB diagnosis include repeated falls, syncope, transient loss of consciousness, autonomic dysfunction, depression, systematized delusions, or hallucinations. In brain MRI, atrophy of the cortical or hippocampus is lower in DLB patients than in AD patients. In ^{18}F-FDG PET or SPECT, maximal hypometabolism was noted in the parieto-occipital area in DLB patients; however, maximal hypoperfusion was noted in the tempo-parietal cortex in AD patients.

Serial DAT with I-[123] β-CIT brain SPECT also demonstrated progressive striatal dopaminergic loss in DLB and Parkinson's disease with dementia, but not in AD. These findings have a high specificity (94%) in distinguishing between DLB and AD.

A brain DAT with TRODAT-1 SPECT also demonstrated a decreased uptake in the striatum, including the putamen and caudate regions, but the DLB patients had relatively symmetric lesions and IPD patients had asymmetric lesions.

4.4.3 Frontotemporal dementia with parkinsonism-17 (FTDP-17)

Frontotemporal dementia (FTD) can be divided into 3 major subtypes, including frontotemporal lobe dementia (FTLD), semantic dementia (SD), and progressive nonfluent aphasia (PNFA). The characteristic behavior changes include disinhibition, social withdrawal, diminished insight, loss of empathy, perseverance, and stereotypic behaviors. Semantic dementia may present with progressive loss of semantic knowledge, and although speech remain fluent, it becomes empty. Semantic dementia usually manifests as a fluent

	VaD	DLB	FTDP-17
Clinical features			
Parkinsonism	+	+	+
Rigidity	+	+	+
Tremor	-	-	-
Bradykinesia	+	+	+
Lose of postural reflex	+	+	+
Language problem	+	-	+
Focal sign	+	-	+
Dysarthria	+	-	-
Dysphagia	+	-	-
Dementia	+	+	+
Hallucination	+	+	-
Cognitive fluctuation	-	+	-
Personality changes	+	+	+
Syncope	-	+	-
Autonomic dysfunction	-	+	-
Response to levodopa	Poor	Poor	Poor
Neuroimages			
CT/MRI	Abn/Abn	Abn/Abn	Abn/Abn
DAT-TRODAT	Normal	Abn	NA
FDG-PET	Abn	Abn	Abn
6FD-PET	NA	Abn	NA

+: Presence; -: absence; Abn: abnormal; NA: not available

Table 4. Clinical features and DAT findings in dementia syndromes

dysphasia with impairment in semantic verbal memory and an associative agnosia in individuals with more left temporal lobe involvement. Prosopagnosia may occur with right temporal damage. Progressive non-fluent aphasia is characterized by aphasia with stuttering and agrammatism. The executive function and working memory are usually impaired. The typical neuroimaging findings are asymmetrical atrophy of the anterior temporal lobe in SD and atrophy of the left inferior frontal lobe and anterior insular cortex in PNFA. In addition, there is overlap of clinical manifestations between AD and FTD. These 3 subtypes of FTD often overlap motor syndromes such as amyotrophic lateral sclerosis (ALS) and parkinsonism.

FTDP-17 is a distinct disease characterized by personality changes, executive dysfunction, memory deterioration, and parkinsonism. Motor disturbances include bradykinesia, axial and limb rigidity, and postural instability. Early manifestations include behavioral changes such as disinhibition, impaired social function, judgment and planning, and global dementia. Parkinsonism in FTDP-17 is unresponsive to levodopa. Table 4 summarizes the clinical manifestations in vascular parkinsonism, DLB, and FTDP-17.

5. Conclusion

The clinical features of IPD and PM are very similar, but some manifestations differ. The treatment and prognosis also differ. The response to treatment with levodopa is variable; therefore, definite diagnosis is very important. Early and accurate differentiation between IPD and PM has been markedly improved by recent developments in neuroimaging, particularly the ^{99m}Tc-TRODAT-1 SPECT, which is not only easy and economical to prepare and use in a wide variety of applications but also reliable in understanding the role of DAT in various neurological diseases. Most importantly, early and correct diagnosis leads to earlier and, therefore, more effective treatment with levodopa, when appropriate.

Abbreviations:

CBS: corticobasal syndrome
β-CIT: (1r) 2β-carbomethoxy-3β-(4-iodophenyl) tropane
CO: carbon monoxide
CS_2: carbon disulfide
DAT: dopamine transporter
DRD: dopa-responsive dystonia
DLB: dementia with Lewy bodies
6-FD: 6-fluorodopa
FDG: fluorodeoxyglucose
FTD: frontotemporal dementia
FTDP-17: frontotemporal dementia with parkinsonism linked to chromosome 17
HD: Hungtington's disease
^{123}I-IBZM scan: I-123–iodobenzamide D_2 receptor scan
IPD: idiopathic Parkinson's disease
MJD: Machado–Joseph disease
Mn: manganese
MPTP: 1-methyl-4-phenyl-1,2,3,6-tetrahydropyridine

MSA: multiple system atrophy
MSA-C: multiple system atrophy-cerebellar subtype
MSA-P: multiple system atrophy-parkinsonism subtype
PET: positron emission tomography
PM: Parkinsonism
PSP: progressive supranuclear palsy
PSP-P: progressive supranuclear palsy-parkinsonism
RS: Richardson syndrome
SCA: spinocerebellar atrophy
SPECT: single photon emission computed tomography
^{99m}Tc-TRODAT-1: Tc-99m labeled radiotracer for imaging DAT
VP: vascular parkinsonism
WD: Wilson's disease

6. References

Idiopathic Parkinson's disease

[1] Parkinson J (Sir James). "An essay on the shaking palsy" Whittingham and Rowland for Sherwood, Neely and Jones. London: 1817.

[2] Lee CS, Schulzer M, Mak EK, Hammerstad JP, Calne S, Calne DB. Patterns of asymmetry do not change over the course of idiopathic parkinsonism: implication for pathogenesis. Neurology 1995; 45: 435-439.

[3] Braak H, Del Tredici K, Rub U, de Vos RA, Jansen Stear EN, Braak E. Staging of brain pathology related to sporadic Parkinson's disease. Neurobiol Aging 2003; 24: 197-211.

[4] Robottom BJ, Weiner WJ, Shulman LM. Parkinsonism In: Lisak RP, Truong DD, Carroll WM, Bhidayasiri R. eds. International Neurology: A Clinical Approach. London: Wiley-Blackwell; 2009: 152-158.

[5] Fahn S, Przedborski S. Parkinson disease. In Rowland LP, Pedley TA, eds. Merritt's Neurology. 12th ed. Philalelphia, Lippincott Williams & Wilkins 2010: 751-769.

[6] Schapira AHV. Parkinson's disease. BMJ 1999;318:311-314.

[7] Innis RB, Seiby JB, Scanley BE, et al. Single photon emission computed tomographic imaging demonstrates loss of striatal dopamine transporters in Parkinson disease. Proc Natl Acad Sci USA 1993;90:11965-11969.

[8] Booji J, Tissingh G, Boer GJ, et al. [123I]FP-CIT SPECT shows a pronounced decline of striatal dopamine transporter labeling in early and advanced Parkinson's disease. J Neurol Neurosurg Psychiatry 1997;62:133-140.

[9] Kao PF, Tzen KY, Yen TC, Lu CS, Weng YH, Wey SP, Ting G. The optimal imaging time for [^{99m}Tc]TRODAT-1/SPECT in normal subjects and patients with Parkinson's disease. Nucl Med Comm 2001; 22: 151-154.

[10] Seibyl JP, Marek KL, Quinlan D, et al. Decreased single-photon emission computed tomographic [123I]-CIT striatal uptake correlates with symptom severity in Parkinson's disease. Ann Neurol 1995;38:589-598.

[11] Marek KL, Seibyl JP, Zoghbi S, et al. [123I]-CIT/SPECT imaging demonstrates bilateral loss of dopamine transporters in hemi-Parkinson's disease. Neurology 1996;46:231-237.

[12] Polymeropoulos MH, Lavedan C, Leroy E, et al. Mutation in the alpha-synuclein gene identified in families with Parkinson's disease. Science 1997;276:2045-2047.

[13] Parkes JD, Marsden CD, Rees JE, et al. Parkinson's disease, cerebral arteriosclerosis, and senile dementia. Q J Med 1974;43:49-61.

[14] Tissingh G, Booij J, Winogrodzka A, van Royen EA, Wolters EC. IBZM- and CIT-SPECT of the dopaminergic system in parkinsonism. J Neural Transm 1997;50(suppl):31-37.

[15] Morrish PK, Rakshi JS, Bailey DL, Sawle GV, Brooks DJ. Measuring the rate of progression and estimating the preclinical period of Parkinson's disease with [18F]dopa PET. J Neurol Neurosurg Psychiatry 1998;64:314-319.

[16] Brooks DJ. The early diagnosis of Parkinson's disease. Ann Neurol 1998;44(suppl):S10-S18.

Manganism

[17] Barbeau A. Manganese and extrapyramidal disorders (a critical review and tribute to Dr. George C. Cotzias). Neurotoxicology 1984;5:13-36.

[18] Huang CC, Chu NS, Lu CS, et al. Chronic manganese intoxication. Arch Neurol 1989;46:1104-6.

[19] Mena I, Court J, Fuenzalida S, Papavasiliou PS, Cotzias GC. Modification of chronic manganese poisoning treatment with L-dopa or 5-OH tryptophane. N Engl J Med 1970;282:5-10.

[20] Calne DB, Chu NS, Huang CC, Lu CS, Olanow W. Manganism and idiopathic parkinsonism: similarities and differences. Neurology 1994;44:1583-1585.

[21] Wolters EC, Huang CC, Clark C, et al. Positron emission tomography in manganese intoxication. Ann Neurol 1989;26:647-651.

[22] Shinotoh H, Snow BJ, Chu NS, et al. Presynaptic and postsynaptic striatal dopaminergic function in patients with manganese intoxication: a positron emission tomography study. Neurology 1997;48:1053-1056.

[23] Huang CC, Lu CS, Chu NS, et al. Progression after chronic manganese exposure. Neurology 1993;43:1479-483.

[24] Huang CC, Chu NS, Lu CS, Chen RS, Calne DB. Long term progression in chronic manganism: ten years follow up. Neurology 1998;50:698-700.

[25] Huang CC, Weng YH, Lu CS, Chu NS, Yen TC. Dopamine transporter binding in chronic manganese intoxication. J Neurol 2003; 250: 1335-1339.

Carbon disulfide

[26] Aaserud O, Hommeren OJ, Tvedt B, Nakstad P, Mowe G, Efskind J, Russel D, Jörgensen EB, Nyber-Hansen R, Rootwelt K, Gjerstad L. Carbon disulfide exposure and neurotoxic sequelae among viscose rayon workers. Am J Ind Med 1990;18:25-37.

[27] Hageman G, van der Hoek J, van Hout M, van der Laan G, Steur EJ, de Bruin W, Herholz K. Parkinsonism, pyramidal signs, polyneuropathy, and cognitive decline after long-term occupational solvent exposure. J Neurol 1999;246:198-206.

[28] Huang CC, Chu CC, Chen RS, Lin SK, Shih TS. Chronic carbon disulfide encephalopathy. Eur Neurol 1996;36:364-368.

[29] Huang CC, Chu CC, Chu NS, Wu TN. Carbon disulfide vasculopathy: a small vessel disease. Cerebrovasc Dis 2001;11:240-250.

[30] Huang CC, Yen TC, Shih TS, Chang HY, Chu NS. Dopamine transporter binding study in differentiating carbon disulfide-induced parkinsonism from idiopathic parkinsonism. Neurotoxicology 2004;25:341-347.

[31] Chuang WL, Huang CC, Chen CJ, Hsieh YC, Kuo HC, Shih TS. Carbon disulfide encephalopathy: cerebral microangiopathy. NeuroToxicology 2007; 28: 387-393.

Carbon monoxide intoxication

[32] Kim JH, Chang KH, Song IC, et al. Delayed encephalopathy of acute carbon monoxide intoxication: diffusivity of cerebral white matter lesions. AJNR 2003; 24: 1592-1597.

[33] Hampson NB, Hauff NM. Risk factors for short-term mortality from carbon monoxide poisoning treated with hyperbaric oxygen. Crt Care Med 2008; 36: 2523-2527.

[34] Chu K, Jung KH, Kin HJ, et al. Diffusion-weighted MRI and 99mTc-HMPAO SPECT in delayed relapsing type of carbon monoxide poisoning: evidence of delayed cytotoxic edema. Eur Neurol 2004; 51: 98-103.

[35] Hsiao CL, Kuo HC, Huang CC. Delayed encephalopathy after carbon monoxide intoxication – long-term prognosis and correlation of clinical manifestations and neuroimages. Acta Neurol Taiwan 2004; 13: 64-70.

Dopa responsive dystonia

[36] Segawa M, Nomura Y, Tanaka S, Hakamada S, Nagata E, Soda M, Kase M. Hereditary progressive dystonia with marked diurnal fluctuation on its pathophysiology based on the characteristics of clinical and polysomnographical findings. In: Fahn S, Marsden CD, Calne DB (eds) Advances in Neurology, vol. 50, Dystonia 2, Raven Press, New York; 1988:367-376.

[37] Nygaard TG, Marsden CD, Fahn S. Dopa-responsive dystonia: long-term treatment response and prognosis. Neurology 1991;41:174-181.

[38] Nygaard TG, Takahashi H, Heiman GA, Snow BJ, Fahn S, Calne DB. Long-term treatment response and fluorodopa positron emission tomographic scanning of parkinsonism in a family with dopa-responsive dystonia. Ann Neurol 1992;32:603-608.

[39] Ichinose H, Ohye T, Takahashi E, et al. Hereditary progressive dystonia with marked diurnal fluctuation caused by mutations in the GTP cyclohydrolase gene. Nat Genet 1994;8:236-242.

[40] Furukawa Y, Shimadzu M, Rajput AH, et al. GTP cyclohydrolase I gene mutations in hereditary progressive and dopa-responsive dystonia. Ann Neurol 1996;39:609-617.

[41] Ludecke B, Knappskog PM, Clayton PT, et al. Recessively inherited L-DOPA-responsive parkinsonism in infancy caused by a point mutation (L205P) in the tyrosine hydroxylase gene. Hum Mol Genet 1996;5:1023-1028.

[42] Snow BJ, Nygaard TG, Takahashi H, Calne DB. Positron emission tomographic studies of dopa-responsive dystonia and early-onset idiopathic parkinsonism. Ann Neurol 1993;34:733-738.

[43] Huang CC, Yen TC, Weng YH, Lu CS. Normal dopamine transporter binding in dopa responsive dystonia. J Neurol 2002; 249: 1016-1020.

Progressive supranuclear palsy

[44] Burn DJ, Lees AJ. Progressive supranuclear palsy: where are we now? Lancet Neurol 2002;1:359-369.

[45] Williams DR, De Silva R, Paviour DC, Pittman A, Watt HC, Kilford L, et al. Characteristics of two distinct clinical phenotypes in pathologically proven progressive supranuclear palsy: Richardson's syndrome and PSP-parkinsonism. Brain 2005;128:1247-1258.

[46] Williams DR, Holton JL, Strand C, Pittman A, De Silva R, Lees AJ, et al. Pathological tau burden and distribution distinguishes progressive supranuclear palsy-parkinsonism from Richardson's syndrome. Brain 2007;130:1566-1576.

[47] Kim YJ, Ichise M, Ballinger JR, Vines D, Erami SS, Tatschida T, et al. Combination of dopamine transporter and D2 receptor SPECT in the diagnostic evaluation of PD, MSA, and PSP. Mov Disord 2002;17:303-312.

[48] Antonini A, Benti R, De Notaris R, Tesei S, Zecchinelli A, Sacilotto G, et al. 123I-Ioflupane/SPECT binding to striatal dopamine transporter (DAT) uptake in patients with Parkinson's disease, multiple system atrophy, and progressive supranuclear palsy. Neurol Sci 2003;24:149-150.

[49] Pirker W, Asenbaum S, Bencsits G, Prayer D, Gerschlager W, Deecke L, et al. [123I]beta-CIT SPECT in multiple system atrophy, progressive supranuclear palsy, and corticobasal degeneration. Mov Disord 2000;15:1158-1167.

[50] Burn DJ, Sawle GV, Brooks DJ. Differential diagnosis of Parkinson's disease, multiple system atrophy, and Steele–Richardson–Olszewski syndrome: discriminant analysis of striatal 18F-dopa PET data. J Neurol Neurosurg Psychiatry 1994;57:278-284.

[51] Oyanagi C, Katsumi Y, Hanakawa T, Hayashi T, Thuy DD, Hashikawa K, et al. Comparison of striatal dopamine D2 receptors in Parkinson's disease and progressive supranuclear palsy patients using [123I] iodobenzofuran single-photon emission computed tomography. J Neuroimaging 2002;12:316-324.

Multiple system atrophy

[52] Hierholzer J, Cordes M, Venz S, Schelosky L, Harisch C, Richter W, et al. Loss of dopamine-D2 receptor binding sites in Parkinsonian plus syndromes. J Nucl Med 1998;39:954-960.

[53] Arnold G, Schwarz J, Tatsch K, Kraft E, Wachter T, Bandmann O, et al. Steele–Richardson–Olszewski–syndrome: the relation of dopamine D2 receptor binding and subcortical lesions in MRI. J Neural Transm 2002;109:503-512.

[54] Schwarz J, Tatsch K, Arnold G, Ott M, Trenkwalder C, Kirsch CM, et al. 123I-iodobenzamide-SPECT in 83 patients with de novo parkinsonism. Neurology 1993;43:S17-S20.

[55] Lin WY, Lin KJ, Weng YH, Yen TZ, Shen LH, Liao MH, Lu CS. Preliminary studies of differential impairments of the dopaminergic system in subjects of progressive supranuclear pslay. Nucl Med Commun 2010;31:974-980.

[56] Wenning GK, Tison F, Ben-Shlomo Y, et al. Multiple system atrophy: a review of 203 pathologically proven cases. Mov Disord 1997;12:133-147.

[57] Wenning GK, Ben-Shlomo Y, Hughes A, Deniel SE, Lees A, Quinn NP. What clinical features are most useful to distinguish definite multiple system atrophy from Parkinson's disease? J Neurol Neurosurg Psychiatry 2000;68:434-440.

[58] Gilman S, Low PA, Quinn N, et al. Consensus statement on the diagnosis of multiple system atrophy. J Neurol Sci 1999;163:94-98.

[59] Wenning GK, Ben-Shlomo Y, Magalhaes M. Clinicopathological study of 35 cases of multiple system atrophy. J Neurol Neurosurg Psychiatry 1995;58:160-166.

[60] Brooks DJ, Ibanez V, Sawle GV, et al. Differing patterns of striatal 18F-dopa uptake in Parkinson's disease, multiple system atrophy, and progressive supranuclear palsy. Ann Neurol 1990;28:547-555.

[61] Gilman S, Koeppe RA, Junck L, et al. Decreased striatal monoaminergic terminals in multiple system atrophy detected with positron emission tomography. Ann Neurol 1999;45:769-777.

[62] Lu CS, Weng YH, Chen MC, Chen RS, Tzen KY, Wey SP, Ting G, Chang HC, Yen TC. [99mTc]-TRODAT-1 imaging of multiple system atrophy. J Nucl Med 2004;1:49-55.

Spinocerebellar degeneration

[63] Gispert S, Twell R, Orozco G, et al. Chromosomal assignment of the second locus for autosomal dominant cerebellar ataxia (SCA2) to chromosome 12q23-24.1. Nat Genet 1993;4:295-299.

[64] Pulst SM, Nechiporuk A, Nechiporuk T, et al. Moderate expansion of a normally biallelic trinucleotide repeat in spinocerebellar ataxia type 2. Nat Genet 1996;14:269-276.

[65] Cancel G, Durr A, Didierjean O, et al. Molecular and clinical correlation in spinocerebellar ataxia 2: a study of 32 families. Hum Mol Genet 1997;6:709-715.

[66] Sasaki H, Wakisaka A, Sanpei K, et al. Phenotype variation correlates with CAG repeat length in SCA2—a study of 28 Japanese patients. J Neurol Sci 1998;159:202-208.

[67] Lu CS, Wu Chou YH, Yen TC, Tsai CH, Chen RS, Chang HC. Dopa-responsive Parkinsonism phenotype of spinocerebellar atokia type 2. Mov Disord 2002; 17: 1046-1051.

[68] Onoders O, Idezuka J, Igarashi S, et al. Progressive atrophy of cerebellum and brainstem as a function of age and the size of expanded CAG repeats in the MJD1 gene in Machado-Joseph disease. Ann Neurol 1998;43:288-296.

[69] Kawaguchi Y, Okamoto T, Taniwaki M, et al. CAG expansions in a novel gene for Machado-Joseph disease at chromosome 14q32.1. Nat Genet 1994;8:221-227.

[70] Murata Y, Tamaguchi S, Kawakami H, et al. Characteristic magnetic resonance imaging findings in Machado-Joseph disease. Arch Neurol 1998;55:33-37.

[71] Ishibashi M, Sakai T, Matsuishi T, et al. Decreased benzodiazepine receptor binding in Machado-Joseph disease. J Nucl Med 1998;39:1518-1520.

[72] Shinotoh H, Thiessen B, Snow BJ. Fluorodopa and raclopride PET analysis of patients with Machado-Joseph disease. Neurology 1997;49:1133-1136.

[73] Soong BW, Liu RS. Positron emission tomography in asymptomatic gene carriers of Machado-Joseph disease. J Neurol Neurosurg Psychiatry 1998;64:499-504.

[74] Yen TC, Tzen KY, Wey SP, Ting G. Decreased dopamine transporter binding in Machado-Joseph disease. J Nucl Med 2000;41:994-998.

[75] Yen TC, Tzen KY, Chen MC, et al. Dopamine transporter concentration is reduced in asymptomatic Machado-Joseph disease gene carriers. J Nucl Med 2002;43:153-159.

[76] Matilla T, McCall A, Subramony SH, Zoghbi HY. Molecular and clinical correlations in spinocerebellar ataxia type 3 and Machado-Joseph disease. Ann Neurol 1995;38:68-72.

[77] Lu CS, Chang HC, Kuo PC. The parkinsonian phenotype of spinocerebellar ataxia type 3 in a Taiwanese family. Parkinsonism Rel Disord 2004; 10: 369-373.

Corticobasal syndrome

[78] Gibb WR, Luthert PJ, Marsden CD. Corticobasal degeneration. Brain 1989;112:1171-1192.

[79] Lang AE, Riley DE, Bergeron C. Cortical-basal ganglionic degeneration. In: Calne DB, ed. Neurodegenerative Diseases. Philadelphia: W.B. Saunders; 1994:877-894.

[80] Eidelberg D, Dhawan V, Moeller JR, et al. The metabolic landscape of cortico-basal ganglionic degeneration: regional asymmetries studied with positron emission tomography. J Neurol Neurosurg Psychiatry 1991;54:856-862.

[81] Grimes DA, Lang AE, Bergeron CB. Dementia as the most common presentation of cortical-basal ganglionic degeneration. Neurology 1999;53:1969-1974.

[82] Grisoli M, Fetoni V, Savoiardo M, Girotti F, Bruzzone MG. MRI in corticobasal degeneration. Eur J Neurol 1995;2:547-552.

[83] Lutte I, Laterre C, Bodart JM, De Volder A. Contribution of PET studies in diagnosis of corticobasal degeneration. Eur Neurol 2000;44:12-21.

[84] Pirker W, Asenbaum S, Bencsits G, et al. [123I]-β-CIT SPECT in multiple system atrophy, progressive supranuclear palsy, and corticobasal degeneration. Mov Disord 2000;15:1158-1167.

[85] Lai SC, Tsai CC, Yen TC, Lu CS. 18F-FDG PET and 99mTc-TRODAT-1 SPECT observations in a case of corticobasal degeneration. Ann Nucl Med Sci 2002; 15: 93-96.

Wilson's disease

[86] Walshe JM. Wilson's disease In: Vinken PJ, Bruyn GW, Klawans HL, eds. Handbook of Clinical Neurology. Vol 49. Extrapyramidal Disorders. Amsterdam: North-Holland; 1986:223-238.

[87] Marsden CD. Wilson's disease. Q J Med 1987;248:959-966.

[88] Williams JB, Walshe JM. Wilson's disease: an analysis of the cranial computerized tomographic appearances found in 60 patients and the changes in response to treatment with chelating agents. Brain 1981;104:735-752.

[89] Roh JK, Lee TG, Wie BA, et al. Initial and follow-up brain MRI findings and correlation with the clinical course in Wilson's disease. Neurology 1994;44:1064-1068.

[90] Huang CC, Chu NS. Acute dystonia with thalamic and brainstem lesions after initial penicillamine treatment in Wilson's disease. Eur Neurol 1998;39:32-37.

[91] Morgan JP, Preziosi TJ, Bianchine JR. Ineffectiveness of L-DOPA as a supplement to penicillamine in a case of Wilson's disease. Lancet 1970;ii:659.

[92] Snow BJ, Bhatt M, Martin WRW, Li D, Calne DB. The nigrostriatal dopaminergic pathway in Wilson's disease studied with positron emission tomography. J Neurol Neurosurg Psychiatry 1991;54:12-17.

[93] Oertel WH, Tatsch K, Schwavz J, et al. Decrease of D2 receptors indicated by ^{123}I-Iodobenzamide single-photon emission computed tomography relates to neurological deficit in treated Wilson's disease. Ann Neurol 1992;32:743-748.

[94] Oder W, Brucke T, Kollegger H, Spatt J, Asenbaum S, Deecke L. Dopamine D2 receptor binding is reduced in Wilson's disease: correlation of neurological deficits with striatal ^{123}I-iodobenzamide binding. J Neural Trans 1996;103:1093-1103.

[95] Jeon B, Kim JM, Jeong JM, Kim KM, Chang YS, Lee DS, Lee MC. Dopamine transporter imaging with [^{123}I]-β-CIT demonstrates presynaptic nigrostriatal dopaminergic damage in Wilson's disease. J Neurol Neurosurg Psychiatry 1998;65:60-64.

[96] Barthel H, Sorger D, Kuhn HJ, Wagner A, Kluge R, Hermann W. Differential alteration of the nigrostriatal dopaminergic system in Wilson's disease investigated with [^{123}I]-β-CIT and high-resolution SPET. Eur J Nucl Med 2001;28:1656-1663.

[97] Huang CC, Chu NS, Yen TC, Wai YY, Lu CS. Dopamine transporter binding in Wilson's disease. Can J Neurol Sci 2003; 30: 163-167.

Vascular parkinsonism

[98] Tzen KY, Lu CS, Yen TC, et al. Differential diagnosis of Parkinson's disease and vascular parkinsonism by 99mTc-TRODAT-1. J Nucl Med 2001;42:408-413.

Dementia with Lewy body

[99] Mckeith IG, Dickson DW, Lowe J, et al. Diagnosis and management of dementia with Lewy bodies: third report of DLB consortium. Neurology 2005; 65: 1863-1872.

[100] Burn DJ. Cortical Lewy body disease and Parkinson's disease dementia. Curr Opin Neurol 2006; 19: 572-579.

Frontotemporal dementia

[101] Mesulam MM. Primary progressive aphasia. Ann Neurol 2001; 49: 425-432.

[102] Cairns NJ, Bigio EH, Mackenzie IR, et al. Neuropathologic diagnostic and nosolgic criteria for frontotemporal lobar degeneration: consensus of the consortium for frontotemporal lobar degeneration. Acta Neuropathol 2007; 114: 5-22.

[103] Scarmeas N, Honig LS. Frontotemporal degenerative dementias. Clin Neurosci Res 2004; 3: 449-460.

[104] Foster NL, Heidebrink JL, Clark CM, et al. FDG-PET improves accuracy in distinguishing frontotemporal dementia and Alzheimer's disease. Brain 2007; 130: 2616-2635.

[105] Rabinovici GD, Frust AJ, O'Neil JP, et al. ^{11}C-PIB PET imaging in Alzheimer's disease and frontotemporal lobar degeneration. Neurology 2007; 68: 1205-1212.
[106] Hutton M, Lendon CL, Rizzu P. Association of missense and 5'-splice-site mutations in tau with the inherited dementia FTDP-17. Nature 1998; 393: 702-705.

Non-Conventional MRI Techniques in Neurophychiatric Systemic Lupus Erythematosus (NPSLE): Emerging Tools to Elucidate the Pathophysiology and Aid the Diagnosis and Management

Efrosini Z. Papadaki[1] and Dimitrios T. Boumpas[2]
[1]*Department of Radiology*
[2]*Internal Medicine and Rheumatology,*
University of Crete School of Medicine, Heraklion
Greece

1. Introduction

Systemic Lupus Erythematosus (SLE) is an autoimmune inflammatory disorder affecting multiple organ systems. 30-40 % of the patients manifest variable neuropsychiatric symptoms leading to significant morbidity and mortality. CNS involvement could be primary if directly related to SLE activity in the CNS or secondary to treatment, infections, metabolic abnormalities or other systemic manifestations such as hypertension (Futrell et al,1992). Primary NPSLE is divided into focal and diffuse disease. Focal NPSLE is characterized by focal neurologic deficits and is strongly associated with the occurrence of thromboembolic events. Diffuse primary NPSLE is a group of neurologic, psychiatric, and cognitive syndromes that vary from overt neurologic and psychiatric symptoms (eg. seizures, psychosis) to more subtle signs such as headache, mood disturbances, anxiety disorders or mild cognitive dysfunction. Neuropsychiatric lupus (NPSLE) manifestations can occur in the absence of either serologic activity or other systemic disease manifestations (Sibbit et al., 1999). Thus, in clinical practice the diagnosis of primary NPSLE is rather presumptive, after the exclusion of alternative causes of the neuropsychiatric symptoms.

There is no single diagnostic test that is sensitive and specific for SLE-related neuropsychiatric manifestations. The assessment of individual patients is based on clinical, neurologic and rheumatologic evaluation, immunoserologic testing, brain imaging, and psychiatric and neuropsychological assessment. These examinations are used to support or refute the clinical diagnostic impression, rule out alternative explanations, and form the basis for prospective monitoring of clinical evolution and response to treatment interventions. The lack of a diagnostic gold standard makes the correct diagnosis of primary NPSLE a challenge. This realization has led us in developing under the auspices of the European League Against Rheumatology (EULAR) evidence and expert based recommendations for the management of NPSLE (Bertsias et al, 2010).

Magnetic resonance imaging (MRI) is the current modality of choice in the imaging assessment of NPSLE patients, due to its high sensitivity in detecting even small alterations in tissue water content (Sibbitt et al., 1999). However, the variable pathologic substrate of the NPLSE lesions result in low MRI specificity. Conventional MRI reveals lesions in about 50-75% of NPSLE patients, depending on the disease activity and the severity and kind of the neurological manifestations (focal or diffuse). In patients with focal symptoms conventional MRI commonly detects small, discrete, frontal–parietal subcortical or periventricular white matter lesions, hyperintense on T2 sequences, that usually represent small acute or chronic infarcts, or even microhemorrhages. Unfortunately, these lesions are not specific for NPSLE and exhibit no clinical correlation. Additional intravenous Gadolinium administration is helpful in differentiating acute from chronic lesions. Mild-to-moderate cerebral atrophy could also be detected by T1 sequences, associated with both generalized and focal brain injury.

In NPSLE patients with diffuse neurological manifestations conventional neuroimaging usually fails to demonstrate abnormalities that explain these symptoms. Additionally, histopathological studies confirm the presence of extensive diffuse parenchymal and cerebrovascular injury that could not be identified by the conventional MRI techniques. On the contrary, brain tissue microscopic structural, hemodynamic or metabolic changes could be assessed by advanced, non-conventional quantitative neuroimaging techniques, such as Diffusion Weighted Imaging (DWI), Diffusion Tensor Imaging (DTI), Perfusion Weighted Imaging (PWI), Magnetization Transfer Imaging (MTI) and Magnetic Resonance Spectroscopy (MRS). Although not available in the current daily practice, these techniques are promising for the better understanding of the NSPLE, and improvement of the diagnostic work-up and treatment.

We critically review the literature on brain imaging in NPSLE, with special emphasis on non-conventional neuroimaging techniques in order to access their contribution to diagnosis, understanding of the pathophysiology and clinical management.

2. Histopathological changes in NPSLE

The underlying pathologic basis of NP-SLE is still under investigation (Bertsias GK, Boumpas DT, 2010). Pathological studies revealed multiple microinfarcts, noninflammatory thickening of small vessels with intimal proliferation, small-vessel occlusion, and intracranial embolism or hemorrhage (Van Dam et al., 1991). True vasculitis, with inflammatory infiltrate and fibrinoid necrosis is relatively rare, occurring in 6-9% of cases (Van Dam et al., 1991). Vasculopathy is most common. SLE vasculopathy affects predominantly arterioles and capillaries, resulting in vessel tortuosity, vascular hyalinization, endothelial proliferation, and perivascular inflammation or gliosis. This vasculopathy could be related to both acute inflammation and ischemia (Hanly et al., 1992; Van Dam et al., 1991).

According to a recent histopathological study (Sibbit et al., 2010) the basic underlying pathologic process of NPSLE is cerebrovascular injury associated with disease activity and thromboembolism, resulting in focal and diffuse brain ischemia, small and large brain infarcts, focal and diffuse brain edema, brain hemorrhage, and focal and diffuse parenchymal injury. Multiple coexisting pathogenic mechanisms including, thromboembolism by cardiac valvular lesions, hypercoagulability, diffuse endothelial injury, and excitotoxicity could not be excluded (Roldan et al., 2006, 2008).

Four patterns of cerebrovascular disease NPSLE have been suggested: (1) an antiphospholipid antibody cerebrovasculopathy characterized by bland thromboses, thrombotic microangiopathy, and arterial intimal fibrous hyperplasia; (2) a diffuse cerebrovasculopathy characterized by endothelial injury associated with increased SLE disease activity, glomerulonephritis, hypertension, and perhaps neuroexcitotoxic antibodies; (3) thromboembolic NPSLE directly caused by cardiac valvular lesions; and (4) mixed cerebrovascular NPSLE with simultaneous aspects of antiphospholipid- associated thrombosis, increased disease activity, and thromboembolic valvular lesions (Sibbit et al.,2010).

3. Conventional MRI

Conventional pre- and postcontrast-enhanced brain MRI appears normal in approximately one-third of both symptomatic and asymptomatic NPSLE patients (Chinn et al., 1997; Jennings et al., 2004). Hyperintense white matter lesions are revealed in up to 70% of SLE patients. In the majority of MRI studies in which white matter lesions were quantified, patient groups with NPSLE (active and inactive) showed a significantly higher number and total volume of white matter hyperintensities compared to non-NPSLE (Appenzeller et al., 2008; Castellino et al., 2008).

According to a recent study (Luyendijk et al, 2011), that reviewed retrospectively the MRI exams of the first episode of active NPSLE in 74 patients, 4 types of findings were observed : 1) focal hyperintensities in white matter (49% of all patients and 84% of patients with abnormalities on MRI) or both white matter and gray matter (5%), suggestive of vasculopathy or vasculitis (Figure 1), 2) more widespread, confluent hyperintensities in the WM, suggestive of chronic hypoperfusion due to the same mechanisms, 3) diffuse cortical GM lesions (12%), compatible with an immune response to neuronal components or post-seizure vasogenic edema, and 4) absence of MRI abnormalities, despite active signs and symptoms (42%). Small punctate focal white matter lesions, the most common imaging finding, are followed in prevalence by cortical atrophy, ventricular dilation and diffuse white matter changes.

The small focal lesions- hyperintense on T2-weighted or FLAIR imaging- typically occur in periventricular and subcortical white matter, especially in the frontoparietal regions. They usually represent small resolved infarcts or focal areas of reduced neuronal density, but in some cases they may be the result of acute infarcts, focal edema, or even acute microhemorrhages (Sibbitt et al., 2010).The corresponding T1-weighted images often appearing normal (Ainiala et al, 2005), while FLAIR images have been shown to be more sensitive for detecting these lesions than T2 images. Periventricular lesions have been particularly associated with the antiphospholipid syndrome (APS) and can be impossible to differentiate on MRI from multiple sclerosis (Peterson et al., 2005).

Although the focal hyperintense white matter lesions are often considered nonspecific- since they are indistinguishable from age-related small vessel disease -they may occur much earlier and in greater numbers in SLE subjects. These findings also seem to be more common in patients with NP-SLE in the presence of antiphospholipid antibodies, although no clinical correlation was observed in most studies (Ainiala et al., 2005). In a large prospective population-based study involving healthy individuals, the presence of focal hyperintense white matter lesions was associated with cognitive impairment (Vermeer et al., 2003). In addition, correlations have been observed between white matter hyperintensities and both cumulative SLE related injury scores, including neuropsychiatric damage (SLICC/ACRDI), and separate neuropsychiatric component scores of SLE-injury indices (neuro-SLEDAI and neuro-SLICC) (Appenzeller et al., 2008; Ainiala et al., 2005).

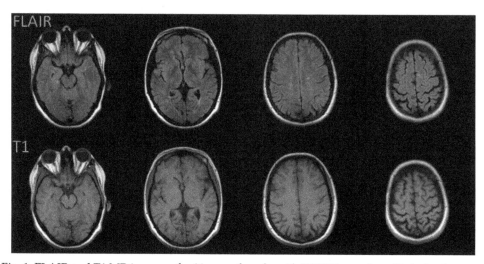

Fig. 1. FLAIR and T1 MR images of a 44 years female with NPSLE reveal multiple focal punctuate lesions-hyperintense on FLAIR and hypointense or isointense on T1- at the periventricular and subcortical white matter, semioval center and the cortex of the left frontal lobe.

Besides aging, white mater hyperintensities are also associated with hypertension, valvular heart disease, and migraine, conditions that commonly occur secondary or concomitantly to NPSLE. Consequently, it is not possible to differentiate NPSLE from other vasculopathies using conventional MRI. The differentiation of acute active disease from old chronic lesions is also difficult. It has been noted that the presence of indiscrete lesion borders, intermediate intensity of T2 lesions and grey matter lesions are all indicative of active disease (Sibbitt et al., 1999). The use of gadolinium has also been shown to be helpful in delineating active inflammatory lesions that usually enhance (Miller et al., 1992). Quantitation of T2 values has also been shown to be helpful in distinguishing active from chronic lesions (Sibbitt et al., 1995). T2 values appear to be increased in the normal appearing frontal grey matter of patients with active diffuse neurological syndromes.

MRI studies may show extensive bilateral, potentially reversible, white matter abnormalities in the cerebral hemispheres, the brainstem, or the cerebellum usually associated with active NPSLE—the so-called "acute posterior leukoencephalopathy,"(Sibbitt et al., 1999). The reversible lesions of acute leukoencephalopathy of NPSLE have been attributed to focal cerebral edema associated with blood vessel injury and microhemorrhages (Sibbitt et al, 2010).

Atrophy was described in 6–12% of SLE patients (Appenzeller et al., 2005,2008) and is associated with multiple factors such as disease duration (Cauli et al., 1994), corticosteroid use (Appenzeller et al., 2005; Ainiala et al, 2005), older age (Appenzeller et al, 2005),

Non-Conventional MRI Techniques in Neurophychiatric Systemic Lupus Erythematosus (NPSLE):
Emerging Tools to Elucidate the Pathophysiology and Aid the Diagnosis and Management

73

antiphospholipid antibodies (Appenzeller et al., 2008; Provenzale et al., 1996) and the presence of hyperintense white matter lesions (Appenzeller et al., 2005; Chinn et al., 1997). The loss of tissue within the brain is thought to result from a combination of both myelin damage and axonal loss, followed by Wallerian degeneration, and the loss of extracellular space and vascular compartments. The histopathological findings associated with MRI-visible cerebral atrophy were highly variable and included multiple infarcts and reduced neuronal density, suggesting that atrophy in NPSLE may be associated with both generalized and focal brain injury. However, normal histological appearance was also noted in some atrophic brains (Sibbitt et al., 2010).

Cerebral atrophy is usually measured from T1-weighted MRI scans, where good contrast between the cerebral spinal fluid (CSF) and the brain parenchyma is observed (Appenzeller et al., 2008). Because high spatial resolution images allow brain volume measurement with the greatest accuracy and precision, three-dimensional gradient methods are generally preferred. As cerebral atrophy can be measured serially on MRI scans of the brain by linear or volumetric measurements, it has been proposed as a means of monitoring the progression of SLE (Appenzeller et al., 2005, 2008).

Regional atrophy in SLE patients has also been described involving cortical and subcortical regions, with particular clinical significance. Selective involvement of the amygdala in patients with SLE and anti-NMDAR antibodies has been found (Emmer et al., 2006). Cognitive impairment may be present more frequently in both corpus callosum and hippocampal atrophy (Appenzeller et al., 2006, 2008). Mild or clinically insignificant spinal cord pathology has also been described in SLE, which might be secondary to Wallerian degeneration of long tract fibers passing through damaged areas of the brain (Benedetti et al., 2007).

MR Angiography detects medium-to-large vessels involvement. Since a small vessel vasculopathy represents the major histopathological background of brain involvement in NPSLE angiographic techniques are usually negative, although angiographic arterial stenoses or occlusions are rarely reported (Weiner et al., 1991). Multiple mechanisms for angiographic arterial stenosis or occlusion have been considered, including coagulopathy, cardiogenic embolism, atherosclerosis from long-term steroid use and anticoagulant or antiplatelet therapy, vasculitis due to SLE or infection, or a combination of these processes (Devinsky et al., 1998).

Conventional MRI techniques are particularly useful in NPSLE patients with acute focal neurologic deficits, although they cannot always differentiate lesions indicating active acute NPSLE from chronic lesions that represent past NPSLE. The differential diagnosis usually includes thromboembolic events due to vasculopathy, lupus-related CNS vasculitis, antiphospholipid antibodies (APL-Ab)- mediated thrombosis, microangiopathy (including thrombotic thrombocytopenic purpura), Libman-Sacks endocarditis, and accelerated atherosclerosis. The pathogenesis in many patients is probably multifactorial. Accurate assessment is crucial, as treatment for these alternative diagnoses differs. Immunosuppressive agents are typically used for suspected vasculitis, while lifelong anticoagulation is the mainstay of therapy for APL-Ab-mediated thromboembolic events.

In diffuse NPSLE presentation conventional MRI could be unremarkable since it doesn't give information about damage in normal-appearing tissue (Sibbitt et al., 1999). Non-conventional MRI techniques, sensitive to microstructural, hemodynamic and biochemical characteristics of the tissues have been developed, that could detect gray and white matter abnormalities in NPSLE patients, otherwise occult by conventional imaging.

4. Advanced MRI methods

4.1 Diffusion–weighted imaging

Diffusion-weighted imaging (DWI) is a magnetic resonance technique that is based on the random, incoherent (brownian) motion of protons on the molecular scale. In free water, proton-containing molecules move unrestricted in all directions, a situation that is referred to as isotropy. In highly structured tissue, such as the corticospinal tract, molecules encounter fewer barriers when moving in a craniocaudal direction than in directions perpendicular to it. This situation gives rise to preferential molecular movement in a certain direction, which is known as anisotropy. DWI can be used to measure diffusivity in the brain, providing signal proportional to the molecular diffusion of water molecules (Schaefer et al., 2000).

Diffusion Tensor Imaging (DTI) is a DWI technique that permits assessment of the preferential direction of proton diffusivity (Ulug et al., 1999). DTI offers increased resolution compared to conventional MRI regarding white matter microstructure by measurement of water diffusion through cellular compartments in vivo (Pierpaoli et al., 1996). Compared to more isotropic movement of water in gray matter, water diffusion in white matter moves anisotropically, meaning that water diffuses preferentially along the length of the axon compared to perpendicular to the axon. This anisotropic diffusion of water appears to be due to the highly structured axonal membranes and their associated myelin sheaths (Cascio et al., 2007). By tracking the diffusion of water in the brain, the measure fractional anisotropy (FA) and mean diffusivity (MD) can be derived. Higher FA (and lower MD) suggests greater axonal coherence and myelination. Measures of FA are usually considered to be overall measures of axonal integrity, reflecting either increased axonal caliber, increased myelin thickness, increased fiber coherence in a given direction, or some combination of these factors. In contrast, MD, is a measure of the average molecular motion independent of the constraints of tissue boundaries, and is affected by cellular size and degradations in tissue integrity (Pierpaoli et al., 1996). One way to assess the magnitude of diffusion is by calculating the apparent diffusion coefficient (ADC), an index of mean diffusivity, for individual pixels on average apparent diffusion coefficient (ADC) maps. Average diffusion coefficient (ADC) maps provide information on the microstructure of tissue and can be very useful in the detection of disease ADC values that can be assessed locally in regions of interest (ROIs). Another way is the generation of ADC histograms for the whole brain (Nusbaum et al., 2000). Such measures consisted of mean ADC values of the whole brain volume and descriptive parameters of ADC histograms of the whole brain, such as peak height. Relatively few studies have emerged showing water diffusivity changes in NPSLE. DWI was first used by Moritani and co-workers (Moritani et al., 2001) who detected acute or subacute lesions in 9 of 20 patients with SLE (45%). Two main patterns of acute or subacute brain parenchymal lesions were described. The first include hyperintense lesions with decreased ADC indicating acute or subacute infarction due to primary or secondary arterial stenosis or occlusion (Figure 2) and the second isointense or slightly hyperintense lesions on diffusion-weighted images with increased ADC representing vasogenic edema, with or without microinfarcts, due to small-vessel vasculopathy or hypertensive encephalopathy (Figure 3).

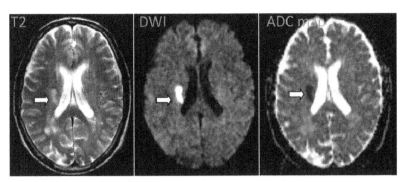

Fig. 2. Hyperintense lesion at the right corona radiata with increased signal intensity on DWI and decreased signal intensity on ADC map due to acute infarction.

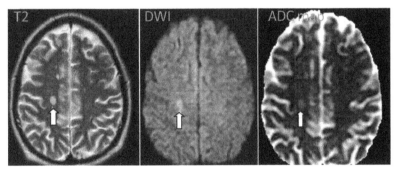

Fig. 3. Hyperintense lesion at the right semioval center with increased signal intensity on DWI and increased signal intensity on ADC map, due to vasogenic edema.

DWI then was used in NPSLE patients to provide quantitative measures of the integrity of the entire brain (Bosma et al., 2003). Using ADC histograms of the whole brain, in a group of 11 patients with a history of non focal NPSLE and 10 healthy volunteers they found changes in NPSLE patients who had no relevant changes on conventional MRI, that correlated with their clinical symptoms. The ADC histograms of the NPSLE group were, on average, significantly lower and broader, with a significant decrease of the peak height and a significant increase in the number of pixels with higher ADC values compared to the healthy subjects. The flatter and broader histograms in the NPSLE group indicate that, in these patients, widespread increased motility of free-water protons occurs. The subtle white matter hyperintensities that were visible on conventional MR images seemed unlikely to be responsible for the significantly different diffusion pattern in NPSLE because their number and sizes were small. These findings suggest that widespread damage exists in the brain parenchyma of NPSLE patients, invisible with conventional MRI. However, the method used in that study did not permit assessment of which parts of the brain were responsible for the observed changes in the ADC histograms of the whole brain.

Welsch and co-workers investigated 21 acute NPSLE patients and 21 healthy volunteers using also ADC histograms (Welsch et al., 2007).Whole-brain histograms, gray matter only histograms, and white matter only histograms were calculated for each subject. They found increased mean ADC values in acute NPSLE, not only in the whole-brain histograms, but also in the gray matter only and white matter only, indicating that the cerebral alterations is not limited to one tissue compartment.

Zhang and co-workers used a region of interest (ROI) approach for ADC and FA measurements to assess a cohort of 34 patients diagnosed with SLE, and 29 healthy volunteers (Zhang et al., 2007). They found early diffusion changes (higher diffusion values and lower FA values) in the frontal lobe, the genu of the corpus callosum, and the anterior internal capsule in patients with SLE, although routine MRI findings were negative. Another group (Hughes et al., 2007) compared 8 female NPSLE patients, with new onset of symptoms, to 20 healthy controls using diffusion tensor imaging (DTI) and an ROI approach. They found that these patients differed from controls in a wide range of normal appearing gray and white matter regions including the insular cortex, thalamus, parietal and frontal white matter, and corpus callosum. These findings are suggestive of the presence of subtle and widespread damage in the brain parenchyma in NPSLE patients.

Recently Jung and co-workers (Jung et al., 2010) using DTI and the tract-based spatial statistics (TBSS) analysis technique assessed white matter abnormalities in 17 NPSLE patients, 16 SLE patients without NPSLE, and 20 age- and gender-matched controls. According to their findings there were no significant FA or MD differences observed between the SLE patients without NPSLE and the matched controls, although many of the SLE patients had subcortical white matter and periventricular lesions. In contrast, when comparing the acute NPSLE patients to controls, or the acute NPSLE patients to patients with SLE without NPSLE they found decreased FA and increased MD values especially at the corpus callosum and the left anterior corona radiata reflecting diffuse white matter abnormalities. They suggest that either the acute effects of the NPSLE disease, or its treatment, results in white matter changes discernable with conventional MRI techniques. This study provides new evidence that FA and MD may have diagnostic use in NPSLE by demonstrating, for the first time, regional brain specificity, and by distinguishing NPSLE from SLE patients, further indicating the potential diagnostic specificity of this technique for patients in the acute stage of this difficult disease.

Using the same analysis technique Emmer and co-workers (Emmer et al., 2010) investigated 12 patients with SLE (7 with NPSLE) and 28 healthy controls with DTI and found reduction in the FA values of patients with SLE as compared with normal subjects, indicating reduced integrity at particular white matter tracts. The integrity of the subcortical white matter tracts of the occipital, parietal and posterior frontal lobe was relatively preserved, whereas the frontobasal and temporal regions including the inferior fronto-occipital fasciculus, the fasciculus uncinatus, as well as the fornix, the posterior limb of the internal capsule (corticospinal tract), and the anterior limb of the internal capsule (anterior thalamic radiation) seem to be predominantly involved.

The increased ADC values, as well as the decreased FA values, could be explained by reduced structural integrity of the brain parenchyma with permanent loss of neurons and demyelination in patients with NPSLE. This will allow the interstitial water molecules to move freely in a less restricted environment. Normally, the ADC values decrease and the FA values increase by the restriction of motion in a particular direction, for example, due to the boundaries of myelin sheets. Alternatively, loss of structural brain integrity would allow interstitial water molecules to move in a more unrestricted environment, thus resulting in an increase in ADC and decrease in FA. A breakdown of the myelin sheets, as in demyelination, would result in less restricted movement of the water molecules transverse to the fiber tracts. The observed increase in gray matter ADC can be interpreted as consistent with inflammation and/or vasculitis of the gray matter.

It has been suggested that the abnormal diffusion findings seen in the brain of NPSLE patients are not mainly related to hypoxic/anaerobic events, but, rather, indicate a host response to injury, such as an inflammatory reaction, membrane activation, or demyelination (Sibbitt et al., 1997). Such a theory can be supported by histopathology studies in which gliosis and demyelination has been described in the brain parenchyma of patients with NPSLE (Hanly et al., 1992). Immune-mediated vascular or neuronal injury was postulated and subsequent neuronal and metabolic dysfunction resulting in edematous processes that increase water content in WM regions of the brain.

The white matter damage in NPSLE could be the indirect result of subtle noxious influences in NPSLE, such as repeated episodes of acute inflammation in small vessels. This could cause priming or activation of the wall of these small vessels by complement and/or antiendothelial antibodies. Priming or activation of the vessel wall could subsequently lead to vasculopathy and microinfarcts or subtle hypoperfusion in the small vessels of the brain (Zvaifler et al., 1982). Altered cerebral blood flow was previously demonstrated with PET and SPECT in NPSLE patients (Kuschner et al., 1990; Kao et al., 1999). If hypoperfusion occurs, it might be responsible for the metabolic abnormalities reported in NPSLE patients, as suggested by decreased high energy phosphate levels in phosporus-31 MR spectroscopic studies and decreased brain oxygen consumption in PET studies. The end stage of this process might be axonal loss and associated demyelination. It is also possible that antibodies aimed directly against myelin, leading to direct white matter damage through a pervasive attack on axonal myelin sheaths or the oligodendrocytes from which they are derived. The involvement of the white matter could be, finally, the reflection of axonal damage through Wallerian degeneration caused by damage to the gray matter (Emmer et al., 2010).

Diffusion differences affecting acute NPSLE patients could also be related to therapy, whereby the introduction of corticosteroids, or other immunosuppression drugs (i.e. cyclophosphamide), and/or disease modifying antirheumatic drugs, can affect water content in the brain parenchyma. Another possible mechanism may be related to platelet or fibrin macro- or microembolism from Libman-Sacks endocarditis or anticardiolipin antibodies causing multiple areas of macroscopic or microscopic ischemia, infarctions, and microhemorrhages with surrounding edema (Roldan et al., 2006).

Undoubtedly, one of the more useful applications of DWI in clinical practice is the assessment of cerebro-vascular accidents; in these conditions DWI allows early detection (within 1 h) of acute ischemic insult showing a reduction of ADC due to cytotoxic edema which occurs rapidly after the onset of ischemia (Figure 2). DWI also permits to discriminate between recent (with restricted diffusivity) and old (with normal diffusivity) hyperintense ischemic lesions which can be otherwise undistinguishable with conventional MRI. Furthermore, for its ability to differentiate between vasogenic and cytotoxic edema, DWI could be also useful in SLE patients to discriminate between inflammatory and ischemic lesions (Iguchi et al., 2007). Increased diffusion occurs although conventional MRI findings are negative in some cases, which suggests that DTI is more sensitive and that quantitative diffusion measurements can be used in detecting early signs of SLE or, furthermore, monitoring disease evaluations. The findings of diffusion-weighted imaging may help guide the choice of treatment and predict patient outcome in patients with SLE and CNS involvement.

4.2 Perfusion weighted imaging

A variety of imaging techniques have been used to assess cerebral perfusion, beginning with positron emission tomography (PET). PET is a nuclear medicine technique which explores both brain glucose metabolism and cerebral blood flow (CBF). In patients with NPSLE multiple areas of hypometabolism were detected in both MRI normal-appearing white and grey matter regions (Otte et al., 1997). Although PET has high sensitivity (abnormal in 100% of patients with active NPSLE), it lacks specificity and due to its high radiation dose, high cost and limited availability, is rarely applied in the daily clinical practice.

Over the past two decades, two more perfusion imaging techniques, single photon emission computed tomography (SPECT), and perfusion-weighted MRI (PWI), were introduced. These techniques have been used to evaluate a variety of disease states, most commonly acute and chronic ischemia. SPECT is based on the radio-tracer uptake by viable neuronal cells and explores brain perfusion that is the result of both CBF and neuronal integrity. The most commonly observed abnormalities detected by SPECT in patients with NPSLE are diffuse, focal or multifocal areas of decreased uptake corresponding to hypoperfusion, which -according to some authors- correlates with NP disease severity and activity (Colamussi et al., 1995). Other SPECT studies reported CBF abnormalities in NPSLE without correlation to disease activity or serological parameters. There is also no significant associations between perfusion parameters and NP symptoms (Waterloo et al., 2001). A recent voxel-based SPECT study found no difference in perfusion parameters between healthy controls and SLE patients with inactive NP involvement. However the authors found a global hypoperfusion in active NPSLE patients compared to healthy controls, which was mainly located in the cortical gray matter (Appenzeller et al, 2008). Although SPECT has high sensitivity (abnormal in 86–100% of patients with major NPSLE) it lacks specificity (abnormal in 10–50% of SLE patients without NPSLE) and has limited anatomic resolution.

The most commonly used MR perfusion technique is dynamic susceptibility contrast (DSC) imaging. This is a non-invasive dynamic process based on the MR signal changes during the first pass of the intravenously injected contrast agent (a gadolinium chelate) through the vasculature. The change in signal intensity is then measured and perfusion maps are generated, most commonly encountering cerebral blood volume (CBV), cerebral blood flow (CBF), time to peak (TTP), or mean transit time (MTT)values. Nowadays PWI is widely used in the acute stroke, for evaluation of the salvageable tissue and the brain neoplasms to detect neoangiogenesis. This technique could be useful in NPSLE and antiphospholipid syndrome (APS) patients (Figure 4) at risk of cerebro-vascular ischemic events, but reports on the use of PWI in NPSLE are still very few and limited.

The first multimodality approach in patients with SLE was performed by Borelli and co-workers (Borelli et al., 2003) using simultaneously MRI, DWI, PWI and SPECT in 20 SLE patients. They found that SPECT was more sensitive than PWI in detecting brain hypoperfused areas, probably due to the different aspects of brain perfusion explored by these two techniques. PWI is a dynamic process related to the blood supply to the anatomical districts of the brain, while SPECT images reflect the distribution of a flow tracer whose uptake at the neuronal level may, however, be in part influenced by the metabolic status of the nervous tissue. Therefore the combination of these techniques might yield more information about the underlying pathogenetic mechanism of brain hypoperfusion.

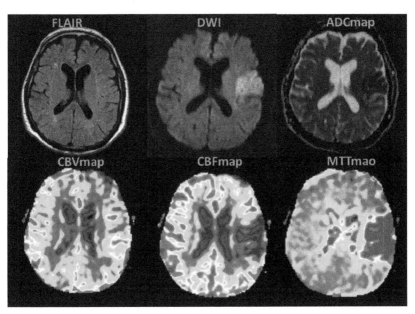

Fig. 4. Imaging of an acute ischemic lesion in a 45 yrs old female with NPSLE and antiphospholipid syndrome (APS), 4 hours after the onset of the symptoms. FLAIR is unremarkable, while the lesion is revealed on DWI and ADC map as hyperintense and hypointense area, respectively, due to cytotoxic edema. Dynamic Susceptibility Contrast (DSC) MR Perfusion technique shows mild increased cerebral blood volume (red on CBV map), decreased cerebral blood flow (dark blue on CBF map) and increased mean transit time (red on MTT map)

Two recent studies with application of dynamic susceptibility contrast perfusion MRI in SLE patients have opposite results. In the first study 15 active NPSLE, 26 inactive NPSLE and 11 control subjects were investigated and no signs of focal or global abnormalities in the perfusion parameters of the patients were found (Emmer et al., 2010). Furthermore, no significant differences were found when comparing patients with a specific SLE criterion (lupus anti-coagulant LAC, anti-cardiolipin antibodies or APS).The main limitation of this study is the fact that the CBF and CBV values have been calibrated to normal white matter, assuming that perfusion in the contralateral white matter is normal. This assumption could be erroneous in SLE patients with diffuse NP symptoms, like cognitive dysfunction or headache.

In the second study (Gasparovic et al., 2010)the DSCMRI technique was performed in 42 SLE patients and 19 healthy controls. They demonstrated higher CBV and CBF throughout cortical and white matter regions in the SLE patients (with or without lesions) relative to the control group. According to the authors the higher global CBF and CBV values may be due to reactive physiologic or pathogenic factors underlying SLE, such as vasomotor instability, compensatory mechanisms for resolving injury, low-grade excitotoxicity due to antibody impairment of N-methyl D-aspartate (NMDA) receptors, or inflammatory factors. This global hyperperfusion in SEL patients is in contrast with most SPECT studies that reveal patchy hypoperfused areas in SLE patients. More studies should be performed to SLE and NPSLE patients with application of both SPECT and MRI perfusion techniques to further delineate this issue.

4.3 Magnetization Transfer Imaging (MTI)

MTI is a quantitative MRI technique that is sensitive to macroscopic and microscopic brain tissue changes (Grossman et al., 1994; Wolff et al., 1994) and more sensitive to the presence of disease than conventional MRI. In MRI, the magnetic characteristics of free-water protons determine the contrasts of the images. MTI is based on the magnetization transfer that occurs between the bound pool of macromolecule-related protons in biologic tissues and the pool of free water protons. In MTI, a saturating RF pulse selectively reduces the magnetization of the bound pool. Due to the interactions between the two proton pools, the magnetization of the free-water pool is also reduced, which is called the MT effect. Tissue factors that affect the amount of this magnetization transfer are the concentration of macromolecules and the surface chemistry and biophysical dynamics of the macromolecules (Wolff et al., 1994). Macromolecules that contribute to the MT effect in the brain are the cholesterol component of myelin, cerebrosides, and phospholipids (Koenig et al., 2001). The amount of MT is expressed by the magnetization transfer ratio (MTR) value. MTR values can be easily calculated in regions of interest (ROIs) to assess local tissue composition. In most diseases affecting the brain, MTR values are reduced, presumably due to dilution or destruction of macromolecules (Finelli et al., 1998). Using this approach it has been proved that MTI could detect abnormalities in brain tissue that are not visible in conventional MRI in cases of multiple sclerosis (Rovaris et al., 2000).Whole brain assessment can be also performed using MTR histograms for quantification of the disease burden of the whole brain (van Buchem et al., 1997). According to this volumetric method, the intracranial volume (ICV) is segmented, and the MTR values of the segmented brain are displayed as a histogram. Gray and white matter have different mean MTRs, which is probably mainly due to different concentrations of myelin. Still, the histograms for gray matter and white matter overlap substantially. The summation of these 2 histograms results in a histogram that is characteristic of the whole brain. The shape of this whole-brain histogram reflects conditions that affect the gray and white matter. MTR histograms of normal brains are characterized by the presence of a single, sharp peak, indicating that most normal brain voxels have approximately the same MTR values due to relative homogeneous tissue composition and microstructure. Demyelination, edema, atrophy and gliosis could impair MTR and the MTR histograms shape become flattened with decreased peak height reflecting dyshomogeneity of the brain tissue. In this way MTI allows the evaluation of brain tissue integridy, while simultaneously permits quantification of structural damage.

Studies that compared MS patients with normal controls using MTI revealed that the MTR histogram peak height was the volumetric MTI parameter that differed most significantly (van Buchem et al., 1998). This peak height was found to be decreased in MS patients. It was suggested that the peak height was a measure of the amount of residual normal brain tissue, and therefore inversely reflected the disease burden of the brain (van Buchem et al., 1998). In

Non-Conventional MRI Techniques in Neurophychiatric Systemic Lupus Erythematosus (NPSLE):
Emerging Tools to Elucidate the Pathophysiology and Aid the Diagnosis and Management

81

several MS studies, this measure was found also to correlate with measures of cognitive and neurologic functioning (van Buchem et al., 1998).

MTI has been applied in NPSLE patients without visible abnormalities on conventional MRI. All these studies used MTR histograms for the quantitative assessment of the whole brain abnormalities. Bosma and co-workers (Bosma et al., 2000) applied the MTI technique to 11 patients with NPSLE, 11 patients with SLE without history of NPSLE (non-NPSLE) and 10 healthy volunteers. In this study, for every patient, an MTR histogram was created after correction for the ICV and another was created after correction for brain volume. In MTR histograms that are adjusted for the ICV, the peak height reflects both the integrity of brain parenchyma and the extent of atrophy. A different distribution of the brain voxels, in terms of changes in MTR values due to disorders of brain parenchyma or a reduction in the total number of brain voxels due to atrophy, can cause a decrease in the peak height. The peak height of the MTR histograms corrected for brain volume is affected only by the aspect of brain parenchyma, and not by the volume of the brain and atrophy (van Buchem et al., 1998). In the group of NPSLE patients, the average peak height of the histograms corrected for intracranial volume and the peak height normalized for brain volume were significantly lower than in either the non-NPSLE patients or the healthy controls at the same position of the peaks. This suggests the presence, in NPSLE, not only of atrophy, but also of an abnormality of the remaining brain parenchyma. The latter disorder in NPSLE is probably primarily present in the normal appearing parenchyma, since the low number and small size of hyperintense lesions observed in these patients cannot solely account for the decreased peak height of the histograms. Since myelin is a major contributing factor to the MT effect in the brain, the decreased peak heights of the MTR histogram corrected for brain volume might have originated from demyelination along with axonal loss. Edema and gliosis are also considered to give rise to abnormal MTRs (Dousset et al., 1992).

In another study (Bosma et al., 2000) MTI was performed to 9 patients with active nonthromboembolic NPSLE, 10 patients with chronic NPSLE, 10 patients with SLE and no history of NPSLE (non-NPSLE), 10 patients with inactive MS, and 10 healthy control subjects, to investigate whether volumetric MTI analysis with MTR histograms can demonstrate abnormalities in patients in the acute stage of diffuse NPSLE and compare these findings with those from chronic SLE, non-SLE and MS. The MTR histograms of both the non-NPSLE group and the healthy controls were similar. There was flattening of the histograms in the active NPSLE group, but with a shift toward higher MTRs. These changes indicate that the uniformity of the brain in patients with active NPSLE is lower than that in SLE patients with no history of NPSLE as well as that in healthy controls, suggesting that patients with active NPSLE can be distinguished from SLE patients with no history of NPSLE by use of MTR histogram analysis. The shift of the MTR histogram peak to the right that was observed in active NPSLE suggest an all-over improvement in the exchange of saturation from the pool of bound protons to that of the free water protons. Increased MTRs were also found in an experimental model of acute inflammation in MS, experimental allergic encephalomyelitis, during the early phase of inflammation in that disease (Dousset et al., 1992). Similar processes may occur during the active phase of NPSLE. In this study, all MTR histogram parameters in chronic NPSLE and MS were identical. Since NPSLE and MS are diseases with a different biologic behavior, it is unlikely that these similarities suggest a similar pathogenesis. Instead, the similarities indicate that different diseases may give rise to a common final pathway (i.e., gliosis and demyelination) that results in similar changes in the MTR. These results also demonstrate that in the chronic stage of diffuse brain diseases, MTR histograms may not be able to differentiate between different diseases.

The same group (Bosma et al., 2002) further investigated the relationship between quantitative estimates of global brain damage based on magnetization transfer imaging (MTI) and the cerebral functioning, as measured by neurologic, psychiatric, and cognitive assessments, as well as the disease duration in patients with NPSLE. They performed MTI to 24 patients with NPSLE and found significant correlations between the descriptive measures of the MTR histograms and: a) the neurologic functioning quantified by the Kurtzke's Expanded Disability Status Scale (EDSS) b) the cognitive functions with the Wechsler Adult Intelligence Scale Revised (WAIS-R), a standardized psychometric test for assessing intelligence and c) the psychiatric functioning by the Hospital Anxiety and Depression Scale (HADS) questionnaire. Since the EDSS score mainly assesses motor skills, these findings suggest that atrophy and diffuse microscopic damage of the remaining brain parenchyma in NPSLE affect, among other areas, brain regions that are responsible for motor skills. Atrophy and diffuse microscopic cerebral damage also contribute the development of psychiatric symptoms, like anxiety and depression and cognitive impairment. There is no correlation between the quantitative estimates of global brain damage and age, SLE duration, or time elapsed since the first occurrence of neuropsychiatric symptoms suggesting that the accumulation of brain damage over time has a nonlinear aspect.

Dehmeshki and co-workers (Dehmeshki et al., 2002) developed an alternative way of analyzing and globally characterizing MTR histograms by using multivariate discriminant analysis (MDA) and correctly assigned patients with MS to clinical subgroups. The same group proceed to a study in SLE patients in order to explore the diagnostic potential of MDA for assigning patients with SLE to different subgroups of patients with on the basis of MTR histograms (Dehmeshki et al., 2002). MTI was performed to 9 patients with active NPSLE, 10 patients with chronic NPSLE, 10 patients with SLE and no history of NPSLE (non-NPSLE), 10 patients with inactive MS, and 10 healthy control subjects. Three binary comparisons were made: First, comparison of active NPSLE versus past NPSLE groups which is important because in patients with NPSLE, a new episode of neuropsychiatric symptoms could be due to an active intrinsic SLE-related brain process—that is, a recurrent active phase of NPSLE—or to extrinsic processes such as the side effects of drug use. Secondly, comparison of active NPSLE from non-NPSLE which is also important because an acute episode of neuropsychiatric symptoms could be due to active NPSLE or to extrinsic processes in patients with SLE. Finally, comparison of patients with active and/or past NPSLE with those who have MS which important because in patients who present with neuropsychiatric symptoms, the differential diagnosis includes SLE and MS, and these diseases are notoriously difficult to differentiate. In this study, MDA proved to be effective in assigning the majority of individual patients to disease categories in the given binary comparisons. In addition, MDA was shown to be considerably more effective for categorizing patient groups on the basis of MTR histograms than the conventional method of analyzing MTR histograms and might be of help in clinical practice.

Steens and co-workers (Steens et al., 2004) performed MTI in 24 SLE patients with a history of diffuse neuropsychiatric symptoms and 24 healthy controls to assess the distribution of

Non-Conventional MRI Techniques in Neurophychiatric Systemic Lupus Erythematosus (NPSLE):
Emerging Tools to Elucidate the Pathophysiology and Aid the Diagnosis and Management

83

MTI abnormalities over gray matter (GM) and white matter (WM) in SLE patients without explanatory MRI evidence of focal disease. MTR maps were calculated for GM and WM separately, and GM and WM MTR histograms were generated. Significantly lower peak height and mean MTR of the gray matter were found in NPSLE patients as compared with healthy controls indicative of parenchymal brain damage specifically in the GM in SLE patients with a history of NP symptoms and without explanatory focal abnormalities seen on MRI. This observation supports the model of neuronal damage in diffuse NPSLE, and can be explained by the greater susceptibility of GM to the sequelae of small-vessel disease and hypoperfusion. Small-vessel disease itself may also increase blood–brain barrier permeability, which facilitates the entrance of antineuronal antibodies. In either case, because of the higher concentration of neurons in GM, the GM will be particularly affected.

The same group (Steens et al., 2006) examined the correlation between gray and white matter magnetization transfer ratio (MTR) parameters and the presence of IgM and IgG anticardiolipins antibodies (aCLs) and lupus anticoagulant in 18 patients with NPSLE, but without cerebral infarcts on conventional magnetic resonance imaging. Lower gray and white matter mean MTR and peak location were observed in IgM aCL-positive patients than in IgM aCL-negative patients. No significant differences were found in MTR histogram parameters with respect to IgG aCL and lupus anticoagulant status, nor with respect to anti-dsDNA or anti- ENA (extractable nuclear antigen) status.

Various autoantibodies have been implicated in the pathogenesis of NPSLE, including anticardiolipin antibodies (aCLs) .Because of their prothrombotic tendency, aCLs may cause cerebral infarctions and as such they are correlated with focal neurological syndromes (Denburg, Denburg, 2003). In a study of Steens and co-workers (Steens et al., 2006) MTI parameters demonstrated brain damage in aCL-positive SLE patients in the absence of cerebral infarcts on conventional MRI. These findings suggest that, apart from giving rise to macroscopic cerebral infarctions, aCLs may play a role in the pathogenesis of diffuse microscopic brain damage in NPSLE. According to the authors there are at least three possible explanations for how aCLs could be involved to diffuse microscopic brain damage in NPSLE. First, the thrombotic tendency of antiphospholipid antibodies, including aCLs, may cause aggregation of thrombocytes and an increase in blood viscosity (Scolding, Joseph 2002; Connor, Hunt 2003). This may affect blood flow in small cerebral blood vessels in particular and cause widespread hypoperfusion, which subsequently causes ischaemic damage to brain tissue. Second, aCLs may activate endothelial cells and cause a diffuse small-vessel vasculopathy – a neuropathological finding that was reported as long ago as 1968 (Connor, Hunt 2003; Scolding, Joseph 2002). The resulting increase in blood–brain barrier permeability permits entrance to the brain parenchyma of substances such as circulating antibodies. Third, it has been shown in vitro that IgG aCLs themselves may interfere with glutamatergic pathways by a mechanism involving over-activation of the N-methyl-d-aspartate receptor (Andreasi et al., 2001).

Emmer and co-workers (Emmer et al., 2006) proved that changes in the clinical status of individual NPSLE patients correspond to changes in the MTR peak height and MTI is a valuable objective measure for following a clinical course in NPSLE. 19 active or inactive NPSLE patients underwent MTI on at least two separate occasions. Their neuropsychiatric status between the first and the second MRI sessions was classified as deteriorated, stable, or improved. In all clinically deteriorated patients the MTR peak height decreased between the first and second scans. In all clinically improved patients the MTR peak height increased between the first and second scans, indicating that brain involvement in NPSLE patients, as detected by MTI, is at least partly reversible. The nature of the pathophysiological substrate of the reversible MTR changes in NPSLE patients is unclear. According to the authors reversible changes in the integrity of the parenchyma are probably due to edema, since neuronal loss would not show such a degree of reversibility, and neuronal apoptosis is not a common finding in postmortem studies of NPSLE. Inflammation influences the vessel walls and permits extravasation of fluid and inflammatory mediators into the brain tissue that leads to inflammatory brain edema

4.4 Magnetic Resonance Spectroscopy

Proton Magnetic Resonance Spectroscopy (MRS) is an MRI technique that permits study of the metabolites in tissue and provides qualitative and quantitative information about some brain metabolites displayed as spectra. The position of metabolites peaks in the spectrum is determined by its molecular characteristics. Studies in humans have used hydrogen –MRS (H-MRS) and rarely phosphorous-MRS (P-MRS). In normal water-suppressed, localized H-MRS of human brain at echo times (TEs) between 135 msec and 270 msec 3 major neurometabolites are revealed: 1. **N-acetylaspartate (NAA)** with peak at 2.0 parts per million, which can be used as a neuronal marker, because is found exclusively in neurons. NAA is reduced in conditions associated with neuronal loss, such as stroke or neuronal degenerative disorders. However, several studies have shown reversible decreases in NAA in a number of conditions have also been recognized, emphasizing that neuronal dysfunction can also lead to a decrease in NAA (Rudkin, Arnold, 1999). 2. **Choline (Cho)**. Choline peak consists of choline, phosphocholine and glycerocholine. Cho is increased during increased cell -membrane turn over or during active myelin breakdown when these choline-containing membrane phospholipids are released. Increase Cho is detected in demyelination, remyelination, inflammation or gliosis (Rudkin, Arnold, 1999). 3. **Creatine and phosphocreatine (Cr)**.Total creatine concentration is relatively constant throughout the brain , and is used as an internal reference to normalize NAA and choline. Nevertheless there is loss of creatine in tissue necrosis (Rudkin, Arnold, 1999).

When performing MRS with short TE (30-35 msec) some other metabolites could also be revealed, such as **myo-inositol (mI)**, which is an osmolyte and astrocyte marker and is usually increased in demyelination, inflammation and gliosis. **Lactate** is elevated in anaerobic glycolysis and is not seen in normal brain spectra. The lactate peak is above the baseline when the TE is low (20–35 msec) or high (270–288 msec). At an intermediate TE (135–144 msec), the lactate peak inverts to project below the baseline, a feature that enables its distinction from lipids and some macromolecules seen at a similar location on the spectrum (1.35 parts per million).

Commonly used spectroscopic techniques include the single- voxel spectroscopy which allows evaluation of only small volumes of tissue, and the multivoxel technique that allows examination of different areas of the brain at the same time and also permits the derivation of metabolite maps. The selection of appropriate MRS techniques, including measurement parameters such as repetition time (TR) and TE, depends on the clinical question. Short TE (20-35 msec) evaluations are required when there is a need for detection of metabolites with short relaxation times, such as glutamine, glutamate or mI, whereas studies with long TE (135–270 msec) are sufficient for the detection of the major metabolites such as NAA, Cho, Cr, and lactate/lipids (Rudkin, Arnold, 1999)

Several studies have been performed using MRS in patients with SLE with or without neuropsychiatric manifestations. Most of them used single voxel MRS and proved reduction of the NAA/Cr and NAA/Cho ratios and elevation of Cho/Cr ratio in patients with SLE, not only in lesions, but also in normal-appearing white matter, when compared to controls. Nevertheless no dinstiction between acute and chronic disease has been demonstrated (Sibbit et al., 1997; Davie et al., 1995; Friedman et al., 1998). The NAA/Cr ratio was negatively correlated to the degree of atrophy in SLE patients, suggesting that cerebral atrophy in SLE in associated with neuronal damage (Sibbit et al., 1994; Chinn et al., 1997).

Decreased NAA/Cr ratio was found in white mater lesions of patients with NPSLE with no correlation with neurololgic or psyschiatric involvement (Davie et al., 1995). Patients with white matter lesions also had a more pronounced reduction in NAA/Cr ratio, when compared with patients without lesions, suggesting that neurophychiatric manifestations are associated with a complex multifocal and diffuse neurotoxic process (Brooks et al., 1999). Cerebrovascular abnormalities with small vessel injury, that underlie diffuse cerebral injury in SLE, (small focal lesions), are primarily associated with a decrease NAA/Cr ratio, while medium vessel injury is primarily associated with an increased Cho/Cr ratio (Friedman et al., 1998). It is well known that small focal lesions are also observed in healthy adults, often associated with older age. However, if neurometabolic changes are observed within these lesions, it could be inferred that these white matter lesions represent a serious pathologic process resulting in focal neuronal death or injury (Brooks et al., 1997).

The amount of reduction in NAA/Cr ratio is associated with disease activity and the severity of clinical manifestations (Sibbitt et al., 1997).The same group failed to demonstrate lactate even in severely ill patients with major NPSLE, suggesting that extensive , anaerobic metabolism is not a fundamental characteristic of NPSLE, although this was contraindicated by others (Sundgren et al., 2005).They also found that increased lipid-macromolecules peaks at 1,2 ppm is an indicator of disease activity representing inflammatory cell infiltration, membrane activation, degradation or demyelination. Appenzeller and co-workers (Appenzeller et al., 2005) also demonstrated that the reduction in NAA /Cr ratio correlated with disease activity, independently of CNS manifestations, and that NAA/ Cr ratio in normal-appearing white matter returned to normal range after remission.

Sabet and co-workers (Sabet et al., 1998) proved that NAA/Cr ratio was lower and Cho/Cr was higher in SLE patients with antiphospholipid antibody syndrome (aPLS) compared to those without aPLS . However thrombotic phenomena are most closely associated with the Cho/Cr ratio elevation in patients with SLE. Elevated Cho/Cr ratio was observed in focal lesions and normal-appearing tissues of patients with SLE-aPLS consistent with infarct, activation of cellular membranes, catabolism of myelin, or inflammation. Cho/Cr ratio was increased in normal-appearing tissues, suggesting exaggerated injury to normal-appearing tissue in patients with SLE-aPLS consistent with widespread microinfarction.

Reduction of NAA/Cr ratio and elevation of Cho/Cr ratio seem to reflect the cerebral metabolic disturbance related to the severity of neuropsychiatric symptoms regardless of the presence of abnormal MRI findings (Lim et al., 2000). In that study metabolic changes at the basal ganglia, besides the normal appearing white matter, was also found, indicating small vessel injury. Reduction of NAA/Cr ratio and elevation of Cho/Cr ratio in normal appearing white matter, related to the severity of neuropsychiatric symptoms was also proved by others (Axford et al., 2001; Handa et al., 2003; Castellino et al., 2005). Axford and co-workers also performed quantitative absolute assessment of the metabolites and found increased absolute concentration of mI in NPSLE patients symptoms, that could be the result of inflammation, with a trend to be reversible in patients with minor. The authors suggest that raised mI, but normal NAA, that characterized SLE minor, may be due to result of vasculitis and inflammatory sequelae, which may be reversible if treated early enough. In contrast with the patients with SLE minor, the patients with SLE major had both increased mI and decreased NAA that may reflect gliosis and irreversible neuronal loss.

Castellino and co-workers (Castellino et al., 2005) assessed metabolites at hypoperfused and normoperfused brain areas according to SPECT finding and found that NAA/Cr ratio was reduced in hypoperfused areas, and Cho/Cr ratio was elevated in normoperfused areas, while new white matter lesions were developed on previous areas of hypoperfusion and NAA/Cr ratio reduction indicating that increased Cho/Cr ratio in normal-appearing white matter may predict the appearance of white matter lesions.

The NAA reduction has been also correlated with cognitive dysfunction and extent of brain damage (Sibbit et al., 1997; Lim et al., 2000). Increased choline was also associated with the presence of cognitive dysfunction in patients with SLE (Kozora et al., 2005) a finding that was further proved by other studies (Lapteva et al., 2006; Filley et al., 2009). Significant correlation was found between cognitive scores and higher Cho/Cr ratio of the dorsolateral prefrontal cortex and white matter (Lapteva et al., 2006) or the left frontal white matter (Filley et al., 2009).

A recent study (Brooks et al, 2010) investigated most-mortem histopathological changes at autopsy in NPSLE patients and matched them voxel-by-voxel with the neurometabolites. They found that neurometabolite abnormalities were closely associated with underlying histopathological changes in the brain. Elevated choline levels were independently associated with gliosis, vasculopathy, and edema, while reduced creatine levels were associated with reduced neuronal–axonal density and gliosis. Reduced NAA levels were associated with reduced neuronal–axonal density and the presence of lactate was associated with necrosis, microhemorrhages, and edema. They suggest that altered neurometabolites in NPSLE patients, as determined by MRS, are a grave prognostic sign, indicating serious underlying histologic brain injury.

Few studies incorporated a multisequence MRI approach in patients with NPSLE to investigate the relationship between the different non-conventional MRI techniques. Emmer and co-workers (Emmer et al., 2008) applied MTI and MRS in SLE and NPSLE patients and healthy controls and found that there was significant association between the MTR histogram peak height of the whole brain parenchyma and the white and gray matter and the NAA/Cr ratio, indicating that demyelination and neuronal/axonal damage often occur together in patients with a history of NPSLE. The Cho/Cr ratio showed no significant association with any MTR parameters. According to another study that investigated the relationship between magnetization transfer imaging (MTI), diffusion weighted imaging (DWI), proton magnetic resonance spectroscopy (H-MRS), and T2 relaxometry findings in patients with primary neuropsychiatric systemic lupus erythematosus (NPSLE) (Bosma et al., 2004), significant correlations were found between the different metrics and cerebral atrophy. The correlations between MTI and DWI parameters indicate that demyelination in NPSLE patients is associated with increased diffusivity, due to either to a breakdown of myelin or a discrete increase of CSF spaces-including perivascular changes-associated with cerebral atrophy. The association between prolonged T2 relaxation time and increased diffusivity could be based not only on atrophy, but also on the presence of gliosis.

5. Conclusion

NPSLE is characterized by variable, focal or diffuse, neuropsychiatric symptoms, leading to significant morbidity and mortality. NPSLE manifestations can occur in the absence of either serologic activity or other systemic lupus manifestations and there is no single sensitive and specific diagnostic test. Thus, in clinical practice the diagnosis of primary NPSLE is rather presumptive, after the exclusion of alternative causes of the neuropsychiatric symptoms. In patients with focal symptoms conventional MRI commonly detects small, discrete, hyperintense, frontal–parietal subcortical or periventricular white matter lesions, or even microhemorrhages, which are not specific for NPSLE and exhibit no clinical correlation. In diffuse NPSLE presentation conventional MRI could be totally unremarkable.

Non- conventional MRI techniques, namely diffusion weighted imaging (DWI), diffusion tensor imaging (DTI), perfusion weighted imaging (PWI), Magnetization transfer imaging (MTI) and magnetic resonance spectroscopy (MRS) have been developed. These techniques are sensitive to microstructural (DWI, DTI,MTI), hemodynamic (PWI) and biochemical (MRS) characteristics of the tissues, and could detect gray and white matter abnormalities in NPSLE patients, otherwise occult by conventional imaging. Vasculopathy is the most common pathologic finding in NSPLE, while true vasculitis is rather uncommon. SLE vasculopathy affects predominantly arterioles and capillaries and could be related to both acute inflammation and hypoperfusion resulting in ischemia, demyelination, axonal loss and gliosis. These pathologic findings lead to particular changes of the non-conventional MRI metrics, such as reduced increased diffusivity, decreased fractional anisotropy, decreased MTR values , decreased NAA levels, and elevated choline levels, not only in focal lesions but mostly in normal appearing white and gray matter in patients with NPSLE. These quantitative changes are related to disease activity and severity, cognitive performance, and also the presence of antiphospholipid antibody syndrome and/or anticardiolipin antibodies, while could affect with the prognosis of new lesions and clinical deterioration. Although there are some inconsistencies in the various reports published thus far reflecting heterogeneity in patient selection, sample size and diagnostic criteria used, , we believe that there is enough data to support the use in daily clinical practice at tertiary care centers of non- conventional MRI techniques for the diagnostic work up of SLE patients with neuropsychiatric manifestations. For places whereby these modalities are not available the EULAR guidelines recommend at a minimum an MRI protocol (brain and spinal cord) that includes conventional MRI sequences (T1/T2, FLAIR), diffusion-weighted imaging (DWI), and gadolinium-enhanced T1 sequences (Bertsias et al., 2010).

6. References

Ainiala H, Dastidar P, Loukkola J, Lehtimaki T, Korpela M &Peltola J (2005) Cerebral MRI abnormalities and their association with neuropsychiatric manifestations in SLE: apopulation-based study. Scand J Rheumatol ; 34:376–382

Andreassi C, Zoli A, Riccio A, Scuderi F, Lombardi L, Altomonte L &Eboli ML(2001). Anticardiolipin antibodies in patients with primary antiphospholipid syndrome: a correlation between IgG titre and antibody-induced cell dysfunctions in neuronal cell cultures. Clin Rheumatol; 20:314-318.

Appenzeller S, Rondina JM, Li LM, Costallat LT &Cendes F (2005) Cerebral and corpus callosum atrophy in systemic lupus erythematosus. Arthritis Rheum; 52:2783–2789

Appenzeller S, Carnevalle AD, Li LM, Costallat LT & Cendes F (2006) Hippocampal atrophy in systemic lupus erythematosus. Ann Rheum Dis; 65:1585–1589

Appenzeller S, Amorim BJ, Ramos CD, Rio PA, de C Etchebehere EC, Camargo EE, Cendes F & Costallat LT (2007) Voxel-based morphometry of brain SPECT can detect the presence of active central nervous system involvement in systemic lupus erythematosus. Rheumatology (Oxford); 46:467–472.

Appenzeller S, Bonilha L, Rio PA, Min Li L, Costallat LT & Cendes F (2007) Longitudinal analysis of gray and white matter loss in patients with systemic lupus erythematosus. Neuroimage 34:694–701

Appenzeller S , Pike BG , Clarke AE, (2008) Magnetic Resonance Imaging in the Evaluation of Central Nervous System Manifestations in Systemic Lupus Erythematosus Clinic Rev Allerg Immunol; 34:361–366

Axford JS, Howe FA, Heron C & Griffiths JR. (2001) Sensitivity of quantitative (1)H magnetic resonance spectroscopy of the brain in detecting early neuronal damage in systemic lupus erythematosus. Ann Rheum Dis; 60:106–11.

Benedetti B, Rovaris M, Judica E, Donadoni G, Ciboddo G & Filippi M (2007) Assessing "occult" cervical cord damage in patients with neuropsychiatric systemic lupus erythematosus using diffusion tensor MRI) J Neurol Neurosurg Psychiatry. J Neurol Neurosurg Psychiatry 78:893–895

Bertsias GK, Ioannidis JP, Aringer M, Bollen E, Bombardieri S, Bruce IN, Cervera R, Dalakas M, Doria A, Hanly JG, Huizinga TW, Isenberg D, Kallenberg C, Piette JC, Schneider M, Scolding N, Smolen J, Stara A, Tassiulas I, Tektonidou M, Tincani A, van Buchem MA, van Vollenhoven R, Ward M, Gordon C.& Boumpas DT.(2010) EULAR recommendations for the management of systemic lupus erythematosus with neuropsychiatric manifestations: report of a task force of the EULAR standing committee for clinical affairs. Ann Rheum Dis.;69(12):2074-82.

Bertsias GK,Boumpas DT. (2010) Pathogenesis, diagnosis and management of neuropsychiatric SLE manifestations. Nat Rev Rheumatol. Jun;6(6):358-67.

Bosma GP, van Buchem MA & Rood MJ, (2000),: Comparison of ADC histograms of patients with neuropsychiatric systemic lupus erythematosus and healthy volunteers. Proc Intl Soc Mag Res Med 8:1244.

Bosma GP, Rood MJ, Zwinderman AH, Huizinga TW & van Buchem MA.(2000) Evidence of central nervous system damage in patients with neuropsychiatric systemic lupus erythematosus, demonstrated by magnetization transfer imaging. Arthritis Rheum;43:48–54.

Bosma GPTh, Rood MJ, Huizinga TWJ, De Jong BA, Bollen ELEM & van Buchem MA. (2000) Detection of cerebral involvement in patients with active neuropsychiatric systemic lupus erythematosus using magnetization transfer imaging. Arthritis Rheum; 43: 2428-36.

Bosma GP, Middelkoop HA, Rood MJ, Bollen EL, Huizinga TW & van Buchem MA. (2002) Association of global brain damage and clinical functioning in neuropsychiatric systemic lupus erythematosus. Arthritis Rheum;46:2665-72

Bosma GP, Huizinga TW, Mooijaart SP & van Buchem MA. (2003) Abnormal brain diffusivity in patients with neuropsychiatric systemic lupus erythematosus. AJNR;24: 850-4.

Bosma GP, Steens SC, Petropoulos H, Admiraal-Behloul F, van den Haak A, Doornbos J,Huizinga TW, Brooks WM, Harville A, Sibbitt WL Jr & van Buchem MA. (2004) Multisequence magnetic resonance imaging study of neuropsychiatric systemic lupus erythematosus. Arthritis Rheum;50:3195–202.

Borrelli M, Tamarozzi R, Colamussi P, Govoni M, Trotta F,& Lappi S. (2003) Evaluation with MR, perfusion MR and cerebral flow SPECT in NPSLE patients. Radiol Med;105:482-9.

Brooks WM, Sabet A, Sibbitt WL Jr, Barker PB, van Zijl PC, Duyn JH & Moonen CT. (1997) Neurochemistry of brain lesions determined by spectroscopic imaging in systemic lupus erythematosus. J Rheumatol;24:2323–9.

Brooks WM, Jung RE, Ford CC, Greinel EJ & Sibbitt WL Jr.(1999) Relationship between neurometabolite derangement and neurocognitive dysfunction in systemic lupus erythematosus. J Rheumatol;26:81–5.

Brooks WM, Sibbitt WL, Mario Kornfeld M,Jung RE,Bankhurst AD & Roldan CA (2010) The Histopathologic Associates of Neurometabolite Abnormalities in Fatal Neuropsychiatric Systemic Lupus Erythematosus Arthritis and Rheumatism; 62: 2055–2063

Cascio CJ, Gerig G & Piven J (2007) Diffusion tensor imaging: Application to the study of the developing brain. J Am Acad Child Adolesc Psychiatry;46(2):213-223.

Castellino G, Govoni M, Padovan M, Colamussi P, Borrelli M & Trotta F. (2005)Proton magnetic resonance spectroscopy may predict future brain lesions in SLE patients: a functional multiimaging approach and follow up. Ann Rheum Dis;64:1022–7.

Castellino G, Padovan M, Bortoluzzi A, Borrelli M, Feggi L, Caniatti ML Trotta F & Govoni M. (2008) Single photon emission computed tomography and magnetic resonance imaging evaluation in SLE patients with and without neuropsychiatric involvement. Rheumatology (Oxford); 47(3):319-23.

Cauli A, Montaldo C, Peltz MT, Nurchis P, Sanna G, Garau P Pala R, Passiu G & Mathieu A. (1994) Abnormalities of magnetic resonance imaging of the central nervous system in patients with systemic lupus erythematosus correlate with disease severity. Clin Rheumatol 13:615–618

Chinn RJ, Wilkinson ID, Hall-Craggs MA, Paley MN, Shortall E, Carter S Kendall BE, Isenberg DA, Newman SP,& Harrison MJ. (1997) Magnetic resonance imaging of the brain and cerebral proton spectroscopy in patients with systemic lupus erythematosus. Arthritis Rheum 40:36–46

Colamussi P, Giganti M, Cittanti C, Dovigo L, Trotta F, Tola MR, Tamarozzi R, Lucignani G & Piffanelli A. (1995) Brain single-photonemission tomography with 99mTc-HMPAO in neuropsychiatric systemic lupus erythematosus: relations with EEG and MRI findings and clinical manifestations. Eur J Nucl Med;22:17–24.

Connor P, Hunt BJ. (2003): Cerebral haemostasis and antiphospholipid antibodies. Lupus, 12:929-934.

Davie CA, Feinstein A, Kartsounis LD, Barker GJ, McHugh NJ, Walport MJ, Ron MA, Moseley IF, McDonald WI & Miller DH. (1995).Proton magnetic resonance spectroscopy of systemic lupus erythematosus involving the central nervous system. J Neurol;242:522–8.

Dehmeshki J , Van Buchem MA, Bosma GPT, Huizinga TWJ & Tofts PS, (2002) Systemic
    Lupus Erythematosus: Diagnostic Application of Magnetization Transfer Ratio
    Histograms in Patients with Neuropsychiatric Symptoms—Initial Results
    Radiology; 222:722–728
Devinsky O, Petito CK & Alonso DR. (1998) Clinical and neuropathological findings in
    systemic lupus erythematosus: the role of vasculitis, heart emboli and thrombotic
    thrombocytopenic purpura. Ann Neurol; 23:380–384.
Denburg SD, Denburg JA: (2003) Cognitive dysfunction and antiphospholipid
antibodies in systemic lupus erythematosus. Lupus; 12:883–890.
Emmer BJ, van der Grond J, Steup-Beekman GM, Huizinga TWJ & van Buchem MA(2006)
    Selective Involvement of the Amygdala in Systemic Lupus Erythematosus PLoS
    Med;3(12): e499.
Emmer BJ, Steens SC, Steup-Beekman GM, van der Grond J, Admiraal-Behloul F, Olofsen H,
    Bosma GP, Ouwendijk WJ, Huizinga TW & van Buchem MA.(2006)Detection of
    change in CNS involvement in neuropsychiatric SLE: a magnetization transfer
    study. J Magn Reson Imaging;24:812–6.
Emmer BJ. Steup-Beekman GM, Steens SCA, Huizinga TWJ,van Buchem MA. & van der
    Grond J(2008) Correlation of Magnetization Transfer Ratio Histogram Parameters
    With Neuropsychiatric Systemic Lupus Erythematosus Criteria and Proton
    Magnetic Resonance Spectroscopy Association of Magnetization Transfer Ratio
    Peak Height With Neuronal and Cognitive Dysfunction Arthritis and
    Rheumatism;58(5): 1451–1457
Emmer BJ, Veer IM, Steup-Beekman GM, Huizinga TWJ, van der Grond J & van Buchem
    MA (2010)Tract-Based Spatial Statistics on Diffusion Tensor Imaging in Systemic
    Lupus Erythematosus Reveals Localized Involvement of White Matter Tracts
    Arthritis Rheum; 62 (12): 3716–3721
Emmer BJ, Osch MJ, Wu O, Steup-Beekman GM, Steens SC, Huizinga TW, van Buchem MA.
    & van der Grond J. (2010) Perfusion MRI in Neuro-Psychiatric Systemic Lupus
    Erthemathosus J Magn Reson Imaging;32:283–288
Filley CM, Kozora E, Brown MS, Miller DE ,West SG, David B. Arciniegas DB, Grimm A. &
    Zhang L. (2009) White Matter Microstructure and Cognition in Non-
    neuropsychiatric Systemic Lupus Erythematosus Cog Behav Neurol;22:38–44
Finelli DA.(1998) Magnetization transfer in neuroimaging. Magn Reson Imaging Clin North
    Am;6:31–52.
Friedman SD, Stidley CA, Brooks WM, Hart BL. & Sibbitt WL Jr (1998). Brain injury and
    neurometabolic abnormalities in systemic lupus erythematosus. Radiology;209:79–
    84.
Futrell N, Schultz LR. & Millikan C.(1992) Central nervous system disease in patients with
    systemic lupus erythematosus. Neurology.;42:1649-57.
Gasparovic CM, Roldan CA, Sibbitt WI Jr, Qualls CR, Mullins PG, Sharrar JM, Yamamoto JJ,
    & Bockholt JH(2010)Elevated Cerebral Blood Flow and Volume in Systemic Lupus
    Measured by Dynamic Susceptibility Contrast Magnetic Resonance Imaging. J
    Rheumatol;37;1834-1843
Grossman RI, Gomori JM, Ramer KN, Lexa FJ & Schnall MD.(1994) Magnetization transfer:
    theory and clinical applications in neuroradiology.Radiographics;14:279–90.

Grunwald F, Schomburg A, Badali A, Ruhlmann J, Pavics L. & Biersack HJ. (1995) 18FDG
    PET and acetazolamide-enhanced 99mTc- HMPAO SPET in systemic lupus
    erythematosus. Eur J Nucl Med;22:1073–7.
Handa R, Sahota P, Kumar M, Jagannathan NR, Bal CS, Gulati M, Tripathi BM & Wali JP.
    (2003);In vivo proton magnetic resonance spectroscopy (MRS) and single photon
    emission computerized tomography (SPECT) in systemic lupus erythematosus
    (SLE). Magn Reson Imaging;21:1033–7.
Hanly JG, Walsh NM & Sangalang V.(1992) Brain pathology in systemic lupus
    erythematosus. J Rheumatol;19:732–741.
Hoeffner EG, (2005) Cerebral Perfusion Imaging(J Neuro-Ophthalmol;25: 313–320)
Hughes M, Sundgren PC, Fan X, Foerster B, Nan B, Welsh RC, Williamson JA,Attwood J,
    Maly PV, Chenevert TL, McCune W & Gebarski S. (2007). Diffusion tensor imaging
    in patients with acute onset of neuropsychiatric systemic lupus erythematosus: a
    prospective study of apparent diffusion coefficient, fractional anisotropy values,
    and eigenvalues in different regions of the brain. Acta Radiol; 48(2):213-222.
Jennings JE, Sundgren PC, Attwood J, McCune J & Maly P (2004) Value of MRI of the brain
    in patients with systemic lupus erythematosus and neurologic disturbance
    Neuroradiology; 46: 15–21
Jung RE, Caprihan A, Chavez RS, Flores RA, Sharrar J,Qualls CR, Sibbitt W, Roldan CA
    (2010) Diffusion tensor imaging in neuropsychiatric systemic lupus erythematosus
    BMC Neurology, 10:65
Kao CH, Lan JL, ChangLai SP, Liao KK, Yen RF, & Chieng PU.(1999).The role of FDG-PET,
    HMPAO-SPECT and MRI in the detection of brain involvement in patients with
    systemic lupus erythematosus. Eur J Nucl Med 26:129–134.
Kelly MC, Denburg JA. (1987) Cerebrospinal fluid immunoglobulins and neuronal
    antibodies in neuropsychiatric systemic lupus erythematosus and related
    conditions. J Rheumatol;14:740-4.
Koenig SH. (1991) Cholesterol of myelin is the determinant of gray-white contrast in MRI of
    brain. Magn Reson Med;20:285–91.
Kodama K, Okada S, Hino T, Takabayashi K, Nawata Y, Uchida Y, Yamanouchi N, Komatsu
    N, Ikeda T. & Shinoda N (1995).Single photon emission computed tomography in
    systemic lupus erythematosus with psychiatric symptoms. J Neurol Neurosurg
    Psychiatry;58:307–11.
Kozora E, Arciniegas DB, Filley CM, Ellison MC, West SG, Brown MS. & Simon JH. (2005).
    Cognition, MRS neurometabolites, and MRI volumetrics in non-neuropsychiatric
    systemic lupus erythematosus: preliminary data. Cogn Behav Neurol; 18:159–62.
Kushner MJ, Tobin M, Fazekas F, Chawluk J, Jamieson D,Freundlich B, Grenell S, Freemen
    L. & Reivich M (1990). Cerebral blood flow variations in CNS lupus.
    Neurology;40:99–102.
Lapteva L, Nowak M, Yarboro CH, Takada K, Roebuck-Spencer T, Weickert T, Bleiberg J,
    Rosenstein D, Pao M, Patronas N, Steele S, Manzano M, van der Veen JW, Lipsky
    PE, Marenco S, Wesley R, Volpe B, Diamond B. & Illei GG.(2006) Anti-N-methyl-D-
    aspartate receptor antibodies, cognitive dysfunction, and depression in systemic
    lupus erythematosus. Arthritis Rheum.;54(8):2505-14.

Lim MK, Suh CH, Kim HJ, Cho YK, Choi SH, Kang JH, Park W & Lee JH. (2000).Systemic lupus erythematosus: brain MR imaging and single voxel hydrogen 1 MR spectroscopy. Radiology;217: 43–9

Luyendijk J, Steens SC, Ouwendijk WJ, Steup-Beekman GM, Bollen EL, van der Grond J, Huizinga TW, Emmer BJ. & van Buchem MA(2011) Neuropsychiatric systemic lupus erythematosus: lessons learned from magnetic resonance imaging. Arthritis Rheum. ;63(3):722-32.

Miller DH, Buchanan N, Barker G Morrissey SP, Kendall BE, Rudge P, Khamashta M, Hughes GR,. & McDonald WI. (1992). Gadolinium enhanced magnetic resonance imaging in the central nervous system in systemic lupus erythematosus. J Neurol; 239: 460–464.

Nusbaum AO, Tang CY, Wei T, Buchsbaum MS & Atlas SW.(2000): Whole-brain diffusion MR histograms differ between MS subtypes. Neurology, 54:1421–1427.

Otte A, Weiner SM, Peter HH, Mueller-Brand J, Goetze M, Moser E, Gutfleisch J, Hoegerle S, Juengling FD & Nitzsche EU. (1997). Brain glucose utilization in systemic lupus erythematosus with neuropsychiatric symptoms: a controlled positron emission tomography study. Eur J Nucl Med;24:787–91.

Peterson PL, Axford JS. & Isenberg D (2005) Imaging in CNS lupus Best Practice & Research Clinical Rheumatology; 19(5): 727–739.

Pierpaoli C, Jezzard P, Basser PJ, Barnett A. & Di Chiro G (1996): Diffusion tensor MR imaging of the human brain. Radiology; 201(3):637-648.

Provenzale JM, Barboriak DP, Allen NB. & Ortel TL (1996) Patients with antiphospholipid antibodies: CT and MR findings of the brain. Am J Roentgenol ;167: 1573–1578

Roldan CA, Gelgand EA, Qualls CR. & Sibbitt WL Jr. (2006) Valvular heart disease is associated with nonfocal neuropsychiatric systemic lupus erythematosus. J Clin Rheumatol; 12(1):3-10.

Roldan CA, Qualls CR, Sopko KS. & Sibbitt WL Jr.(2008) Transthoracic versus transesophageal echocardiography for detection of Libman- Sacks endocarditis: a randomized controlled study. J Rheumatol;35:224-9.

Rovaris M, Viti B, Ciboddo G Gerevini S, Capra R, Iannucci G, Comi G. & Filippi M. (2000) Brain involvement in systemic immune mediated diseases: magnetic resonance and magnetization transfer imaging study. J Neurol Neurosurg Psychiatry; 68:170–177

Rudkin TM, Arnold DL. (1999) Proton magnetic resonance spectroscopy for the diagnosis and management of cerebral disorders. Arch Neurol;56:919–26.

Sabet A, Sibbitt WL Jr, Stidley CA, Danska J. & Brooks WM.(1998)Neurometabolite markers of cerebral injury in the antiphospholipid antibody syndrome of systemic lupus erythematosus. Stroke;29:2254–60

Scolding NJ, Joseph FG (2002) The neuropathology and pathogenesis of systemic lupus erythematosus. Neuropathol Appl Neurobiol; 28:173-189.

Schaefer PW, Grant PE. & Gonzalez RG (2000) Diffusion-weighted MRimaging of the brain. Radiology; 217:331–345.

Sibbitt Jr.WL, BrooksWM, Haseler LJ & Griffey RH. (1995) Spin-spin relaxation of brain tissues in systemic lupus erythematosus. A method for increasing the sensitivity of magnetic resonance imaging for neuropsychiatric lupus. Arthritis Rheum; 38(6): 810–818.

Sibbitt Jr WL, Haseler LJ, Griffey RR, Friedman SD& Brooks WM. (1997)Neurometabolism
    of active neuropsychiatric lupus determined with proton MR spectroscopy. AJNR
    Am J Neuroradiol;18: 1271-1277.
Sibbitt WL Jr, Sibbitt RR. &Brooks WM.(1999)Neuroimaging in neuropsychiatric SLE.
    Arthritis Rheum;42:2026-38.
Sibbitt WL Jr, Brooks WM, Kornfeld M, Hart BL, Bankhurst AD,& Roldan CA (2010)
    Magnetic Resonance Imaging and Brain Histopathology in Neuropsychiatric
    Systemic Lupus Erythematosus. Semin Arthritis Rheum; 40:32-52
Steens SC, Admiraal-Behloul F, Bosma GP, Steup-Beekman GM, Olofsen H, le Cessie S,
    Huizinga TWJ & van Buchem MA.(2004) Selective gray matter damage in
    neuropsychiatric lupus: a magnetization transfer imaging study. Arthritis Rheum ;
    50:2877-81.
Steens SC, Bosma GP, Steup-Beekman GM , le Cessie S , Huizinga TWJ. & van Buchem MA
    (2006)Association between microscopic brain damage as indicated by
    magnetization transfer imaging and anticardiolipin antibodies in neuropsychiatric
    lupus Arthritis Research & Therapy; 8 : 1186-1892.
Stojanovich L, Zandman-Goddard G, Pavlovich S & Sikanich N (2007) Psychiatric
    manifestations in systemic lupus erythematosus. Autoimmun Rev 6:421-426
Sundgren PC, Jennings J, Attwood JT, Nan B, Gebarski S, McCune WJ, Pang Y. & Maly P.
    (2005) MRI and 2D-CSI MR spectroscopy of the brain in the evaluation of patients
    with acute onset of neuropsychiatric systemic lupus erythematosus.
    Neuroradiology;47:576-85.
Ulug AM, Moore DF, Bojko AS.& Zimmerman RD.(1999) Clinical use of diffusion-tensor
    imaging for diseases causing neuronal and axonal damage. AJNR Am J
    Neuroradiol ;20:1044-8.
Van Buchem MA, Grossman RI, Armstrong C, Polansky M, Miki Y, Heyning FH Boncoeur-
    Martel MP, Wei L, Udupa JK, Grossman M, Kolson DL & McGowan JC.(1998)
    Correlation of volumetric magnetization transfer imaging with clinical data in MS.
    Neurology;50:1609-17.
Van Dam AP (1991) Diagnosis and pathogenesis of CNS lupus. Rheumatol Intl 11: 1-11
Vermeer SE, Priens ND, den Heijer T, Hofman A, Koudstaal PJ. & Breteler MB (2003) Silent
    brain infarcts and the risk of dementia and cognitive decline. N Engl J Med
    348:1215-1222
Waterloo K, Omdal R, Sjoholm H, Koldingsnes W, Jacobsen EA, Sundsfjord JA, Husby G. &
    Mellgren SI. (2001). Neuropsychological dysfunction in systemic lupus
    erythematosus is not associated with changes in cerebral blood flow. J Neurol;248:
    595-602.
Weiner DK, Allen NB. (1991)Large vessel vasculitis of the central nervous system in
    systemic lupus erythematosus: report and review of the literature.J Rheumatol;
    18:748-751
Welsh RC, Rahba H, Foerster B, Thurnher M & Sundgren PC. (2007)Brain Diffusivity in
    Patients with Neuropsychiatric Systemic Lupus Erythematosus with New Acute
    Neurological Symptoms J of Magnetic Resonance Imaging ;26:541-551
Wolff SD, Balaban RS.(1994) Magnetization transfer imaging: practical aspects and clinical
    applications. Radiology;192:593-9.

Yuh WTC, Ueda T. & Male YJE.(1999) Diagnosis of microvasculopathy in CNS vasculitis: value of perfusion and diffusion imaging. J Magn Reson Imaging;10:310–3.

Zhang L, Harrison M, Heier LA, Zimmerman RD, Ravdin L, Lockshin M. & Ulug AM: (2007) Diffusion changes in patients with systemic lupus erythematosus. Magn Reson Imaging; 25(3):399-405.

Zvaifler NJ, Bluestein HG.(1982) The pathogenesis of central nervous system manifestations of systemic lupus erythematosus. Arthritis Rheum;25:862–6.

5

Central Nervous System Tuberculosis

Shahina Bano[1], Vikas Chaudhary[2] and Sachchidanand Yadav[3]
[1]Department of Radiodiagnosis, G.B. Pant
Hospital & Maulana Azad Medical College, New Delhi
[2]Department of Radiodiagnosis, Employees' State Insurance
Corporation (ESIC) Model Hospital, Gurgaon, Haryana
[3]Department of Radiodiagnosis, Dr. Ram Manohar
Lohia Hospital & PGIMER, New Delhi,
India

1. Introduction

Tuberculosis is a formidable disease worldwide because of its highly infectious nature and propensity for latency. The increasing prevalence of tuberculosis in both immunocompetent and immunocompromised individuals in recent years makes this disease a topic of universal concern. The disease has insidious onset and can affect virtually any organ system in the body, including the central nervous system (CNS). The CNS tuberculosis can mimic a number of other disease entities, and therefore it is important to be familiar with the various radiologic features of CNS tuberculosis to ensure early, accurate diagnosis. In this chapter we discuss various possible presentation of central nervous system tuberculosis involving the brain and spine.

2. Pathophysiology

Most tuberculous infections of the central nervous system are caused by *Mycobacterium tuberculosis,* as a result of hematogenous spread from a primary location, either the lung or gastrointestinal tract. Initially, small tuberculous lesions (Rich's foci) develop in the CNS, either during the stage of bacteraemia of the primary tuberculous infection or shortly afterwards. These initial tuberculous lesions may be inoculated in the meninges; the subpial and subependymal surface of the brain or the spinal cord, and may remain dormant for years. Later, rupture or growth of one or more of these small tuberculous lesions produces various types of CNS tuberculosis. The type and extent of lesion depend upon the number and virulence of bacilli and the immune response of the host.[1] A tubercular rupture into the subarachnoid space results in TB meningitis; where as deep lesions cause tuberculoma or abscesses. TB meningitis may cause inflammatory changes in cranial/spinal nerves and the blood vessels. The inflammation of blood vessels (vasculitis) subsequently results in thrombosis and infarction. Hydrocephalous can occur secondary to impedance of CSF circulation and absorption. The inflammatory exudates may also surround the spinal cord producing tuberculous arachnoiditis. Infrequently, infection spreads to the CNS from a site of discal TB, tuberculous otitis, or osteogenic tubercular foci in the spine or cranial vault.[2]

Pathologically, a tuberculoma is composed of central core of caseous necrosis surrounded by a capsule of collagenous tissues and an outer layer of mononuclear inflammatory cells (including plasma cells & lymphocytes), epitheloid cells and multinucleated Langerhans' giant cells. A tuberculoma harbours few tubercular bacilli within the necrotic center and the capsule. Outside the capsule, there is parenchymal edema and astrocyte proliferation. Unlike caseous tuberculoma, a tubercular abscess has purulent center rich in tubercular bacilli, and lacks epithelioid giant cell granulomatous reaction in its wall.[3]

3. Clinical features

CNS TB usually has signs and symptoms of increased intracranial pressure or space-occupying lesions in the brain or spine. Signs of meningitis includes constitutional symptoms (such as low grade fever, headache, nausea, vomiting, lethargy), meningismus, confusion, seizure, papilloedema, cranial nerve palsies (commonly second, third, fourth, sixth and seventh nerves), focal neurological deficits, stupor and coma. Patients with brain and spinal cord tuberculomas will have physical signs and symptoms consistent with the location of the lesion, which may include altered mental status, visual changes, hemiparesis/hemiplegia or seizure as seen with brain lesions; while weakness of extremities or bowel and bladder symptoms as seen with spinal cord lesions.[4,5]

4. Classification of cns tuberculosis

The manifestations of CNS tuberculosis are highly variable; however we have tried to include various possible presentations of CNS tuberculosis in this chapter as summarized in the box 1 given below:

• Tubercular Meningitis(TBM) & its complications • Hydrocephalus • Vasculitis causing infarction • Cranial Neuropathies • Pachymeningitis • Granulomatous basal meningitis • Parenchymal Tuberculosis • Parenchymal Tuberculomas • Tubercular abscesses • Miliary Tuberculomas • Focal Tubercular Cerebritis • Tubercular Encephalopathy • Tuberculoma en plaque • CNS Tuberculosis in HIV patients • Tubercular Hypophysitis • Tuberculosis of Calvarium and base of skull • Orbital Tuberculosis • Tubercular Otitis Media & temporal bone tuberculosis • Spinal Tuberculosis • Tubercular Spondylitis (Pott's spine) - C1/C2 - Thoracic spine - Thoraco-lumbar spine • Non-osseous spinal tuberculomas • Tubercular arachnoiditis(myeloradiculopathy) • Tubercular myelitis

Box 1. Variable presentation of CNS tuberculosis

5. Imaging features

5.1 Tuberculous meningitis

Tuberculous meningitis (TBM) is the most common presentation of CNS TB and is seen most frequently in children and adolescents. TBM develops when a meningeal, subpial or subependymal tuberculous focus (Rich focus) ruptures into the subarachnoid space or into the ventricular system. Important features of TBM are: [6]

1. Enhancing basal exudates
2. Progressive hydrocephalus
3. Vasculitis & Infarction, and
4. Cranial neuropathies

5.1.1 Basal exudates

In tuberculous meningitis, there is formation of thick, gelatinous exudate as a result of cell-mediated immunity. Initially the exudate is largely confined to basal subarachnoid areas, but rapidly extends to involve the basal cisterns, particularly the interpeduncular and the suprasellar cisterns. From these sites the exudate spreads to the ambient cistern, prepontine cistern, sylvian fissures, cerebral convexities, to the ependymal surfaces of the ventricles and over choroid plexus.[7,8] On noncontrast CT, the most common finding of cranial tuberculous meningitis is obliteration of basal cistern by isodense or slightly hyperdense exudates. Contrast enhanced CT demonstrates thickening and intense homogenous enhancement of the basal meninges, giving characteristic spider leg appearance [figure1]. MRI is more sensitive than CT in depicting these abnormalities. The basal exudates are best appreciated on FLAIR sequences, while the cisternal enhancement is better demonstrated on postgadolinium MRI images [Fgure2].[9] The brain parenchyma immediately beneath the exudate shows various degrees of edema. The meningeal enhancement can extend over the surface of the brain convexities, along tentorium and the sylvian fissures.[6,7] Isolated sylvian fissure involvement by tuberculous meningitis is also known.[10] Extension into the ventricular system may cause ependymitis (abnormal enhancement of ventricular linings), or choroid plexitis (enlarged, enhancing choroid plexus).[7,8]

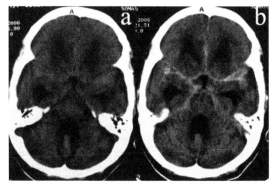

Fig. 1. Tuberculous meningitis. NCCT scan of the brain(a) shows effacement of basal cisterns by isodense exudates. CECT scan(b) shows dense enhancement of thickened and inflamed basal meninges along the basal cisterns (giving characteristic spider leg appearance), tentorium and the sylvian fissure with evidence of hydrocephalus and periventricular ooze.

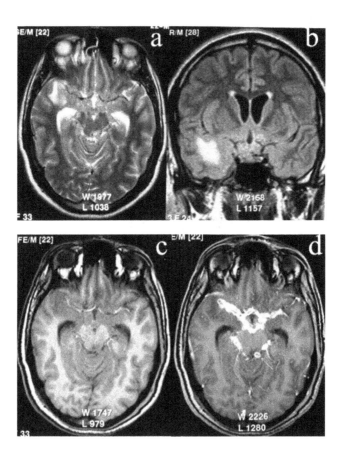

Fig. 2. Tuberculous meningitis. Axial T2W(a), and Fluid attenuated inversion recovery(b) MR images shows abnormal complex hyperintensity in the suprasellar, interpeduncular and perimesencephalic cisterns. Axial T1W(c) and corresponding post contrast image demonstrates diffuse enhancement of the basal cisterns. Few ring-enhancing tuberculomas (arrow) are also noted within the cistern.

5.1.2 Hydrocephalus

Hydrocephalus is the most common sequel of tuberculous meningitis. Communicating hydrocephalus [Figure1,2] is the most frequently observed form, usually caused by obstruction to CSF flow by thick gelatinous inflammatory exudates within the basal cisterns and over the brain convexities.[11,12] Less commonly, the hydrocephalus may be obstructive, due to obstruction of cerebral aqueduct or fourth ventricular foramen by focal parenchymal lesion with mass effect or due to entrapment of the ventricle by granulomatous ependymitis.[13,14] The presence of periventricular ooze suggests high pressure hydrocephalus. The incidence of hydrocephalus increases with the duration of disease and is associated with poor prognosis especially in children. The progress of hydrocephalus may be followed up by sequential CT or MRI scan.[15]

5.1.3 Vasculitis & infarction

In TB meningitis, the basal exudates are maximally localized to the circle of Willis, and produce a vasculitis like syndrome. The vasculitis is initiated by either direct invasion of vessel wall by mycobacteria or may result from secondary extension of adjacent arachnoiditis. Thus a consequent inflammatory change in the arteries and veins may lead to spasm or thrombosis of the vessels with resulting infarction.[6] The vessels at the base of the brain are most severely affected, including the terminal segment of common carotid artery and proximal segment anterior, middle and posterior cerebral arteries.[10,16,17] The middle cerebral and its branches are most often affected, especially the medial striate and thalamoperforating arteries supplying the basal ganglia and thalami.[14,16,17] Cortical infarctions resulting from the involvement of cortical vessels are less common. The infarcts are commonly bilateral, often hemorrhagic, and relatively more common in infants and children than in adults. Although both CT and MRI can demonstrate the infarction, MRI is more sensitive than CT for demonstration of these infarcts. Infarcts appear as low density regions on CT scan, while as areas of prolonged T1 and T2 relaxation on MR images. Diffusion weighted images (DWI) are gold standard for the diagnosis of acute infarction, which appears bright on DWI, and shows decrease signal on corresponding apparent diffusion coefficient(ADC) map[Figure3]. MR angiography is useful in follow-up of patients with vasculitis secondary to TB meningitis. The angiogram demonstrates a triad of narrowing of arteries at the base of the brain, narrowed or occluded small or medium sized arteries with early draining veins, and wide sweep of pericallosal arteries secondary to hydrocephalus [Figure4].[16,17]

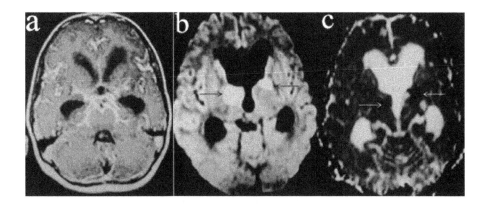

Fig. 3. Tuberculous meningitis with acute infarct. Post contrast axial MR image (a) shows enhancing basal exudates with associated hydrocephalus. Diffusion weighted image(b) and corresponding apparent diffusion coefficient(c) mapping reveals acute infarct in bilateral basal ganglia (due to vasculitis) showing high signal intensity on b1000 and low signal intensity on ADC map.

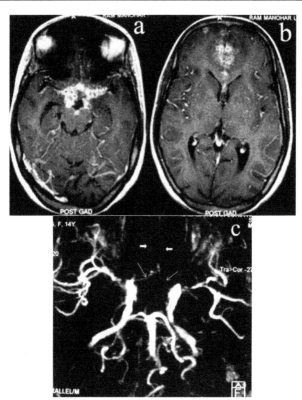

Fig. 4. Basal granulomatous meningitis with vascular changes. Axial T1W post contrast MR images of the brain at two different levels (a,b) shows basal meningitis with multiple conglomerate tuberculomas in suprasellar cistern and along anterior interhemispheric fissure. TOF MR angiogram(c) demonstrates severe narrowing of bilateral anterior cerebral arteries(thin arrows), and splaying of pericallosal arteries (thick arrows) by these conglomerate masses.

5.1.4 Cranial neuropathies

Cranial nerve palsies occurs in 20-40% of patients and may be the presenting feature of TB meningitis. Cranial nerve involvement is partly due to vascular compromise resulting in ischemia of the nerve or may be due to entrapment of the nerves by the exudates. Most commonly affected cranial nerves are II, III, IV, VI, VII. The affected cranial nerves are best evaluated by MRI. They appear thickened and hyperintense on T2-weighted sequences, and show marked enhancement on postgadolinium images. Constructive Interference at Steady State (CISS), which is a T2-weighted, 3D-Gradient echo sequence is particularly used for evaluating cranial nerves around the brain stem. Optochiasmatic arachnoiditis, compression of optic chiasma by third ventricular dilatation (in case of hydrocephalus) and optic nerve granuloma are common factors associated with vision loss in these patients. On MRI optochiasmatic arachnoiditis is characterized by perichiasmal enhancement (of basal exudates), hypertrophy and enhancement of chiasma and cisternal segment of both optic nerves. Associated dilatation of third and lateral ventricles is also evident.[7,8,19,20]

5.2 Pachymeningitis

Chronic tubercular infection of dura mater results in pachymeningitis, a rare manifestation, seen as focal or diffuse thickening and enhancement of the dura. Common sites include cavernous sinus, floor of middle cranial fossa, tentorium and the cerebral convexity. On noncontrast CT, the affected dura has plaque like appearance with or without calcification. On MRI, thickened dura appears hypointense to gray matter both on T1 and T2-weighted images. Post contrast study shows intense homogenous enhancement of thickened pachymeninges [Figure5]. Important differential diagnosis includes neurosarcoidosis, meningioma and lymphoma. [21]

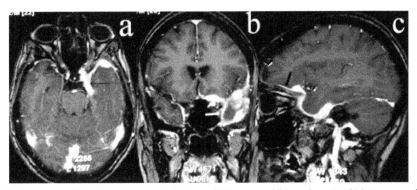

Fig. 5. Pachymeningitis. Post contrast T1W axial(a), coronal(b) and sagittal(c) images of brain show intensely enhancing, thickened pachymeninges(dura mater) encircling the left temporal lobe(thick white arrow), floor of ipsilateral anterior cranial fossa (thick black arrow) and the left cavernous sinus (thin black arrow). The process seems to be progressive with further extension to involve ipsilateral tentorium and cerebral convexity, where dura appears mild thickened.

5.3 Granulomatous basal meningitis

Granulomatous basal meningitis is another, relatively uncommon presentation of intracranial tuberculosis. It is characterised by diffuse or circumscribed granulomatous involvement of meninges at the skull base. It commonly causes compression of optic nerves and the optic chiasma producing visual disturbances. On CT scan, it is seen as an irregular lumpy enhancing mass, superimposed on dense basal enhancement. On MRI, the granulomatous basal mass is hypointense on T2-weighted images and shows intense but heterogeneous postgadolinium enhancement.[9,22]

5.4 Parenchymal tuberculosis
5.4.1 Parenchymal tuberculomas

Tuberculous granuloma (tuberculoma) is the most common form of parenchymal lesion.[6] Tuberculoma can occur at all age group; however, its incidence is higher in pediatric population.[11] These are usually located at corticomedullary junction and periventricular region, as expected for hematogenous dissemination. They are mostly infratentorial in children, and supratentorial in adults.[23,24] Common locations where tubercuomas can be found includes cerebrum, cerebellum, brainstem, basal ganglia, subarachnoid space, cisterns and fissures Rarely, they can be found within the ventricle (lateral ventricle being the most common site), cavernous sinus, sella turcica, hypophysis, hypothalamus, sphenoid sinus and mastoid air cells.[25,26] Parenchymal tuberculomas can be single or multiple, with or without coexisting meningitis.[27] Both the parenchymal and intraventricular tuberculoma may be associated with hydrocephalus.[28]

On CT, the noncaseating granulomas are solid, isodense or hyperdense in attenuation and show homogenous contrast enhancement, while the caseating granulomas enhance peripherally. Moderate to marked perilesional edema is frequently present. The 'target sign' seen on CECT is characterized by a central calcific nidus surrounded by rim of enhancement. This sign is highly suggestive of, but not pathognomonic of tuberculosis.[29,30] Solitary ring enhancing lesion on CT in patients presenting with seizures present a diagnostic dilemma since the granuloma of tuberculosis and cysticerus both may have similar morphological appearances. Some authors have tried to differentiate these two entities on basis of clinical signs and radiological (CT) findings. In patients with tuberculoma there is evidence of raised intracranial tension with progressive neurological deficit. The ring enhancing lesion is usually greater than 20mm in size, show irregular margin and cause midline shift. On contrary, neurocysticercus granuloma is less than 20mm in size, rounded disc like with no significant mass effect. Enlarging lesions on repeat CT after 8-12 weeks of anticonvulsant therapy could be due to different etiologies and should be biopsied.[31]

The MR features of individual tuberculoma will depend on whether the lesion is noncaseating, caseating with a solid center or caseating with a liquid center.[32,33] The Noncaseating granuloma is usually hypointense on T1-weighted images(T1WI), hyperintense on T2-weighted images(T2WI) and shows homogenous nodular enhancement on post gadolinium images. The caseating granuloma(s) with solid center [Figure6]. appears hypointense to isointense on T1WI (may have a slight hyperintense rim) and strikingly hypointense on T2W images. On contrast administration the lesion shows peripheral rim enhancement. The relative hypointensity on T2WI is attributed to high cellular density of central core of tuberculoma. The caseating granuloma with central liquefaction of caseous material appears hypointense on T1WI and hyperintense on T2WI with peripheral hypointense rim which represents the capsule of tuberculoma. The rim enhancement occurs after gadolinium administration. These lesions are indistinguishable from pyogenic abscess on imaging. At this stage, diffusion weighted images(DWI) may reveal diffusion restriction within the tuberculoma [Figure6].[34] A variable degree of vasogenic edema surrounds the lesion, and is relatively more prominent in the early stages of granuloma formation.

MR spectroscopy has been used to differentiate tuberculoma from pyogenic abscesses and neoplasms (both primary and secondary). On proton MRS [Figure6], these lesions show a large lipid peak at 0.9, 1.3, 2.0 and 2.8 ppm, highly specific for tuberculomas, more choline and less NAA and creatine. The choline/creatine ratio is greater than 1 in all tuberculomas. Caseous material typical of tuberculomas has high lipid content.[35] Pyogenic brain abscesses show lipid and lactate peak at 1.3 ppm and amino acid peak (e.g. valine, leucine and isoleucine) at 0.9 ppm.[36] The lesions such as metastases and high grade gliomas may show lipid peak in addition to significantly elevated Choline/NAA ratio.[35]

Magnetization transfer imaging (MTI) improves the detectability of these lesions with more number of tuberculomas detected on precontrast T1-weighted MT-SE images, compared to routine spin echo (SE) sequences and postcontrast T1-weighted MT-SE images.

Conventional SE invisible lesions (isointense on T1-and T2-weighted images) can be easily picked up on MT images because of lower transfer of magnetization in tuberculomas as compared to surrounding brain parenchyma. The presence of lipid within tuberculoma is probably responsible for lowering magnetization transfer. Detection of more lesions on precontrast T1-weighted MT-SE image as compared to postcontrast T1-weighted MT-SE image suggests lack of breach of the blood-brain barrier in some of the lesions. Thus the improved estimate of disease load on precontrast T1-weighted MT-SE images helps to better assess to response to specific therapy. The Quantitative MT (i.e. MT ratio) further helps to differentiate T2 hypointense tubercular granulomas from similar appearing lesions of neurocysticercosis. The MT ratio is significantly lower in tuberculomas as compared to cysticercus granulomas.[37]

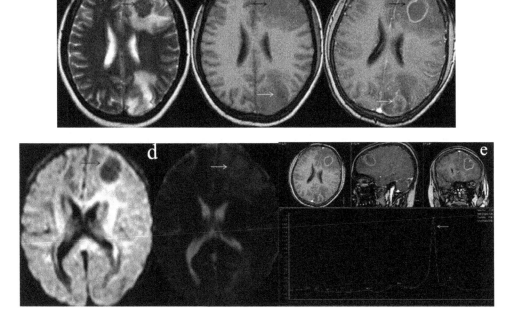

Fig. 6. Caseating tuberculoma. Axial T2W MR image(a) of brain shows profoundly hypointense lesion in left frontal lobe(black arrow) with marked perilesional oedema. The lesion demonstrates isointense core with slight hyperintense rim on T1W image(b), and thin peripheral ring enhancement on gadolinium-enhanced image(c). Multiple similar lesions were present involving both supra and infratentorial compartments, note similar lesion in left occipito-parietal region(white arrow). The solid portion of the lesion shows no diffusion restriction on DWI and corresponding ADC mapping(d). Single voxel MR spectroscopy(e) done at TE=30 shows large lipid peak at 1.33 ppm (arrow), with marked reduction in other metabolites. Large lipid peak corresponds to high lipid content within the caseous material.

Healed tuberculomas and the inflammatory exudates may calcify (in up to 23% cases) and these are more evident on CT [Figure7]. On MRI, the calcifications are better appreciated on gradient recalled echo (GRE- T2*WI) and Susceptibility weighted images (SWI).[30] Multiple conglomerate tuberculomas generally impose no difficulty in making a correct diagnosis; however, a solitary parenchymal tuberculoma needs to be differentiated from neurocysticercosis, pyogenic abcesses, primary or metastatic neoplasm.

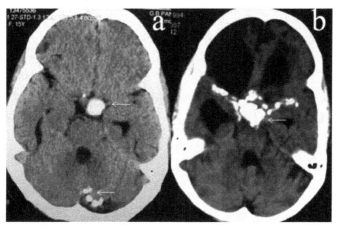

Fig. 7. Healed tuberculomas and basal exudates. Axial NCCT brain of two different patients demonstrate discrete calcified granulomas (arrow) in suprasellar cistern and left cerebellar hemisphere(a), and densely calcified basal exudates(arrow) in suprasellar region and along the M1 segment of bilateral middle cerebral arteries(b).

5.4.2 Tubercular abscesses

Tubercular abscess is a rare manifestation of CNS tuberculosis, occurring in less than 10% cases. They are found more frequently in elderly and immunocompromised patients. The patient is acutely ill with focal neurological deficit. TB abscesses have a more accelerated clinical course.[24]

On imaging, a TB abscess may be indistinguishable from a caseous tuberculoma with central liquefaction or a pyogenic abscess. However, a TB abscess is usually solitary and larger than tuberculoma. Perilesional edema and mass effect is more as compared to tuberculoma. On CT and MRI [Figure 8], it is often multinucleated and shows thin, smooth peripheral wall enhancement on post contrast images.[38] Proton MRS and MTI help to differentiate tuberculous from pyogenic brain abscesses. On MRS, a pyogenic abscess demonstrates amino acid peak at 0.9 ppm, which is characteristically absent in tubercular abscess. On MTI, MT ratio of a tubercular abscess is lower than that found in pyogenic abscess.[36] The role of DWI is conflicting in making correct diagnosis of tuberculoma as well as tubercular abscess. The reports in the literature vary regarding findings on diffusion weighted images with regard to both the tuberculoma and tubercular abscess. Some papers report slightly increased diffusivity in tuberculoma, and significantly higher in tubercular abscesses,[36] others report decreased diffusivity, [39] while still others report diffusion characteristic similar to the normal brain. [40]

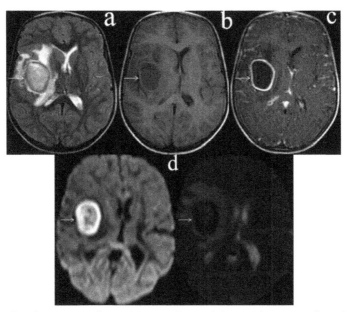

Fig. 8. Tubercular abscess. Axial T2W(a), T1W (b), and CEMR(c) images of another patient shows solitary ring enhancing lesions with liquified center, involving right basal ganglia region(arrow). There is associated marked perilesional edema with mass effect. The lesion demonstrates restriction on DWI and corresponding ADC mapping (d). MRS(not shown) revealed findings consistent with tubercular abscess.

5.4.3 Miliary tuberculomas

Miliary tuberculosis of the brain may be a part of generalized pathological process, with primary focus situated in the lung or elsewhere. The condition is subtle with no clinical evidence of brain involvement. On imaging, these lesions are small, less than 5mm in size;

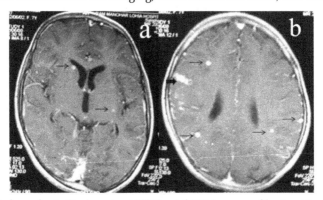

Fig. 9. Miliary tuberculosis. Post contrast T1W axial MR images of brain at two different levels reveal intense nodular enhancing small granulomas (thin arrow) randomly distributed throughout the brain parenchyma. Few larger lesions (thick arrow) were also seen along with these miliary nodules.

located at cortico-medullary junction and in the distribution of perforating vessels. They appear as high signal intensity foci throughout the brain parenchyma on T2WI and show intense nodular enhancement on post gadolinium images [Figure 9]. Contrast enhanced MRI is more sensitive than CECT for detecting these lesions.[41,42]

5.4.4 Focal tubercular cerebritis
This entity was described by Jinskin based on retrospective analysis of five patients. CT imaging shows intense focal gyral enhancement. On MRI, focal tuberculous cerebritis appears hypointense on T1, hyperintense on T2 and shows small areas of patchy contrast enhancement on post gadolinium images.[30]

5.4.5 Tubercular encephalopathy
Tubercular encephalopathy is a diffuse cerebral disorder characterized by convulsion, stupor and coma, without signs of meningeal irritation or focal neurological deficit. It is exclusively seen in infants and children receiving antitubercular treatment. Imaging shows unilateral or bilaterally symmetrical cerebral white matter edema, occasionally with perivascular demyelination or hemorrhagic leukoencephalopathy. A picture resembling post-infectious demyelinating encephalomyelitis may be observed. The pathological basis suggested for TB encephalopathy is an allergic delayed type IV hypersensitivity reaction due to cell mediated immunity to tubercular protein.[43,44]

5.5 Tuberculoma en plaque
An en plaque meningeal tuberculoma is a rare manifestation, seen as dural based, mass-forming localized meningeal process which morphologically resembles en plaque meningioma or meningeal metastases. They are commonly seen along the frontal and parietal convexities, tentorium, interhemispheric fissures and in the posterior fossa. On noncontrast CT, these lesions are hyperdense in appearance. On MRI, they appear isointense on T1WI, hypo to hyperintense on T2WI, and show homogenous or peripheral contrast enhancement, depending on the presence or absence of central caseation [Figure 10]. Prominent feeding meningeal vessels may also be evident.[45,46]

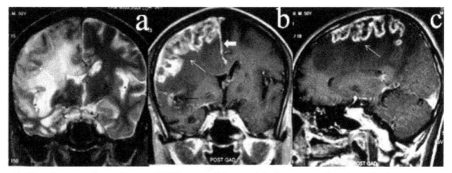

Fig. 10. En-plaque tuberculoma. T2W coronal image(a) shows predominantly hypointense dura based lesion widely spread along the right cerebral convexity, with associated marked vasogenic white matter edema and mass effect. Post contrast T1W coronal(b) and sagittal(c) image shows irregular peripheral rim enhancement of the lesion(thin white arrow). Also note, thickened enhancing dura along the falx (thick white arrow) and right cerebral convexity; and right sylvian fissure meningitis(thin black arrow).

5.6 CNS tuberculosis in AIDS

Although TB infection of CNS in AIDS patients follows a rapidly progressive course, the spectrums of imaging findings are similar to those of the non-immunocompromised patients. Meningitis, cerebral abscesses and tuberculomas are often observed in combination with one another [Figure11]. The differential diagnosis includes other opportunistic infections and primary or secondary CNS lymphoma.[47]

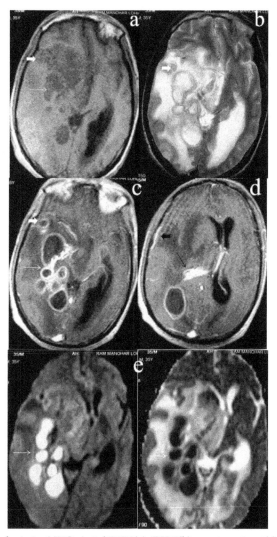

Fig. 11. CNS tuberculosis in AIDS. Axial T1W(a), T2W(b), post contrast(c) and diffusion weighted(d) MR images of brain demonstrate multiple cerebral abscesses (thin white arrows), tuberculomas(thick white arrow), choroid plexitis (thin black arrow) and dural thickening(thick black arrow). Note associated marked perilesional vasogenic edema with significant mass effect.

5.7 Tuberculous hypophysitis

Tubercular hypophysitis is an extremely rare entity that commonly presents with enlargement of pituitary gland, mimicking a pituitary adenoma. On MR imaging, the gland is diffusely enlarged with a thickened stalk, seen infrequently. The thickening and enhancement of stalk and surrounding dura differentiates these lesions from pituitary adenoma[Figure12]. However, these are non-specific findings and are also seen with tuberculous meningitis, sarcoidosis, syphilis and eosinophilic granuloma.[48]

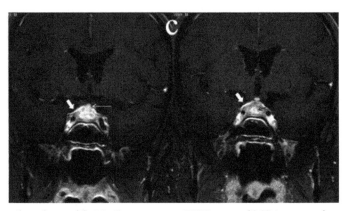

Fig. 12. Tuberculous hypophysitis. Post contrast T1W coronal MR images of a young adult male showing enlarged pituitary gland with intra-glandular ring enhancing tuberculoma (thin black arrow), and thick enhancing pituitary stalk(thin white arrow). Thickening and enhancement of diaphragma sellae (thick white arrow) is also noted. The patient had associated pulmonary tuberculosis and showed complete resolution of the pituitary lesion after a course of antitubercular therapy.

5.8 Tuberculosis of calvarium and base of skull

Isolated calvarial tuberculosis is a rare condition; and commonly occurs secondary to hematogenous spread from primary focus elsewhere. Frontal and parietal bones are most commonly involved followed by occipital and sphenoid bone. Calvarial tuberculosis may present as a subgaleal swelling (Pott's puffy tumor) with a discharging sinus when the outer table is involved. Inner table involvement which is relatively more common is associated with formation of underlying extradural granulation tissue. Both tables involvement is not uncommon. The bony lesions are usually osteolytic, and appear as a well defined punched out defect with central sequestrum. Rarely sclerosis may be seen. Cranial sutures do not prevent the spread of granulation tissue, and hence extensive destruction can occur before a sinus or swelling becomes apparent. Despite the dura mate, which is an effective barrier to the spread of infection, subdural empyema, meningitis, and parenchymal granulomas may be encountered. CT scan of the brain [Figure13] helps in assessing the extent of bone destruction, scalp swelling and extent of intracranial involvement.[49,50]

Tuberculous ostitis of skull base (spheno-clival) is very rare in occurrence. The usual clinical picture is of jugular foramina syndrome. The involvement of skull base may be either by contiguous spread of infection from the adjacent site, or via hematogenous route from primary focus elsewhere. On imaging [Figure14], there is destruction of the skull base with enhancing soft tissue mass that may cause compression of adjacent structures. Associated

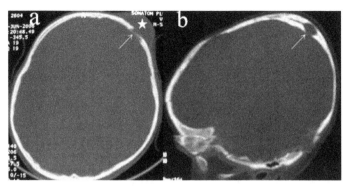

Fig. 13. Calvarial tuberculosis. NCCT head (bone window) of two different patients. First case(a) shows a large subgaleal soft tissue swelling (Pott's puffy tumor)(asterix) with destruction of both outer and inner table(arrow). Second case(b) shows a well defined lytic lesion involving right parietal bone with destruction of inner table but intact outer table(arrow). Both the cases showed no intracranial extension of the lesion.

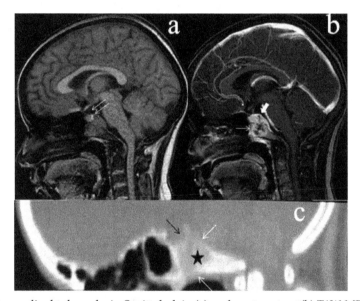

Fig. 14. Spheno-clival tuberculosis. Sagittal plain (a) and post contrast(b) T1W MR image of brain demonstrates an intraosseous soft tissue lesion in anterior part of body of clivus, showing heterogeneous contrast enhancement(thin white arrow). The dura along the superior aspect of the clivus shows thickening and enhancement(thick white arrow). Soft tissue along the inferior margin of the clivus also shows inflammatory changes. Note, the pituitary gland and the stalk(double white arrow) which appears normal in morphology and signal intensity. Sagittal NCCT skull(c) demonstrates destruction of anterior half of the body of clivus(asterix) and erosion of both antero-superior and antero-inferior cortical margin of the clivus(thin white arrow). The floor of sella tursica and the posterior clinoid process also shows rarefaction (thin black arrow).

meningitis may further complicate the disease producing multiple cranial neuropathies. The imaging characteristic mimics a malignant tumor (e.g. Cordoma), making the diagnosis of tuberculosis difficult, hence a high degree of clinical suspicion is mandatory.[51,52]

5.9 Orbital tuberculosis

Tuberculosis of orbit is rare, usually occurring in pediatric age group. Hematogenous spread from a primary tubercular focus or contiguous spread from paranasal sinuses may affect the orbit. The disease is usually unilateral and has slow progressive course. The imaging findings include involvement of bony orbital wall (producing cortical irregularity, destruction, thickening or sclerosis) and lacrimal gland, with extraconal inflammatory mass or frank abscess formation. The patient may present with isolated preseptal thickening. Infratemporal and intracranial extension is not uncommon [Figure15]. MRI is the imaging modality of choice in these cases. Post contrast, fat suppression techniques significantly

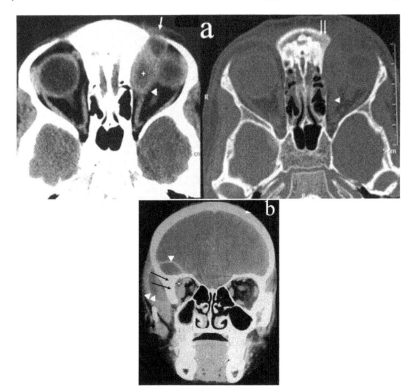

Fig. 15. Orbital tuberculosis. Axial CECT orbit(a) shows a medially situated extraconal orbital abscess(asterix) with extension into preseptal tissue and root of nasion(single thin arrow). Adjacent medial rectal muscle is displaced medially by the extraconal mass(arrow head). Irregularity and destruction of nasion(double thin arrows) is also present. Coronal CECT orbit (b) of another patient shows a laterally situated extraconal lacrimal gland abscess(asterix) which extends intracranially as epidural abscess(single arrow head) and into the infratemporal fossa (double arrow heads). Ipsilateral zygomatic bone appears thickened (double black arrows). (From IJRI 2010; 20:6-10.

improve the visualization of subtle masses. Non-tuberculous infection, vascular malformations and various neoplasms should always be considered in differential diagnosis of orbital masses.[53]

5.10 Tubercular otitis media and tuberculosis of temporal bone

Tubercular otitis media (TOM), a relatively uncommon condition, may be a part of widespread central nervous system disease or hematogenous spread from a primary tubercular focus elsewhere. The disease is more common in infants and children. It may be unilateral or bilateral. The patient usually presents with profuse painless otorrhea. High resolution CT is the modality of choice for imaging the temporal bone. Imaging shows middle ear soft tissue mass with destruction of bony walls. In addition, mucosal thickening of bony external auditory canal (EAC), extension of soft tissue mass into EAC and destruction of osscicles may also be documented. However, the scutum is always preserved in a case of TOM. T1-weighted post gadolinium MR images demonstrate the extent of inflammatory changes, evident as enhancing granulation tissues. Important complications include conductive deafness, facial palsy, cochlear involvement with labyrinthitis, sensory neural hearing loss and intracranial dissemination of infection. Mastoiditis and sinus formation may occur. Important differential includes other bacterial infections, cholesteatoma, fungal granulomas, wegener's granulomatosis, Langerhans cell histiocytosis.[54]

5.11 Spinal tuberculosis
5.11.1 Tuberculous Spondylitis (pott's spine)

Tuberculous Spondylitis is a leading cause of paraplegia. In developing countries, spinal tuberculosis affects younger age groups, including infants and children. In developed countries, it mostly affects the elderly. However, due to HIV epidemic, its incidence has increased among younger age groups. The disease has insidious onset and indolent course. The lower dorsal and lumbar spines are most commonly affected, followed by cervical spine. The atlanto-axial region involvement is relatively uncommon. The disease process results from hematogenous spread of infection to the vertebral body via paravertebral venous plexus of Batson. Infection usually begins in anterior part of vertebral body within the cancellous bone adjacent to the end plate or anteriorly under the periosteum of the vertebral body. Destruction of end plate allows the spread of infection to the adjacent intervertebral disc, and subsequently to the additional spinal segment. Subsequent spread of infection to other vertebral bodies may also occur via subligamentous route, with sparing of intervertebral disc [Figure16]. Thus the classic pattern of involvement of more than one vertebral body together with the intervening disc is seen in TB spine [Figure17]. Skip lesions are not uncommon. Occasionally, tuberculous spondylitis affects only one vertebral body, sparing the adjacent disc. The pedicle and posterior element involvement is rare. The spread of infection into the paraspinal tissues results in the formation of paravertebral soft tissue inflammatory mass (phlegmon) and/or frank abscess [Figure16,17]. Intraspinal extension is also frequent.[55,56,57,58] Neurological deficits are commonly associated with spinal tuberculosis of cervical region, particularly when cranio-vertebral junction or C1-C2 spine is involved [Figure18]. The neurological deficit is usually caused by significant thecal or cord compression by displaced bony fragment, epidural inflammatory mass and/or abscess. Death may occur due to atlanto-axial instability or cervico medullary compression.[59,60]

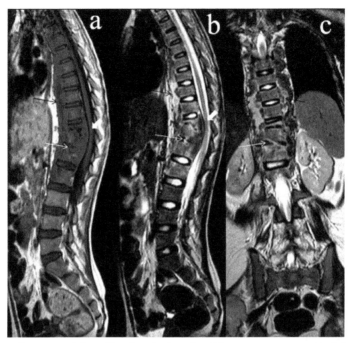

Fig. 16. Tuberculous spondylitis (Pott's spine) with subligamentous spread of the disease. Sagittal T1W(a), T2W(b), and Coronal T2W(c) image of dorso-lumbar spine demonstrates primary involvement of D12-L1 vertebral bodies and the intervening discs (thin white arrow) by the disease process with contiguous spread if the infection cranially (to involve all dorsal vertebrae) and caudally(to involve L2 vertebra) along the subligamentous route(thin black arrow) with sparing of intervening discs(except at D12-L1 level). Note, marrow signal intensity changes in all the involved vertebral bodies, and an epidural phlegmon at D12-L1 level causing localized cord compression (thick white arrow).

Conventional radiograph of spine demonstrates end plate irregularity, destruction of vertebral body and involvement of intervertebral disc. Reactive sclerosis is not a feature on initial presentation. CT scans [Figure19] characteristically demonstrate extensive bone destruction and large paraspinal abscesses. Large paravertebral abscesses and subligamentous spread of infection may produce anterior scalloping of the vertebral bodies. Calcification within the abscess is virtually diagnostic for tuberculosis. If left untreated, the infection eventually results in vertebral collapse and anterior wedging, leading to kyphosis and gibbus formation with healing, fusion of vertebral bodies (bony ankylosis) occurs in most cases. In patients with neurological deficit CT can define the extent of epidural compression, detection of bony fragment within the spinal canal and atlanto-axial instability.[61,62] MRI is the modality of choice for evaluating intraspinal and subligamentous spread of the infection, cervico medullary junction and nerve root compression, intervertebral disc changes and vertebral skip lesions. Contrast enhanced MRI is particularly useful for demonstrating intraosseous, epidural and paraspinal soft tissue involvement.[56,57,58]

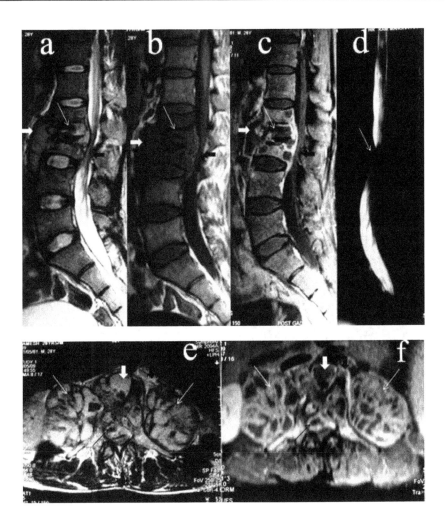

Fig. 17. Tuberculous spondylitis with involvement of intervening disc. Sagittal T2W(a), T1W(b) and post contrast(c) MR of lumbar spine demonstrates involvement of L2-L3 vertebral bodies and the intervening discs by the disease process, showing osseous destruction and heterogeneous contrast enhancement(thin white arrow). Associated heterogeneous enhancing prevertebral soft tissue(thick white arrow) and an epidural phlegmon/abscess(thick black arrow) is also present at the same level. The epidural phlegmon/abscess causes severe lumbar canal stenosis and compression of conus and cauda equina nerve roots, producing a CSF cut off sign on MR myelogram (d) (thin white arrow). Multiple intraosseous lesions (thick white arrow), subligamentous inflammatory mass(thick black arrow), bilateral psoas abscesses (thin white arrow) and epidural phlegmon causing cord compression (thin black arrow) are well appreciated on axial T2W(e) and T1W post contrast image(f).

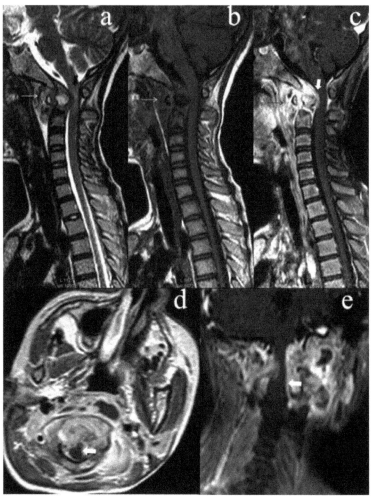

Fig. 18. Tuberculous spondylitis (C1-C2 vertebrae). Sagittal T2W(a), T1W(b) and post contrast(c) image of cervical spine shows enhancing inflammatory soft tissue mass (thin arrows) surrounding the anterior arch of C1 vertebra, tip of odontoid process (os odontoideum) and posterior part of the clivus, appearing isointense to the cord both on T1W and T2W image. Note subligamentous spread of infection along anterior aspect of C2-C3 vertebral body. There is associated atlanto-axial dislocation and cervicomedullary junction compression both by the posteriorly displaced odontoid tip and epidural-intraspinal phlegmonatous inflammatory tissue (thick white arrow), best appreciated on post contrast sagittal(c), axial(d) and coronal(e) images. The compressed cervical cord shows focal T2 hyperintense(thick black) signal suggestive of compressive myelopathy. Intraosseous marrow signal changes involving anterior arch of atlas, odontoid tip and posterior part of clivus is also present. There is severe narrowing of nasopharynx and the oropharynx by the prevertebral inflammatory mass.

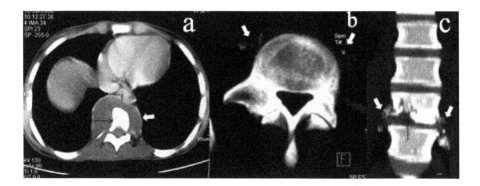

Fig. 19. Tuberculous spondylitis (Pott's spine). Axial (a,b) and coronal (c) noncontrast CT spine demonstrates marked osseous and intervertebral disc destruction(thin black arrow), and calcified/ non-calcified paravertebral abscesses(thick white arrows).

The major differential diagnosis is low grade pyogenic osteomyelitis (e.g. brucellosis), metastatic disease and fungal infections. Tuberculosis is characteristically associated with little or no reactive sclerosis, a feature that helps to distinguish it from pyogenic infections of spine.[58] Tuberculosis rarely affects the posterior vertebral elements, including pedicles, in contrast to metastatic disease.[62] Anterior scalloping of vertebral bodies can also be seen with paravertebral lymphadenopthy, metastatic or lymphomatous deposits.[58,62] CT guided needle biopsy is very useful in establishing the diagnosis in case of uncertainty.

5.11.2 Non-osseous spinal tuberculomas
Spinal tuberculoma are very rare presentation of non-osseous spinal tuberculosis, characterized as extradural (64%), intramedullary (8%), or intradural extramedullary (IDEM) (1%) according to their location.[63] Most of the subdural (IDEM) tuberculomas are detected as a result of paradoxical response to antitubercular therapy for meningitis, ranging from three months to one year.[64] Intramedullary tuberculomas are mostly induced by hematogenous dissemination from primary focus in the lung, or via CSF seeding, and rarely local spread of spinal tuberculosis.[65] MRI is imaging modality of choice for these lesions. IDEM tuberculoma may present as a single, dural based ring enhancing lesion or as a long segment enhancing soft tissue mass. En plaque IDEM tuberculoma may mimic meningioma. IDEM tuberculomas commonly cause spinal cord and nerve root compression; however, may or may not be associated with arachnoiditis [figure20].[64,66] Concurrent IDEM tuberculoma and syringomyelia has also been reported.[67] Intramedullary tuberculomas have specific findings on MRI, and hence can be diagnosed accurately on imaging. T2WI shows a typical "target sign" demonstrating low signal center (caseous material) surrounded by high signal rim (peripheral infective granulation tissue). This "target sign" is a valuable indicator and differentiates tuberculoma from other intramedullary lesions. Intravenous contrast administration shows sharp margin with peripheral rim enhancement. Associated syrinx and/or arachnoiditis may or may not be present with these lesions [Figure21].[65]

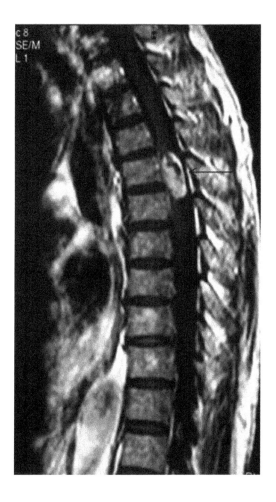

Fig. 20. Intradural extramedullary spinal tuberculoma. Contrast enhanced T1-weighted
Sagittal image demonstrates an intradural extramedullary (arrow) lesion in posterior
subarachnoid space, at mid-dorsal spine level, showing dense nodular enhancement with a
linear non-enhancing area. There is localized spinal cord compression and widening of
dorsal subarachnoid space. No associated syrinx or arachnoiditis is present.

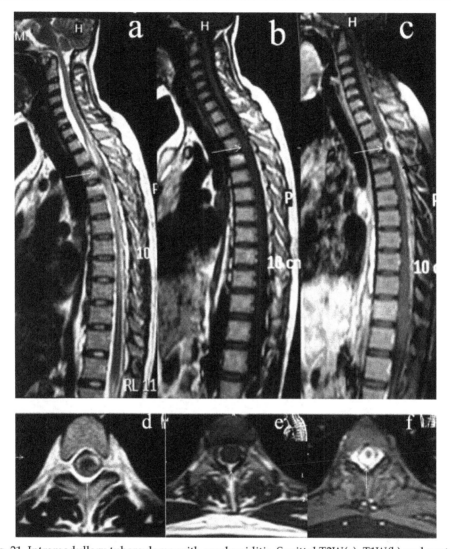

Fig. 21. Intramedullary tuberculoma with arachnoiditis. Sagittal T2W(a), T1W(b) and post contrast(c) image of thoracic spine shows an intramedullary space occupying lesion (thin white arrow) at D3 level with loss of normal cord-CSF interface posteriorly from D1-D11 level and few thin septations within posterior subarachnoid space, best appreciated on T2W image. The intramedullary SOL appears iso-hypointense on T1W image, shows typical "target sign" on T2W image and peripheral rim enhancement on contrast administration. There is obliteration and intense enhancement of posterior subarachnoid space from D1-D11 level with scattered thin CSF loculations consistent with arachnoiditis (thin black arrow). Note, a short segment syrinx situated cranial to the intramedullary lesion and T2 hyperintense signal within the cord caudal to this lesion. Intramedullary tuberculoma is well appreciated on axial T2W(d), T1W(e) and post contrast(f) images.

5.11.3 Spinal tubercular arachnoiditis (myeloradiculopathy)

Spinal tuberculous arachnoiditis is an inflammatory condition that involves the leptomeninges along the spinal tract and often manifests as myeloradiculopathy. Previously, it was known as adhesive spinal arachnoiditis or chronic adhesive arachnoiditis. Clinically patient presents with progressive spinal cord and/or nerve root dysfunction, usually accompanied by constitutional symptoms. This condition may result from downward extension of intracranial tuberculous meningitis (most common) or a tuberculous lesion primarily arising in the spinal meninges, or extension from tuberculous spondylitis. The thoracic region is most commonly affected followed by the lumber and cervical region. The involvement may be focal, multifocal or diffuse. The inflammatory exudate surrounds the spinal cord and the nerve roots, causing obliteration of spinal subarachnoid space (SAS). On imaging [figure22], there is increased CSF signal intensity within the SAS on T1WI due to elevated protein content of CSF with resultant loss of spinal cord outline in cervico-thoracic region. Thickening and clumping of nerve roots in the lumber region is frequently seen with arachnoiditis. Meningeal involvement has been described in patients with arachnoiditis; it represents ongoing meningeal inflammation and may constitute an early sign of arachnoiditis. Contrast enhanced MR images show linear enhancement of surface of spinal cord and nerve roots, or plaque like enhancement of dura-arachnoid mater complex which can obliterate the subarachnoid space.[68] Enhancing subarachnoid space nodular lesions may represents IDEM tuberculoma or vascularized fibrous tissue. In chronic adhesive

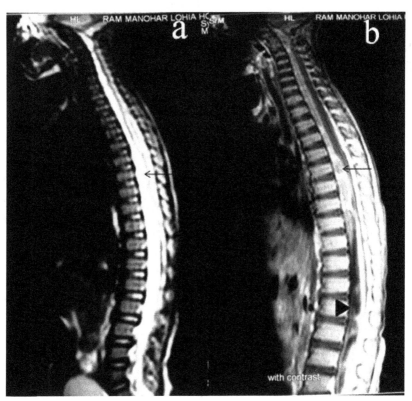

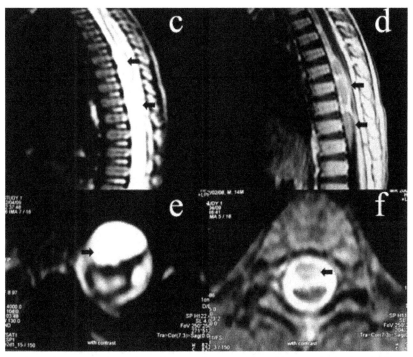

Fig. 22. Tuberculous spinal arachnoiditis with ascending infection to the brain. Sagittal T2W (a) and T1W post contrast(b) MR image of whole spine demonstrates loss of normal cord-CSF interface with obliteration of anterior subarachnoid space(SAS) by thick inflammatory exudates appearing hyperintense on T2W image, and showing intense enhancement on post contrast image (thin black arrow). Few scattered intervening septae are also present within the anterior SAS (at upper cervical and mid thoracic level) forming loculations. These loculations containing the inflammatory tissue have pseudomass appearance (on sagittal and axial T2W/post contrast image-c,d,e,f), which causes severe cord compression (thick black (arrow). Thickening and clumping of cauda equine nerve roots is evident in lumbar region (arrow head). The obliteration and intense enhancement of anterior subarachnoid space along the entire spinal canal, scattered pseudomasses in upper cervical (please see figure5b-sagittal post gad. image) and mid thoracic level, and clumping of cauda equine nerve roots in lumbar region is consistent with spinal arachnoiditis.

arachnoiditis, the spinal SAS is irregularly obstructed with formation of CSF loculations.[32] The CSF loculations usually show normal CSF signal intensity on T1-and T2WI and do not enhance on post contrast images. The recognition of CSF loculation is important as they may cause cord compression, necessitating surgical intervention. The spinal cord changes are frequently seen in these patients and may include myelitis, cord edema, syringomyelia, infarction, myelomalacia, cavitation or atrophy.[32]
Spinal tuberculous arachnoiditis must be distinguished from other possible causes of arachnoiditis, for example subarachnoid hemorrhage or iatrogenic cause.

5.11.4 Tubercular myelitis

Tuberculous myelitis, an important cause of paraparesis, and usually occurs as a secondary event in the course of common forms of tuberculous meningitis. The cervico-thoracic segment of the spinal cord is most commonly involved. MR Imaging features of TB myelitis are similar to those of cerebritis. There is diffuse cord swelling with signal abnormality. Most spinal cord lesions appear as hyperintense on T2, isointense to hypointense on T1-weighted images, and show segmental enhancement on post contrast images [Figure23].

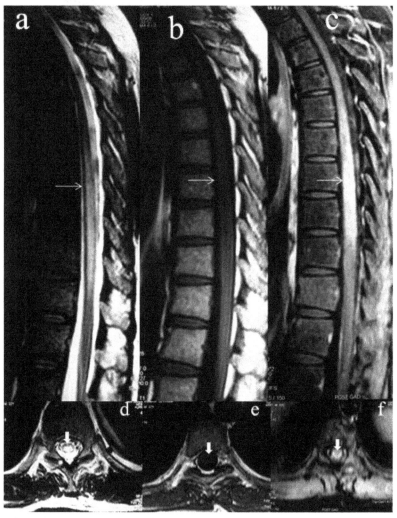

Fig. 23. Tuberculous Myelitis. Sagittal T2W(a), T1W(b) and post contrast(c) MRI of dorso-lumbar spine shows diffuse cord swelling and edema appearing hypointense on T1W and hyperintense on T2W image and showing intense central contrast enhancement on post gadolinium images(thin white arrow). These changes are better appreciated (thick white arrow) on axial T2W(d), T1W(e) and post contrast image(f).

Intramedullary abscess demonstrates central necrotic area with clearly defined marginal enhancement. Cord atrophy, cavitation and syringomyelia may be associated with poor outcome. Differential diagnosis includes cord contusion, cord infarction due to vasculitis, acute transverse myelitis, and demyelinating diseases.[69,70]

6. Differential diagnosis

The important differential diagnosis of CNS tuberculosis has been already discussed with individual manifestations. Broadly, the conditions which may mimic cranial and spinal tuberculosis on imaging include other infectious and non-infectious inflammatory disease such as fungal infection, sarcoidosis, primary and metastatic neoplastic disease.

7. Role of imaging in the evaluation of cns tuberculosis

Role of imaging has been dealt in detail with individual manifestation of CNS tuberculosis (vide supra). In nut shell contrast-enhanced MRI is superior to CT scanning or unenhanced MRI for the demonstration of CNS TB, and is currently the best modality for demonstration of meningeal disease, parenchymal abnormalities, for assessment of complication and monitoring the disease. The multiplanar capability of MRI offers additional advantage for localization of lesions. CT is particularly used for evaluation of osseous changes, calcification, and intracranial shunt in cases of hydrocephalus.

8. Management of cns tuberculosis

Inspite of rapid advances in the management of pulmonary tuberculosis, currently no general agreement about the form of chemotherapy or optimal duration of treatment has been reached. The World Health Organization[71] has put CNS tuberculosis under TB treatment category1, and recommended an initial phase therapy with streptomycin, isoniazid, rifampicin and pyrazinamide for 2-months, followed by a seven month continuation phase with isoniazid and rifampicin. The duration of therapy should be at least 6-months, and in some cases up to 12-months treatment is required. A similar drug regimen has been recommended for all forms of CNS tuberculosis. A four-drug regimen is needed to treat atypical mycobacteria (M avium intracellulare) in persons with HIV infection. Current recommended therapy for HIV patients include azithromycin and clarithromycin in combination with ethambutol or clofazimine.[72,73,74]

Role of corticosteroids in the treatment of CNS tuberculosis is controversial. It is believed that corticosteroids improve both the survival rate and neurological outcome in patients with TB meningitis. However they should be used with caution in pediatric population. The response to corticosteroids may be dramatic with rapid resolution of basal exudates and tuberculomas on serial imaging. The main argument against using corticosteroids is that they decrease meningeal inflammation, and in turn can affect CSF penetration of antituberculous drugs.[74,75]

Surgical procedures in patients with tuberculous meningitis are primarily directed to the treatment of hydrocephalus. Serial lumbar puncture along with diuretics is used as temporary measures to relieve raised intracranial pressure. Ventriculo-peritoneal or ventriculo-atrial shunts are permanent measures, which relieve the signs and symptoms of hydrocephalus and significantly improve the sensorium and neurological deficit. However, these shunts may require replacement due to blockage by high protein content of CSF. Early shunting in combination with drug therapy offers best therapeutic outcome.

Intracranial tuberculoma, which may behave as single space occupying lesion causing midline shift and increased intracranial pressure, and that fail to respond to chemotherapy should be removed surgically.[72,76] In chronic adhesive spinal arachnoiditis, the CSF loculations in SAS may cause cord compression, necessitating surgical intervention.[32]

9. Paradoxical response of tuberculomas to the treatment

Paradoxical enlargement of pre-existing tuberculoma or appearance of new intracranial and spinal tuberculoma in patients receiving effective antituberculous therapy has been noted in the past. This paradoxical phenomenon is thought to be due to result of an immunological reaction. These lesions are usually discovered accidently when follow-up scan is performed routinely or when new neurological signs develop during the course of antitubercular therapy. Concomitant steroid therapy probably has a preventive role against these focal lesions. However, with continuation of antituberculous therapy, eventual resolution of these tuberculoma usually occurs. In case of unresponsiveness to medical therapy, surgery is recommended.[77,78]

10. Prognosis

The single most important factor determining the prognosis in cases of CNS tuberculosis is the stage of tuberculous meningitis at which the treatment has been started. If treatment is started at stage I (prodromal phase with no definite neurological symptoms) the mortality and morbidity is very low, whereas in stage III (loss of sensorium, convulsions, focal neurological deficit, and involuntary movements) almost 50% patient die, and those who recover may have some form of neurological deficit. Stage II patients (signs of meningeal irritation, slight or no clouding of sensorium, minor cranial nerve palsies, and no neurological deficit) have intermediate prognosis.[74,79]

11. Summary

CNS tuberculosis is rare but serious complication and its early recognition and treatment is imperative. Early diagnosis can prevent further deterioration and result in better prognosis. Imaging plays a very important role in establishing the diagnosis of CNS tuberculosis. A radiologist should maintain a high degree of suspicion when patients with tuberculosis risk factors present with neurologic complains. Various imaging modalities, CSF studies, and brain biopsy if necessary, can aid in establishing the diagnosis of CNS tuberculosis. Pharmacological regimen is the mainstay of treatment, although various other options such as addition of corticosteroid and surgical intervention are also recommended as per requirement.

12. References

[1] Rich AR, Mccordock HA. Pathogenesis of tubercular meningitis. Bull John Hopkins Hosp 1933; 52:5-13.

[2] Leonard MK. Tuberculosis: forms of tuberculosis. 2002 Oct 1. Available at: www.medscape.com/viewarticle/534783?rssm Accessed May 25, 2006.

[3] Dastur DK. Neurotuberculosis. In: Minckler J, ed. Pathology of the nervous system, Vol. 3. New York: McGraw-Hill 1972;2412-2422.

[4] Nicolls DJ, King M, Holland D, Bala J, del Rio C. Intracranial tuberculomas developing while on therapy for pulmonary tuberculosis. Lancet Infect Dis. 2005; 5(12):795-801.

[5] Bayindir C, Mete O, Bilgic B. Retrospective study of 23 pathologically proven cases of central nervous system tuberculomas. Clin Neurol Neurosurg. 2006;108 (4):353-357.

[6] Wallace RC, Brutons EM, Beret FF, et al. Intracranial tuberculosis in children. CT appearance and clinical outcome. Pediatric Radiol. 1991;21:241-246.

[7] Barkovich AJ. Infections of the nervous system. In: Barkovich AJ (Ed). Pediatric Neuroimaging (4th edn). Lippincott Williams and Wilkins 2005;801-805.

[8] Synder RD, Bacterial infections of the nervous system. In: Berg BO, ed. Neurologic aspects of pediatrics. Boston: Butterworth-Heinemann, 1992;195-226.

[9] Shah, GV. Central nervous system tuberculosis. Neuroimaging Clin North Am 2000;10(2),355-374.

[10] Klingensmith WC, Datu J, Tuberculous meningitis of the sylvian fissure. Clin Nucl Med. 1978; 3:315-317.

[11] Jamieson DH. Imaging intracranial tuberculosis in childhood. Paediatr Radiol.1995;25:165-170.

[12] Kioumehr F, Dadsetan MR, Rooholamini SA, et al. Central nervos system tuberculosis: MRI. Neuroradiology. 1994;36:93-96.

[13] Rovira M, Romero F, Torrent O, et al. Intracranial tuberculoma. MR Imaging. Neuroradiology. 1989;31:299-302.

[14] Sheller JR, DesPrez RM. CNS tuberculosis. Neurol Clin 1986;4:143-158.

[15] Fischbein N, Dillon W, Barkovich A (Eds). Tuberculosis. In: Teaching atlas of brain imaging. Thieme 2000;165-168.

[16] Hsuh EY, Chi a LG, Shen We. Location of cerebral infarctions in tuberculous meningitis. Neuroradiol 1992;34:197.

[17] Reid H, Fallon RJ. Bacterial infections. In Adams JH Duchen L (Eds). Greenfields Neuropathology (5th edn). New York: Oxford University Press 1992;317-342.

[18] Gupta RK, Gupta S, Singh D, Sharma B, Kohli A, Gujral RB. MR imaging and angiography in tuberculous meningitis. Neuroradiol 1994;36:87-92.

[19] Garg RK, Tuberculosis of central nervous system. Postgrad Med J. 1999;75:133-140.

[20] Silverman IE, Liu GT, Bilaniuk LT, Volpe NJ, Galetta SL. Tuberculous meningitis with blindness and perichiasmal involvement on MRI. Pediatr Neurol. 1995;12(1):65-67.

[21] S. Prabhakar, R. Bhatia, V. Lal, Paramjeet Singh. Hypertrophic Pachymeningitis : Varied Manifestations of a Single Disease Entity. Neurol India. 2002;50: 45-52.

[22] Beşkonakli E, Çayli S, Turgut M, Yalçinlar Y. Primary giant granulomatous basal meningitis: An unusual presentation of tuberculosis. Child Nerv Syst 1998;14:79-81.

[23] Welchman JM. CT of intracranial tuberculomata. Clin Radiol 1979;30:567-579.

[24] Bhargava, Tandon PN. Intracranial tuberculomas: A CT study. Br J Radiol 1980;53:935-945.

[25] Altenbesak S, Baytok V, Alhan E, et al. Suprasellar tuberculoma causing endocrinological disorders and initiating craniopharyngioma. Paeditr Neurosurg 1995;23:328-331.

[26] Esposito V, Fraioli B, Ferrante L, et al. Intrasellar tuberculoma: Case report. Neurosurgery 1987;21:721-723.

[27] Sze G. Infections and inflammatory diseases. In:Stark DD, Bradley WG Jr. Magnetic resonance imaging. St. Louis, MO: CV Mosby, 1988:316-343.

[28] Desai K, Nadkarni T, Bhatjiwale M, Goel A. Intraventricular tuberculoma. Neurol Med Chir (Tokyo) 2002; 42:501-3.

[29] Van Dyk A. CT of intracranial tuberculosis with specific reference to the 'target sign.' Neuroradiology. 1988;30:329-336.

[30] Jinkins JR. Computed tomography of intracranial tuberculosis. Neuroradiology. 1991;33:126-135.

[31] Rajshekhar V, Haran RPO, Prakash GS, et al. Differentiating solitary small cysticercus granulomas and tuberculomas in patients with epilepsy. J Neurosurg 1993;78:402-407.

[32] Jinkins JR. Gupta R, Chang KH, Rodriguez-Carbajal J. MR imaging of central nervous system tuberculosis. Radiol clin North Am 1995;33(4):771-789.

[33] Gupta RK, Jena A, Sharma DK, et al. MR imaging of intracranial tuberculomas. J Comput Assist Tomogr. 1988;12:280-285.

[34] Gupta RK, Prakash M, Mishra AM, et al. Role of diffusion weighted imaging in differentiation of intracranial tuberculoma and tuberculous abscess from cysticercus granulomas - a report of more than 100 lesions. Eur J Radiol. 2005;55(3):384-392.

[35] Gupta RK, Poptani M, Kohli A, et al. In vivo localized proton magnetic resonance spectroscopy of intracranial tubercolomas. Ind J Med Res. 1995;101:19-24.

[36] Gupta RK, Vatsal DK, Husain N, Chawla S, Prasad KN, Roy R, Kumar R, Jha D, Husain M. Differentiation of tuberculous from pyogenic brain abscesses with in vivo proton MR spectroscopy and magnetization transfer MR imaging. Am J Neuroradiol 2001;22:1503-1509.

[37] Gupta RK, Kathuria MK, Pradhan S. Magnetization transfer MR imaging in central nervous system tuberculosis. Am J Neuroradiol 1990;20:867-875.

[38] Whitener DR. Tuberculous brain abscess. Report of a case and review of the literature. Arch Neurol 1978;35:148-155.

[39] Bulakbasi N, Kocaoglu M, Ors F, Ucoz T. Combination of single-voxel proton MR spectroscopy and apparent diffusion coefficient calculation in the evaluation of common brain tumors. AJNR Am J Neuroradiol 2003;24:225-233.

[40] Kaminogo M, Ishimaru H, Morikawa M, Suzuki Y, Shibata S. Proton MR spectroscopy and diffusion weighted MR imagingfor the diagnosis of intracranial tuberculomas. Report of two cases. Neurol Res 2002;24:537-543.

[41] Withman RR, Johnson RH, Roberts DL. Diagnosis of military tuberculosis by cerebral computed tomography. Arch Intern Med 1979;139:479-480.

[42] Gee GT, Bazan C III, Jinkins JR. Miliary tuberculosis involving the brain: MR findings. AJR 1992;159:1075-1076.

[43] Dastur DK, Manghani DK, Udani PM. Pathology and pathogenetic mechanisms in neurotuberculosis. Radiol Clin North Am 1995;33:733–52.

[44] Udani PM, Dastur DK. Tuberculous encephalopathy with and without meningitis: clinical features and pathological correlations. J Neurol Sci 1970;10:541–61.

[45] Ng SH, Tang LM, Lui TN, et al. Tuberculoma en plaque: CT. Neuroradiology 1996; 38:453-5.

[46] Dubey S, Devi BI, Jawalkar VK, Bhat DI. Tuberculoma en plaque: a case report. Neurol India 2002; 50:497-9.

[47] Villoria MF, Fortea F, Moreno S, Munoz L, Manero M, Benito C. MR imaging and CT of central nervous system tuberculosis in the patient with AIDS. Radiol Clin North Am. 1995 Jul:33(4):805-820.

[48] Bhaya A. Granulomatous hypophysitis - A rare entity mimicking pituitary adenoma. Indian J Radiol Imaging 1999;9:203-4.

[49] Diyora B, Kumar R, Modgi R, Sharma A. Calvarial tuberculosis: A report of eleven patients. Neurology India. 2009;57(5):607-612.

[50] Abhijit AR, Arpit MN, Datta M, Ashish JC, Ranjeet SN, Sudhir F and Veena LB. Imaging Features of Calvarial Tuberculosis: A Study of 42 Cases. American Journal of Neuroradiology 25:409-414, March 2004.

[51] Shenoy SN, Raja A. Tuberculous granuloma of the spheno-clival region. Neurology India. 2004; 52(1):129-130.

[52] Indira DB, Tyagi AK, Bhat DI, Santosh V. Tuberculous osteitis of clivus. Neurol India 2003;51:69-70.

[53] Narula MK, Chaudhary V, Baruah D, Kathuria M, Anand R. Pictorial essay: Orbital tuberculosis. Indian J Radiol Imaging. 2010;20:6-10.

[54] M.H. Rho, D.W. Kim, S.S. Kim, Y.S. Sung, J.S. Kwon, S.W. Lee. Tuberculous Otomastoiditis on High-Resolution Temporal Bone CT: Comparison with Nontuberculous Otomastoiditis with and without Cholesteatoma. AJNR Am J Neuroradiol.2007;28:493–496.

[55] McGuinness F. Tuberculous spondylitis. In McGuinness F (ed). Clinical imaging of non-pulmonary tuberculosis. Springer, Berline Heidelberg New York, pp 43-80.

[56] Sharif HS. Role of MR imaging in the management of spinal infections. AJR Am J Roentgenol.1992;158:1333-1345.

[57] Sharif HS, Morgan JL, Al-Shahed MS, et al: Role of CT and MR imaging in the management of tuberculous spondylitis. Radiol Clin North Am. 1995;33:787-804.

[58] Smith AS, Weinstein MA, Mizushima A et al: MR imaging of characteristics of tuberculous spondylitis vs vertebral osteomyelitis. AJNR. 1989;10:619-625.

[59] Akhaddar A, Gourinda H, Gazzaz M, Elmadhi T, Elalami Z, Miri A. Craniocervical junction tuberculosis in children. Rev Rhum Engl Ed. 1999;66(12):739-742.

[60] Allali F, Benomar A, EL Yahyaoui M, Chkili T, Hajjaj-Hassouni N . Atlantoaxial tuberculosis: three cases. Joint bone spine.2000;67(5):481-484.

[61] Zamiati W, Jiddane M, El Hassani MR, Chakir N, Boukkrissi N. Contribution of spiral CT scan and MRI in spinal tuberculosis (Spanish). J of Neuroradiology. J de Neuroradiologe. 1999;26:27-34.

[62] Resnick D. Tuberculous infection. In: Resnick D, ed. Diagnosis of bone and joint disorders. 3rd ed. London, United Kingdom: Saunders, 2002; 2524–2545.

[63] Dastur HM. Diagnosis and neurosusgical treatment of tuberculosis disease of the CNS. Neurosurg Rev 1983; 6: 111-17.

[64] Roca B. Intradural extramedullary tuberculoma of the spinal cord: a review of reported cases. J Infect. 2005;50(5):425-31.

[65] Ming Lu. Imaging Diagnosis of Spinal Intramedullary Tuberculoma:Case Reports and Literature Review. J Spinal Cord Med. 2010;33(2):159–162.

[66] Shim DM, Kyum S, Kim TK, Chae SU. Intradural Extramedullary Tuberculoma Mimicking En Plaque Meningioma Clinics in Orthopedic Surgery 2010; 2:260-263.

[67] Sanser G, Guven C, Murat K, Bektas A. Syringomyelia and Intradural Extramedullary Tuberculoma of the Spinal Cord as a Late Complication of Tuberculous Meningitis. Turkish Neurosurgery 2010; 20: 561-565.

[68] SharmaA, Goyal M, Mishra NK, Gupta V, Gaikwad SB. MR imaging of tubercular spinal arachnoiditis. AJR Am J Roentgenol1997;168(3):807–812.

[69] Mohammad W, Hiba A , Bhojo K, Humera A. Neuroimaging of Tuberculous Myelitis: Analysis of Ten Cases and Review of Literature. Journal of Neuroimaging. 2006;16(3):197-205.

[70] Trivedi R, Saksena S, Gupta RK. Magnetic resonance imaging in central nervous system tuberculosis. Indian J Radiol Imaging. 2009 November; 19(4): 256–265.

[71] Harries A, Maher D. TB: a clinical manual for South East Asia. Geneva:World Health Organisation, 1997.

[72] Berger JR. Tuberculous meningitis. Curr Opin Neurol 1994;7:191–200.

[73] Small PM. Schecter GF, Goodman PC, Sande MA, Chaisson RE, Hopewell PC. Treatment of tuberculosis in patients with advanced human immunodeficiency virus infection. N Engl J Med 1991;324:289–94.

[74] Holdiness MR. Management of tuberculous meninglitis. Drugs 1990;39:224–33.

[75] Schoeman JF, Vanzyl LF, Laubscher JA, Donald PR. Effect of cortico- steroids on intracranial pressure, computed tomographic findings, and clinical outcome in young children with tuberculous meningitis. Pediatrics 1997;99:226–31.

[76] Leonard JM, Des Prez RM. Tuberculous meningitis. Infect Dis Clin North Am 1990;4:769–87.

[77] Afghani B, Lieberman JM: Paradoxical enlargement or development of intracranial tuberculomas during therapy : case report and review. Clin Infect Dis 1994;19:1092–1099.

[78] Nomura S, Akimura T, Kitahara T, Nagomi K, Suzuki M: Surgery for expansion of spinal tuberculoma during antituberculous chemotherapy: a case report. Pediatr Neurosurg 2001;35:153–157.

[79] Medical Research Council. Streptomycin in tuberculosis trials committee. Streptomycin treatment of tuberculous meningitis. Lancet 1948;i:582–96.

6

Imaging of Metabotropic Glutamate Receptors (mGluRs)

Zhaoda Zhang and Anna-Liisa Brownell
Athinoula A. Martinos Biomedical Imaging Center
Massachusetts General Hospital
Harvard Medical School, Charlestown,
Massachusetts
USA

1. Introduction

The ubiquitous amino acid L-glutamate is thought to act as a neurotransmitter at the majority of synapses in the brain. It mediates the major excitatory pathways in the brain, and is referred to as an excitatory amino acid (EAA). The EAA plays a role in a variety of physiological processes, such as long-term potentiation (learning and memory), the development of synaptic plasticity, motor control, respiration, cardiovascular regulation, emotional states and sensory perception (Bliss & Collingridge, 1993).

The excessive or inappropriate stimulation of EAA receptors leads to neural cell damage or loss by a mechanism known as excitotoxicity (Lucas & Newhouse, 1957; Oney, 1978). EAA receptors are classified in two general types (Kornhuber & Weller, 1997). Receptors that are directly coupled to the opening of cation channels in the cell membranes of the neuron are termed 'ionotropic', which include NMDA, AMPA, and kainate receptors. The second type of receptors are the G-protein or second messenger-linked 'metabotropic' EAA receptors. This second type is coupled to multiple second messenger systems that lead to enhanced phosphoinositide hydrolysis, activation of phospholipase D, increase or decrease in cAMP formation, and changes in ion channel function (Kozikowski et al., 1998).

Metabotropic glutamate receptors belong to Class C of a superfamily of G-protein coupled receptors (GPCRs). Class C GPCRs possess a large extracellular domain that is responsible for endogenous ligand recognition (Pin et al., 2003), in addition to the seven strand transmembrane domain, which is characteristic of all GPCRs. The mGluRs possess a large bi-lobed extracellular N-terminus of ~560 amino acids which has been shown by mutagenesis studies to confer glutamate binding, agonist activation of the receptor, and subtype specificity for group selective agonists (Schoepp et al., 1999).

Since mGluRs have neuromodulatory role in the control of both glutamatergic and GABAergic neurotransmission, there has been much interest to develop novel mGluR ligands for therapeutic purposes of a variety of neurological and psychiatric conditions. The mGluRs have been proposed to be involved in physiological and pathophysiological processes of a number of CNS disorders, including anxiety, pain, depression, neurodegenerative disorders, schizophrenia, epilepsy, and drug abuse. In order to characterize the role of mGluRs in different physiological processes there is a need to identify novel compounds, which are highly potent and specific for an mGluR group or a subtype. Such compounds are needed to further investigate mGluR function, and as potential therapeutic agents for a variety of neurological diseases, which are associated with the abnormal activation of mGluRs. A large amount of pharmacological agents acting at metabotropic glutamate receptors have been described in the literature (Guitart & Khurdayan, 2005; Kew, 2004; Layton, 2005; Marino et al., 2005; Rudd & McCauley, 2005; Schoepp et al., 1999; Slassi et al., 2005; Williams & Lindsley, 2005; Yang, 2005). According to the mode of binding, these mGluR pharmacological agents can be classified into competitive and non-competitive agents. Based on the mode of action, they can be classified into agonists, antagonists, and positive/negative/neutral modulators (Layton, 2005). Competitive agonists and antagonists bind to the same orthosteric binding site as endogenous glutamate (Niswender et al., 2005; Ritzen et al., 2005; Rudd & McCauley, 2005), which is a cleft between the two lobes in the extracellular N-terminus. Their binding ability depends on how much they can stabilize the closed conformation (Kew, 2004). These ligands received earliest research interest and have been well developed (Schoepp et al., 1999). They are all glutamate analogs or substituted glycines, which imply that they have poor selectivity within their group. In addition, competitive agonists and antagonists have structural carboxyl and amino groups, which make them too polar to penetrate the blood brain barrier (BBB) (Kew, 2004).

Starting from 1996 (Annoura et al., 1996), a number of different types of non-competitive negative, positive and neutral allosteric modulators have been developed as mGluR ligands (Niswender et al., 2005; Ritzen et al., 2005). These ligands modulate mGlu receptor activity by binding to allosteric binding sites that are located in the seven strand transmembrane domain. The allosteric binding sites are structurally distinct from the classical agonist orthosteric binding site (Williams & Lindsley, 2005). Positive and negative modulators thus offer a potential for improved selectivity for individual mGluR family members compared to competitive agonists and antagonists at the glutamate site (Kew, 2004). Positive allosteric modulators (PAM)s have little or no effect on the receptor but can significantly enhance the effect of endogenous ligand. Correspondingly negative allosteric modulators inhibit the activity of orthosteric agonists in a noncompetitive manner. These ligands are structurally diverse and not amino acid derivatives. They are lipophilic and have much better CNS penetrating ability. Thus, positive and negative modulators with high subtype selectivity, and appropriate lipophilicity are good candidates for mGluR radiotracer development. There will be no competitive binding of this kind of tracers with endogenous glutamate, which might otherwise decrease the availability in vivo, and thus decrease the sensitivity of potential ligands.

During the last fifteen years the subtype selective modulators have been identified for mGluR1, mGluR2, mGluR3, mGluR4, mGluR5, mGluR7 and mGluR8. Based on these modulators, several positron emission tomography radiotracers have been developed for in vivo imaging of specific mGluRs. Presently, three mGluR ligands have been used for human studies. They have been developed as negative allosteric modulators for mGluR5. In this review we intend to summarize the radiotracers which have characteristics to be developed as tracers for in vivo PET imaging to investigate modulation of mGluRs in normal and pathological conditions. Emphasis will also be given to the highly potent and subtype selective allosteric modulators which are candidates for radiolabeling with ^{18}F or [11]C.

2. Metabotropic glutamate receptors and their physiological function

Recent molecular cloning studies have revealed the existence of eight different subtypes of mGluRs. The mGluR subtypes can be divided into three different groups according to their sequence similarities, signal transduction mechanism, and pharmacological profiles to agonists (Pin & Duvoisin, 1995). The first group comprising mGluR1 and mGluR5 is coupled to stimulating of phosphoinositide hydrolysis/Ca2+ signal transduction (Schoepp et al., 1994). The second group, consisting of mGluR2 and mGluR3, is negatively coupled through adenylate cyclase to cAMP formation (Tanabe et al., 1997). The third group, containing mGluR4, mGluR6, mGluR7 and mGluR8, is also negatively linked to adenylate cyclase activity but shows a different agonist preference (Conn & Pin, 1997; Tanabe et al., 1997).

The neuroanatomical localization of Group I and Group II mGluRs in the rodent brain, as assessed by immunohistochemical or *in situ* hybridization techniques, has revealed overlapping, yet distinct patterns of expression of these receptors. In order to better characterize the roles of mGluRs in physiological processes, there is a need to identify novel compounds that are highly potent and specific for an mGluR group or a subtype. Such compounds are needed as pharmacological tools for further investigation of mGluR function, and as potential therapeutic agents for the treatment of diseases or conditions including epilepsy, cerebral ischemia, pain, spinal cord injury, 'neurotoxicity' and chronic neurodegenerative diseases (e.g. Parkinson's and Huntington's disease), which are associated with abnormal activation of mGluRs (Aguirre et al., 2001; Blakely, 2001; Calabresi et al., 1999; Keyvani et al., 2001; Marino et al., 2001; O'Neill, 2001; Popoli et al., 2001; Rao et al., 2000; Rouse et al., 2000).

It is known that glutamate can act as a neurotoxin when energy supplies are compromised. This has stimulated a hypothesis that injury to neurons in some neurological conditions may be caused, partly, by over stimulation of glutamate receptors and/or glutamate transporters. These neurological conditions may be acute insult like stroke or chronic neurodegenerative states like Parkinson's or Huntington's disease or dementia. To better explore the roles of mGluRs in physiological and pathological processes, there is a need to learn more about functional behavior of these receptors *in vivo*.

3. PET radiotracer development

Positron emission tomography (PET) has become an important clinical diagnostic and research modality, and also a valuable technology in drug discovery and development (Cai et al., 2008). PET tracers have been used for the imaging and quantification of biochemical processes. PET tracers play a critical role for assessing *in vivo* distribution of specific receptors in normal and disease conditions to understand underlying mechanisms of physiology and pathology. Moreover, PET tracers serve as invaluable biomarkers during the clinical development of potential therapeutic mGluR modulators, in which the receptor occupancy of potential drug candidates in the brain is measured (Passchier et al., 2002; Sharma & Lindsley, 2007). *In vivo* receptor occupancy can help to answer many vital questions in the drug discovery and development process such as whether potential drugs reach their molecular targets, the relationship between therapeutic dose and receptor occupancy, the correlation between receptor occupancy and plasma drug levels, and the duration of time a drug remains at its target (Passchier et al., 2002). In PET imaging a small amount of tracer is injected into a living object. The tracer is labeled with a short-lived radioisotope, which emits positrons as it decays. The positrons collide with electrons resulting in high-energy photons that escape from the object and are detected by the PET scanner. Carbon-11 ($t_{1/2}$ = 20.4 min) and fluorine-18 ($t_{1/2}$ = 109.7 min) are the most commonly used radionuclides in PET imaging (Miller et al., 2008). The characteristics of successful PET tracers include high affinity, high selectivity over other mGluR subtypes as well as other receptors, suitable pharmacological properties including lipophilicity, metabolic stability, no radiolabeled metabolites that can penetrate into the brain, and the chemical structure of the precursor to allow fast labeling.

3.1 Allosteric modulators and radiotracers for Group I mGluRs
The group I receptors mGluR1 and mGluR5 exhibit different patterns of expression in the CNS. The distribution of mGluR1 is found throughout the human brain with high levels in the olfactory bulb, thalamus, hippocampus, lateral septum, superior colliculus and cerebellum (Olive, 2009). Inhibition of mGluR1 has been suggested as potential treatment for various psychiatric disorders including schizophrenia, anxiety, and neuropathic pain.
The mGluR5 is usually found in postsynaptic neurons with moderate to high density in the frontal cortex, caudate, putamen, nucleus accumbens, olfactory tubercle, and hippocampus, whereas in contrast to expression patterns of mGluR1, the density in the cerebellum is low (Olive, 2009). Dysfunction of mGluR5 is implicated in a variety of diseases in the CNS, including anxiety, depression, schizophrenia, Parkinson's disease, and drug addiction or withdrawal.

3.1.1 Allosteric modulators and radiotracers for mGluR1
A variety of mGluR1 modulators have been reported in the literature. Competitive mGluR1 agonists and antagonists historically have been amino acid derivatives, which display poor potency, lack of selectivity and unsatisfactory BBB penetration (Layton, 2005). Although a number of selective competitive mGluR1 ligands appear in literature, they are not good candidates for potential PET tracers. None of the existing orthosteric ligands has a binding affinity (or potency) of $IC_{50}/K_i/K_d$ less than 20 nM with an acceptable selectivity over other members in the same group. There is a consensus that identification of highly potent and subtype selective competitive mGluR ligands has been difficult due to a high degree of sequence similarity at the orthosteric binding site to which the endogenous agonist binds (Layton, 2005; Williams & Lindsley, 2005). Alternatively, several structural types of mGluR1 allosteric modulators have been reported in literature, including negative and positive allosteric modulators which show high binding affinity, high selectivity and good lipophilicity (Layton, 2005).
CPCCOEt (1) was the first reported mGluR1 negative allosteric modulator (Fig.1). Before 2008, only compound 4 (3,5-dimethyl PPP) (Micheli et al., 2003b) and a quinoline derivative 5 (JNJ16259685) (Lavreysen et al., 2004b; Mabire et al., 2005) had reported binding affinity (or potency) less than 20 nM (Table 1). 2,4-Dicarboxy-pyrrole ester 4 (3,5-dimethyl PPP), as a racemic mixture, is a highly potent and subtype-selective noncompetitive antagonist of mGluR1, having IC_{50} of 16 nM at rat mGluR1 and > 1000-fold selectivity over mGluR 2, 4, and 5 (Micheli et al., 2003b). Pharmacological studies of its two enantiomers showed that the S-enantiomer had the same activity as the racemic mixture, while the R-enantiomer was less potent (40 nM). Although compound 4 had a poor stability to rat plasma esterase ($t_{1/2}$=12 min versus 2.8 h in mice), a good CNS accumulation was observed 5 min after intravenous administration with a brain/plasma ratio of 20 (Micheli et al., 2003b). Compound 5 (JNJ-

16259685) demonstrated high specificity over other mGlu receptor subtypes and a fast brain penetration with high receptor occupancy after subcutaneous administration (Lavreysen et al., 2004b). In addition to **5**, a series of quinoline derivatives have been synthesized. The *in vitro* pharmacological data showed that they are highly potent noncompetitive mGluR1 antagonists (Mabire et al., 2005) with high binding affinity. However, the quinoline derivatives have issues of poor aqueous solubility and poor stability to human liver microsomes (Layton, 2005; Mabire et al., 2005).

Since 2008, many new compounds (Fig. 1 and Table 1) have been reported having binding affinity (or potency) less than 20 nM and high selectivity over other mGluRs. These compounds are diverse heterocyclic compounds including mono-, di- and tri-cyclic structures. Some of these compounds or their derivatives are amenable to radiolabeling with fluorine-18 or carbon-11. For example, a series of potent 2-fluoro-3-pyridyl-triazol derivatives such as FTIDC (**10**) and FPTQ (**11**) have been developed.. These derivatives are relatively easy to label with fluorine-18 at 2-pyridine position. Other compounds such as **12** are amenable to radiolabeling with carbon-11.

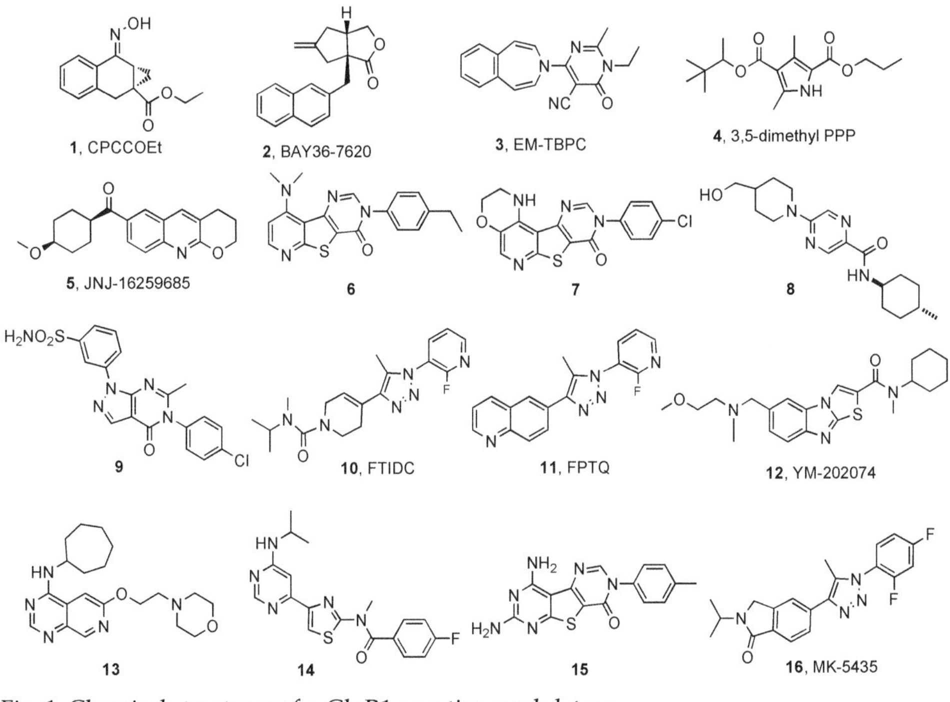

Fig. 1. Chemical structures of mGluR1 negative modulators.

MGluR1 expression is localized throughout the nervous system (Layton, 2005; Spooren et al., 2003). The distribution of mGluR1 in the peripheral nervous system (Bhave et al., 2001; Lesage, 2004; Skerry & Genever, 2001) and in the CNS has been studied using various methods including radioligand autoradiography and immunohistochemical techniques (Lavreysen et al., 2003; Lavreysen et al., 2004a; Shigemoto & Mizuno., 2000; Simonyi et al., 2005). MGlu1 receptors have been observed in the cerebellum, thalamus, hippocampus and

Compound	Rat mGluR1 IC_{50} (nM)	Human mGluR1 IC_{50} (nM)	Selectivity	*In vivo* properties	References
1 (CPCCOEt)		1500-6500	>15 over mGluR2, 4, 5, 7, 8		(Litschig et al., 1999; Ott et al., 2000)
2 (Bay36-7620)	160		>100 over mGluR 2, 3, 4, 5, 7, 8	30% receptor occupancy in cerebellum and thalamus (s.i.)	(Carroll et al., 2001)
3 (EM-TBPC)	130		No binding for rat mGluR5		(Malherbe et al., 2003)
4 (3,5-dimethyl PPP)	16		>1000 over mGluR2, 4, 5	Good CNS exposure with brain/plasma ratio of 20	(Micheli et al., 2003a; Micheli et al., 2003b)
5 (JNJ-16259685)	3	0.55	>400 over rat mGluR5; >20,000 over human mGluR5	Fast brain penetration and high receptor occupancy (s.i.)	(Lavreysen et al., 2004b; Mabire et al., 2005)
6	K_i=5	3	IC_{50}=442 nM for human mGluR5; K_i=194 nM for rat mGluR5	Demonstrated efficacy in various *in vivo* animal models	(Zheng et al., 2005)
7	K_i=0.4	2.9	>1,000 nM for human mGluR5	Demonstrated activity in the rat spinal nerve ligation neuropathic pain model (SNL model) with ED_{50} of 5.1 mg/kg.	(Wu et al., 2007)
8	K_i=9			LogD=3.3; human liver microsomal metabolic stability: Cl_{int}<7 µl/min/mg	(Owen et al., 2007)
9		127	>100,000 nM for human mGluR5	Solubility: 42 µM; microsomal clearance: <2.5 L/h/kg; quantitative bioavailability	(Wang et al., 2007b)

Compound	Rat mGluR1 IC_{50} (nM)	Human mGluR1 IC_{50} (nM)	Selectivity	*In vivo* properties	References
10 (FTIDC)	5.8	5.8	6200 nM for human mGluR5; >1720 over mGluR2, 4, 6, 7, 8	LogD=2.1; demonstrated efficacy in (S)-3,5-DHPG-induced face-washing behavior in mice	(Suzuki et al., 2009; Suzuki et al., 2007a)
11 (FPTQ)	14	3.6			(Suzuki et al., 2009)
12 (YM-202074)	8.6 K_i=4.8		>1000 for rat mGluR2, 3, 4, 6, 7; >100 for rat mGluR5;	Showed efficacy for neuroprotection in rats suffering from transient focal cerebral ischemia;	(Kohara et al., 2008)
13	K_i=6			CSF:C_u=0.5; HLM: Cl_{int}=24 µl/min/mg	(Mantell et al., 2009)
14		5.1	7000 nM for human mGluR5; >10,000 nM for human mGluR2, 8	Mouse brain/plasma concn 0.17 nmol/g/0.19 µM; Rat F: 53%, $T_{1/2}$: 2.3 h, CLp: 28 mL/min/kg; Rat PPI disruption model MED 1.0 mg/kg, PO; Mouse hyperlocomotion model MED 0.3 mg/kg, PO	(Satoh et al., 2009)
15	K_i=9.3	2.1	>3000 nM for human mGluR5	Rat PK, (10 mg/kg), AUC (ng h/mL): 965; Brain concn @ 6 h (ng/g): 100; Brain/plasma: 0.9	(Sasikumar et al., 2010)
16 (MK-5435)		4.3	1500 nM for human mGluR5		(Hostetler et al., 2011)

Table 1. *In vitro* and *in vivo* pharmacological profiles for mGluR1 negative allosteric modulators.

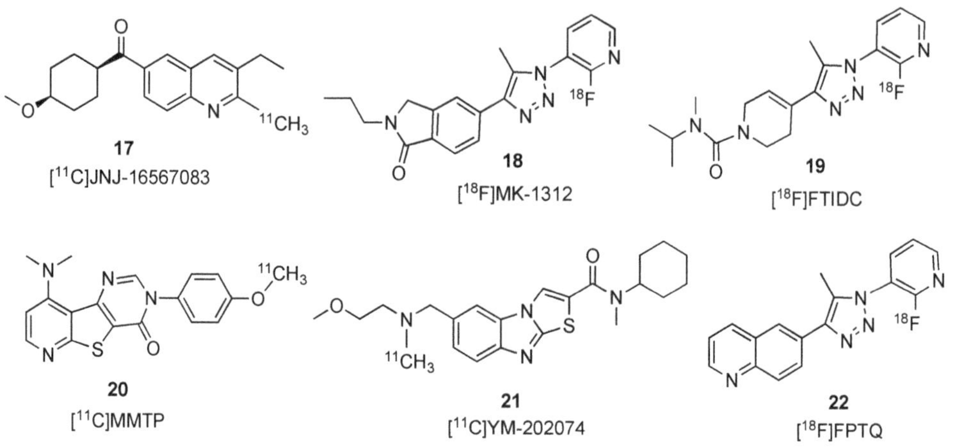

Fig. 2. PET ligands for mGluR1

spinal cord (Karakossian & Otis, 2004; Lavreysen et al., 2003; Shigemoto & Mizuno, 2000; Spooren et al., 2003). Tritium-labeled highly potent and subtype-selective radioligands were used earlier in mapping mGluR1 *ex vivo* (Yang, 2005). Presently, demands on PET radioligands are increasing due to the advantage of *in vivo* noninvasive imaging techniques to investigate pathophysiological processes.

In 2002, a carbon-11 labeled CPCCO-Me analog was described in the literature (Yu & Brownell, 2002), but no animal studies were conducted. In the series of quinoline derivatives (represented by **5**), several compounds are amenable to radiolabeling with either fluorine-18 or carbon-11. Carbon-11 labeling would not be preferred in the methyl ether positions, in spite of methyl ether position is very popular in ^{11}C-methylation, since O-demethylation of the methoxy groups on the quinoline moiety and the cyclohexyl ring are the major metabolic pathways (Mabire et al., 2005). Therefore, practical methods must be developed to label the methyl groups elsewhere in the molecule. Accordingly, Huang et al. successfully labeled a quinoline derivative, providing the first PET tracer, [11C]JNJ-16567083, suitable for *in vivo* imaging of mGluR1 (Huang et al., 2005). [11C]JNJ-16567083 (**17**) is an analog of JNJ-16567083 (**5**). *In vitro* binding experiments showed that JNJ16567083 (cold compound) possesses high affinity for rat mGluR1 ($K_i = 0.87$ nM) and low affinity for mGluR5 ($K_i = 2366$ nM). *Ex vivo* biodistribution studies in rats showed that [11C]JNJ-16567083 has high brain uptake and its binding in brain is specific to mGluR1. MicroPET imaging experiments in rats indicated that radioactivity entered the brain rapidly and was localized over time in brain regions with high densities of mGluR1, such as the cerebellum and striatum. Activity in cerebellum peaked at ~10 min after intravenous injection. Radioactivity uptake was highest in the cerebellum, followed by striatum and hippocampus. However, evaluation of this PET tracer in higher species has not been reported.

Yanamoto et al. have labeled an mGluR1 antagonist YM-202074 (**12**, $K_i = 4.8$ nM) with ^{11}C and evaluated its potential as a PET ligand for mGluR1 (Yanamoto et al., 2010). *In vitro* autoradiographic study demonstrated that [11C]YM-202074 (**21**, Fig.2) had high specific binding with mGluR1 in the rat cerebellum and its regional distribution was consistent with the distribution pattern of mGluR1 in the brain. However, the total accumulation of

[¹¹C]YM-202074 in the brain was very low including lipophilic radiometabolites hampering its usefulness for *in vivo* imaging.

Prahakaran et al. have reported the synthesis for *in vitro* and *in vivo* evaluation of [¹¹C]MMTP (20) as a potential PET ligand for mGluR1 (Prabhakaran et al., 2010). Synthesis of the corresponding desmethyl precursor was achieved by demethylation of the methoxyphenyl compound MMTP in 90% yield. Methylation using [¹¹C]MeOTf in presence of NaOH afforded [¹¹C]MMTP in 30% yield (EOS) with >99% chemical and radiochemical purities and with a specific activity of 3–5 Ci/µmol (n = 6). The total synthesis time was 30 min from EOB. *In vitro* autoradiography using phosphor imaging demonstrated that the radiotracer bound selectively mGlu1 receptors in slide-mounted sections of postmortem human brain containing cerebellum, hippocampus, prefrontal cortex and striatum. PET studies in anesthetized baboon showed that [¹¹C]MMTP penetrates the BBB and accumulates in cerebellum, a region of high expression of mGluR1.

Recently, a ¹⁸F-labeled triazole analog [¹⁸F]FTIDC (19, Ki = 3.9 nM) (Ohgami et al., 2009) was presented for imaging of mGluR1 showing high uptake in the rat brain. In addition, Fujinaga et al. have labeled a triazole analog, FPTQ (11, IC₅₀ = 3.6 nM and 1.4 nM for human and mouse mGluR1, respectively) (Fujinaga et al., 2011). [¹⁸F]FPTQ (22) was synthesized by [¹⁸F]fluorination of the corresponding 2-bromo-3-pyridyl precursor with potassium [¹⁸F]fluoride. At the end of synthesis, 35-50 mCi (n = 8) of [¹⁸F]FPTQ was obtained with >98% radiochemical purity and 3.2-6.4 Ci/µmol specific activity using 89-108 mCi of [¹⁸F]fluoride. *In vitro* autoradiography showed that [¹⁸F]FPTQ had high specific binding with mGluR1 in the rat brain. Biodistribution study using a dissection method and small-animal PET showed that [¹⁸F]FPTQ had high uptake in the rat brain. The uptake of radioactivity in the cerebellum was reduced by unlabeled FPTQ and mGluR1-selective ligand JNJ-16259685 (Fujinaga et al., 2011), indicating that [¹⁸F]FPTQ had *in vivo* specific binding to mGluR1. However, because of a low amount of radiolabeled metabolite present in the brain, this compound may have limiting use for *in vivo* imaging of mGluR1 by PET.

Hostetler et al. have reported a PET radioligand, [¹⁸F]MK-1312 (18), which was radiolabeled with fluorine-18 via nucleophilic displacement of the corresponding 2-chloropyridine precursor with [¹⁸F]potassium fluoride (Hostetler et al., 2011). [¹⁸F]MK-1312 was synthesized (n = 25) in good yield (46 ± 15%) with >98% radiochemical purity and high specific activity (2.5 ± 1.4 Ci/µmol). *In vitro* autoradiographic studies with [¹⁸F]MK-1312 in rhesus monkey and human brain tissue slices revealed an uptake distribution consistent with the known distribution of mGluR1, with the highest uptake in the cerebellum, moderate uptake in the hippocampus, thalamus, and cortical regions, and the lowest uptake in the caudate and putamen. *In vitro* saturation binding studies in rhesus monkey and human cerebellum homogenates confirmed that [¹⁸F]MK-1312 binds to a single binding site with a Bmax/Kd ratio of 132 and 98, respectively. PET studies in rhesus monkey with [¹⁸F]MK-1312 showed high brain uptake and a regional distribution consistent with *in vitro* autoradiography results. Blockade of [¹⁸F]MK-1312 uptake with mGluR1 allosteric antagonist MK-5435 dose-dependently reduced tracer uptake in all regions of gray matter. These results show that [¹⁸F]MK-1312 is a promising PET tracer for clinical studies to determine mGluR1 occupancy of MK-5435.

In summary, several PET radioligands have been developed using highly potent and subtype-selective mGluR1 negative allosteric modulators. Although they showed efficacy in studying the distribution of mGluR1, some compounds may have limited applications because of low brain uptake and/or brain penetrating radiometabolites. [18F]MK-1312 is the most advanced mGluR1 PET tracer, which has demonstrated efficacy in rhesus monkey.

Although all the published mGluR1 PET tracers are radiolabeled mGluR1 negative allosteric modulators, mGluR1 positive allosteric modulators can also be used for developing mGluR1 PET tracers. Several papers have been published about the functional differences between antagonist and agonist tracers in imaging G-protein coupled receptors, including dopamines D2 receptor (Hwang et al., 2004; Wilson et al., 2005), serotonin receptors (Kumar et al., 2006; Prabhakaran et al., 2006) and mGlu receptors. GPCRs have been postulated to exist in interconvertible high-affinity and low-affinity states. The high-affinity sites are G-protein coupled, whereas the low-affinity sites are those uncoupled with G-protein. Antagonist radiotracers bind with equal affinity to both the high- and low-affinity forms of the receptor, and they do not provide information about *in vivo* affinity of the receptor for antagonist. On the contrary, agonist radioligands bind only to high-affinity form of the receptor, thus giving valuable information about *in vivo* affinity of the receptor for agonists in normal and abnormal states. Concerning the binding sites of allosteric modulators in the seven strand transmembrane domain, there is no evidence for difference between negative and positive modulators in terms of their binding to high-affinity or low-affinity states of mGlu receptors (Kew & Kemp, 2005). Fig. 3 illustrates structures of some representative positive allosteric mGluR1 modulators reported (Knoflach et al., 2001; Layton, 2005; Wichmann et al., 2002).

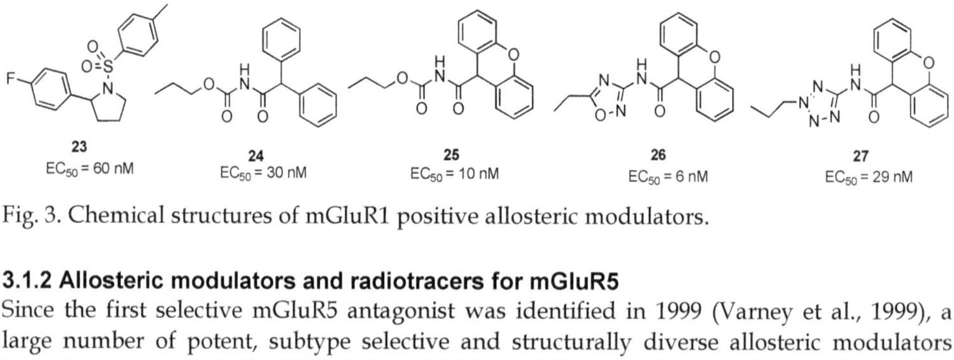

23
$EC_{50} = 60$ nM

24
$EC_{50} = 30$ nM

25
$EC_{50} = 10$ nM

26
$EC_{50} = 6$ nM

27
$EC_{50} = 29$ nM

Fig. 3. Chemical structures of mGluR1 positive allosteric modulators.

3.1.2 Allosteric modulators and radiotracers for mGluR5

Since the first selective mGluR5 antagonist was identified in 1999 (Varney et al., 1999), a large number of potent, subtype selective and structurally diverse allosteric modulators have been described. SIB1757 (**28**) and SB1893 (**29**) were discovered through random screening. Subsequent optimization by replacement of the trans-olefinic tether in SIB1893 (**29**) with a C≡C triple bond led to MPEP (**30**), which demonstrated a dramatically improved mGluR5 antagonist activity (Gasparini et al., 1999). Various structure-activity relationship (SAR) studies have been done on MPEP, in which chemical modifications were done to each of the three regions of the lead molecule, identifying a series of highly potent and selective diaryl (heteroaryl) acetylenes as mGluR5 noncompetitive antagonists. By assumption that the (2-methyl-1,3-thiazo-4-yl)ethynyl group is one of the best structural parts to achieve mGluR5 antagonist activity further SAR studies on MTEP (**31**) identified more high-profile ligands containing thiazole moiety as mGluR5 noncompetitive antagonists such as (**33**) (Iso et al., 2006). Many PET tracers have been synthesized by radiolabeling on the derivatives of MPEP and MTEP.

A major concern with acetylenes in potential drugs is the possibility of chemical or metabolic reactivity (Milbank et al., 2007). Terminal acetylenes are well known to be mechanism-based CYP-inactivators (Testa & Jenner, 1981) and there is an increasing body of information suggesting that internal acetylenes can be activated by CYPs (Fontana et al., 2005; Foroozesh et al., 1997; Shimada et al., 2007) or even undergo uncatalyzed addition of glutathione (Chen et al., 2002; Mutlib et al., 1999). Mutlib et al. reported that incubation of MPEP with triple-labeled glutathione gave compounds with molecular weights and fragmentations consistent with both activated and unactivated addition of GSH to the alkyne (Mutlib et al., 2005). These events are potential sources for hepatic or idiosyncratic toxicity. To avoid a potential metabolic liability, many research groups have designed and synthesized mGluR5 negative allosteric modulators without the acetylene structure. Some structures such as **37** to **48** are given in Fig. 4, which may be useful for development of a new PET tracer.

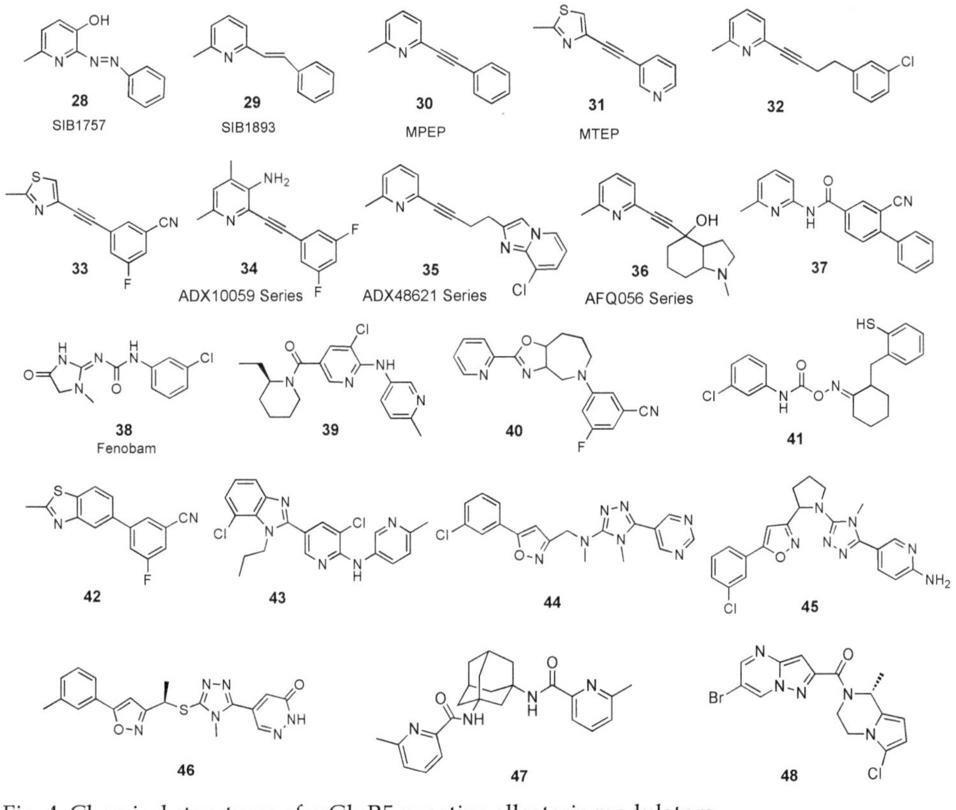

Fig. 4. Chemical structures of mGluR5 negative allosteric modulators

Since the discovery of the first mGluR5 positive modulator, DFB (**49**, Fig. 5) (O'Brien et al., 2003), Merck has reported three series of positive allosteric modulators for mGluR5, which are benzaldazine, benzamide and pyrazole series, exemplified by DFB, CPPHA (**50**) (O'Brien et al., 2004) and CDPPB (**51**) (Kinney et al., 2005; Lindsley et al., 2004), respectively. Subsequent structure-activity relationship study on CDPPB identified several nanomolar potent pyrazole ligands (De Paulis et al., 2006). Although these compounds are potent with an EC_{50} value of less than 20 nM, their poor binding affinity (K_i) and high lipophilicity

Compound	Rat mGluR5 IC_{50} (nM)	Human mGluR5 IC_{50} (nM)	*In vivo* properties	References
28 (SIB1757)				(Varney et al., 1999)
29 (SIB1893)				(Varney et al., 1999)
30 (MPEP)	$K_i = 12$	2		(Cosford et al., 2003)
31 (MTEP)	$K_i = 16$	5	MTEP is more potent than MPEP *in vivo* (rats) in both a receptor occupancy assay and in the fear-potentiated startle model of anxiety.	(Cosford et al., 2003)
32	5			(Bach et al., 2006)
33	0.8 $K_i = 0.9$			(Kulkarni et al., 2009)
34 ADX10059 Series			Positive data from phase II clinical studies in both GERD and acute migraine.	(Keywood et al., 2009; Marin & Goadsby, 2010)
35 ADX48621 Series			Showed efficacy in nonhuman primate model of PD-LID.	(Emmitte, 2011)
36 AFQ056 Series			Reported improvements in certain aberrant behaviors in clinical trial for treating FXS.	(Emmitte, 2011)
37	0.8 $K_i = 22$		Showed efficacy for anxiolytic activity in the Vogel assay.	(Milbank et al., 2007)
38 (Fenobam)			Using prepulse inhibition as an outcome measure for treating FXS, 50% of patients responded according to the predefined criteria of efficacy.	(Berry-Kravis et al., 2009; Porter et al., 2005)
39	32			(Spanka et al., 2010)
40		16	Showed good brain penetration, robust receptor occupancy and short half-life in rodent.	(Burdi et al., 2010)
41	109 $K_i = 9.1$			(Galambos et al., 2010)
42	61		Showed efficacy in the OSS model.	(Lindsley et al., 2011)
43	24		Showed a robust anxiolytic-like effect.	(Carcache et al., 2011)

Compound	Rat mGluR5 IC$_{50}$ (nM)	Human mGluR5 IC$_{50}$ (nM)	*In vivo* properties	References
44	20		Rat B/P ratio=0.16.	(Isaac & Waallberg, 2009)
45	<3		Rat B/P ratio=0.085.	(Granberg & Holm, 2009)
46	19		Rat B/P ratio=0.26.	(Granberg & Holm, 2010)
47	K$_i$=6.7			(Jimenez et al., 2010)
48	7.8	25		(Henrich et al., 2009)

Table 2. *In vitro* and *in vivo* pharmacological profiles for mGluR5 negative allosteric modulators.

(logP) prevent them from being good candidates for radiotracer because high lipophilicity decreases brain penetration. Bessis et al. reported a fourth structural series represented by ADX47273 (**52**) (Bessis et al., 2005). Recently, many mGluR5 positive allosteric modulators, **53–60**, have been reported to have an EC$_{50}$ value below 20 nM (Fig. 5) (Varnes et al., 2011; Williams et al., 2011). However, no PET tracers have been developed from this class of compounds.

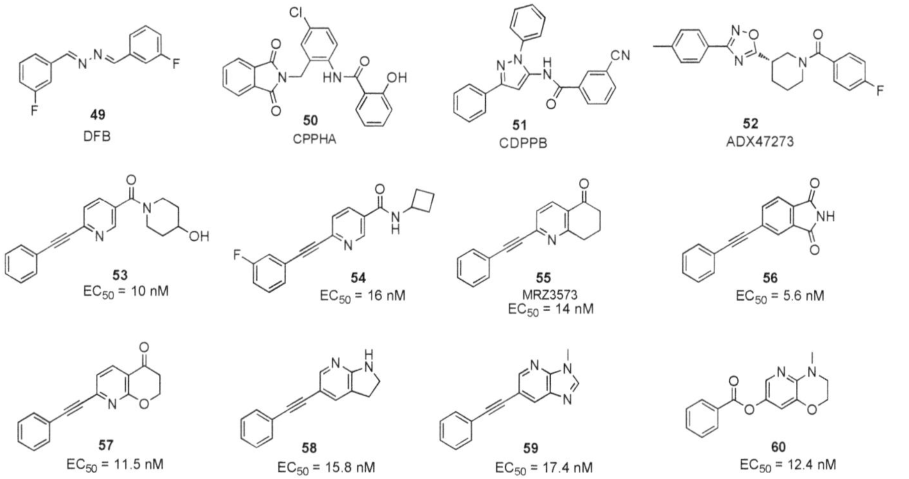

49
DFB

50
CPPHA

51
CDPPB

52
ADX47273

53
EC$_{50}$ = 10 nM

54
EC$_{50}$ = 16 nM

55
MRZ3573
EC$_{50}$ = 14 nM

56
EC$_{50}$ = 5.6 nM

57
EC$_{50}$ = 11.5 nM

58
EC$_{50}$ = 15.8 nM

59
EC$_{50}$ = 17.4 nM

60
EC$_{50}$ = 12.4 nM

Fig. 5. Chemical structures of mGluR5 positive allosteric modulators

The discoveries of noncompetitive allosteric modulators with high binding affinity and subtype-selectivity entitle the exploration of the physiological functions of mGluR5 in normal and pathological states. Although *in vitro* and *ex vivo* studies using selective mGluR5 allosteric antagonists labeled with tritium (Cosford, 2003; Gasparini et al., 2002) have played important roles in elucidating the distribution and functions of mGluR5, PET tracers are needed for the *in vivo* quantitative visualization of mGluR5 in a living body and to conduct longitudinal studies of modulation of mGluR5 expression.

3.1.3 PET imaging studies of mGluR5 function

MPEP and MTEP have provided leads to some radioligand candidates for imaging human mGlu5 receptors with PET *in vivo*. Great effort was done to identify suitable positron-emitting radiotracers for noninvasive imaging of mGluRs. To date, more than 15 mGluR5-selective PET ligands labeled with ^{18}F or ^{11}C have been reported (Fig. 6) (Ametamey et al., 2006; De Paulis et al., 2006; Hamill et al., 2005; Honer et al., 2007; Krause et al., 2003; Musachio et al., 2003; Patel et al., 2005; Sanchez-Pernaute et al., 2008; Simeón et al., 2007; Wang et al., 2007a; Yu, 2005; Zhu et al., 2007).

In 2005, Hamill and colleagues from Merck demonstrated the first successful PET imaging of mGluR5 in rhesus monkeys using [^{18}F]F-MTEB (**61**) (Hamill et al., 2005; Patel et al., 2005). This compound was highly selective and bound with high affinity (IC$_{50}$ = 80 pM) to the receptor. However, the synthesis of this tracer in the cyclotron gave low yields (2-5%), which limited its potential utility as a ligand for clinical trials in humans.

Brownell et al. have synthesized and radiolabeled five noncompetitive antagonists for mGluR5: [^{11}C]M-MPEP (**62**) (Yu et al., 2005), [^{11}C]M-PEPy (**63**) (Sanchez-Pernaute et al., 2008), [^{11}C]MPEP (**64**) (Yu et al., 2005), [^{18}F]FMTEP (**65**) (Zhu et al., 2007) and ^{18}F]FPEB (**66**) (Wang et al., 2007a) and conducted *in vivo* PET imaging studies in different disease models to investigate modulation of mGluR5 function. It was found in these studies that accumulation of pyridine derivatives [^{11}C]M-MPEP (**62**), [^{11}C]M-PEPy (**63**), [^{11}C]MPEP (**64**) and [^{18}F]FMTEP (**65**) into the brain was fast and the highest accumulation was reached in 1-5 min followed by fast washout, suggesting little retention by high affinity receptor binding. This creates limitation to obtain statistically meaningful imaging data without overdosing the object with radiation or saturating the receptor binding sites with accompanying cold compound. These ligands have limitation, due to high lipophilicity, unfavorable brain uptake kinetics, or a high rate of metabolism, though they possess favorable *in vitro* pharmacological profiles. For PET ligands to be used in the central nervous system, a postulated lipophilicity coefficient (logD or logP) value should be between 2 and 3 for good brain accumulation. The compounds [^{11}C]ABP688 (**67**) (Ametamey et al., 2006) and [^{18}F]FPEB (**66**) (Patel et al., 2007; Wang et al., 2007a) have better binding profile for imaging studies of mGluR5. The logD value of 2.3 for [^{11}C]ABP688 and the logP value of 2.8 for [^{18}F]FPEB suggest that the two compounds are sufficiently lipophilic for the BBB penetrating. Both compounds have good binding properties with a K$_i$ Value of 0.2 nM for [^{18}F]FPEB and a K$_d$ value of 1.7 nM for [^{11}C]ABP688. The brain uptake of both compounds is highly selective, with high accumulation in mGluR5-rich brain regions such as the hippocampus, striatum and cortex. Blocking studies by coinjection of [^{11}C]ABP688 and corresponding unlabeled compound revealed up to 80% specific binding in these regions, whereas in cerebellum, a region with negligible mGluR5 density, no significant changes in radioactivity uptake were observed (Ametamey et al., 2006). Specific binding of compounds [^{11}C]ABP688 and [^{18}F]FPEB were also demonstrated with mGluR5-knockout mice which exhibited a homogeneous background level accumulation throughout the brain (Black et al., 2010). The metabolism studies of [^{11}C]ABP688 and [^{18}F]FPEB indicated that more than 95% of the radioactivity found in the brain was parent compound 30 min after injection for [^{11}C]ABP688 and 78% for [^{18}F]FPEB. Both compounds have been translated to human studies to investigate mGluR5 function.

Siméon and colleagues of the NIH reported a new high affinity radioligand, [^{18}F]-SP203 (**68**), for mGluR5 (Simeón et al., 2007). [^{18}F]-SP203 has high affinity (IC$_{50}$ = 36 pM) and potency in a phosphoinositol hydrolysis assay (IC$_{50}$ = 0.71 pM) for mGluR5. It demonstrates a high uptake in mGlu5 receptor rich regions of the rat and rhesus brain. The major advantage of this tracer over [18F]F-MTEB is its high radiochemical yield (87%) and easy radiosynthesis. This ligand is presently in NIH administrated clinical trial.

[11C]M-FPEP (**69**, K_D 1.2 nM and B_{max} 84.5 f_{mol}/mg) has an even biodistribution in all brain regions demonstrating that this tracer lacks specific binding (Ametamey et al., 2003). Compound **70** showed little retention by the receptor (Krause et al., 2003). Compound **71** (rat K_i 0.23 nM) had a good brain uptake and slow washout, with high concentration in striatum, frontal cortex and cerebellum of monkey (Hamill et al., 2005). However, the

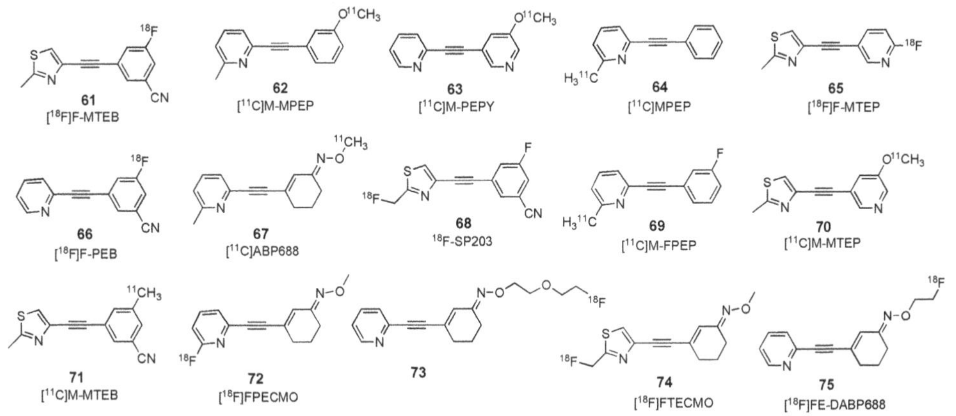

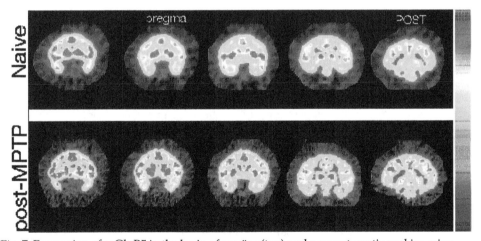

Fig. 6. Chemical structures of mGluR5 PET tracers.

Fig. 7. Expression of mGluR5 in the brain of a naïve (top) and a symptomatic parkinsonian primate, using the highly selective tracer [18F]FPEB (3-[18F]fluoro-5-(2-pyridinylethynyl)benzonitrile). Primate Parkinson's disease (PD) was introduced by low dose long-term systemic administration of MPTP. In PD monkey accumulation of [18F]FPEB was enhanced compared to naïve monkey in several brain areas including caudate, putamen, accumbens and SN/VTA. Distribution of [18F]FPEB accumulation is illustrated at 60-70 min after administration of radioligand (1.2-1.5 mCi iv., specific activity 1.9 Ci/μmol).

cerebellum is an area with fairly low mGluR5 expression indicating that **71** may have non-specific binding.

Four derivatives, **72-75**, were developed of ABP688. PET imaging with **72** (Lucatelli et al., 2009) did not allow visualization of mGluR5-rich brain regions in the rat brain due to fast washout and rapid defluorination. Compound **73** (Baumann et al., 2010a) was reported to have the high binding affinity to mGluR5. Further *in vitro* evaluation and *in vivo* imaging are needed for characterization of this ligand. Baumann et al. (Baumann et al., 2010b) reported that although [18F]-FTECMO (**74**) displayed optimal lipophilicity (log $D_{pH7.4}$ = 1.6 ± 0.2) and high stability in rat and human plasma as well as sufficient stability in rat liver microsomes, PET imaging with [18F]-FTECMO in Wistar rats showed low brain uptake. Uptake of radioactivity into the skull was observed suggesting *in vivo* defluorination. Honer et al. reported that [18F]-FE-DABP688 (**75**) have optimal lipophilicity (logD 2.1±0.1) and high plasma stability (Honer et al., 2007). Saturation assays of [18F]-FE-DABP688 revealed a single high affinity binding site with a dissociation constant (K_d) of 1.6±0.4 nM and a B_{max} value of 119±24 fmol/mg protein. PET scanning indicated radioactivity uptake in mGluR5-rich regions such as the hippocampus, striatum and cortex, and radioactivity accumulation in the cerebellum, a region with negligible mGluR5 density, was significantly lower. Biodistribution studies showed a similar distribution pattern of [18F]-FE-DABP688 binding in the brain. The hippocampus-to-cerebellum and striatum-to-cerebellum ratios were 1.81±0.16 and 1.93±0.36, respectively. Blocking studies using coinjection of [18F]-FE-. DABP688 and unlabeled M-MPEP (1 mg/kg) revealed more than 45% replacement in the hippocampus and striatum, thus demonstrating the *in vivo* specificity of tracer binding. This result shows that [18F]-FE-DABP688 may be a useful PET tracer for imaging mGluR5

3.2 Allosteric modulators and radiotracers for group II mGluRs

Group II mGluRs have been shown to be expressed in several brain areas. The expression patterns of Group II receptors in the rodent brain parallel those of mGluR5, although the overall abundance of mGluR2/3 receptors appears slightly reduced as compared with that of mGluR5 (Olive, 2009). Expression levels of mGluR2/3 receptors are high in the olfactory bulb and hippocampus, and moderate in the dorsal striatum, nucleus accumbens, amygdala, anterior thalamic nuclei, cerebral cortex and cerebellum. Low levels of mGluR2/3 are found in the pallidum, colliculi, ventral midbrain and hypothalamus.

Group II mGluRs act in the hippocampus to decrease synaptic transmission and glutamate release when activated. These receptors have been targeted extensively by potential neuroprotective agents to develop treatments for anxiety, schizophrenia, Alzheimer's disease, Parkinson's disease, pain, drug withdrawal, and epilepsy (Rudd & McCauley, 2005).

3.2.1 Allosteric modulators for mGluR2

Over the past decade, a number of highly potent (EC_{50} in subnanomolar) mGluR2 agonists and antagonists with high binding affinity (K_i < 2 nM) have been identified (Rudd & McCauley, 2005; Yasuhara et al., 2006). However, their mGluR2-selectivity over mGluR3 in the same group is fairly low with the highest potency ratio being 6.5 (Dominguez et al., 2005). A high potency ratio does not necessarily imply a high binding affinity ratio, whereas the specific binding of a radiotracer depends much on the binding affinity ratio. Considering a low subtype-selectivity and unfavorable brain penetration of classical mGluR2 agonists and antagonists, the focus has presently been to develop noncompetitive allosteric modulators. When the allosteric binding sites on glutamate receptors within a group are sufficiently different it is possible to develop subtype selectivity modulators.

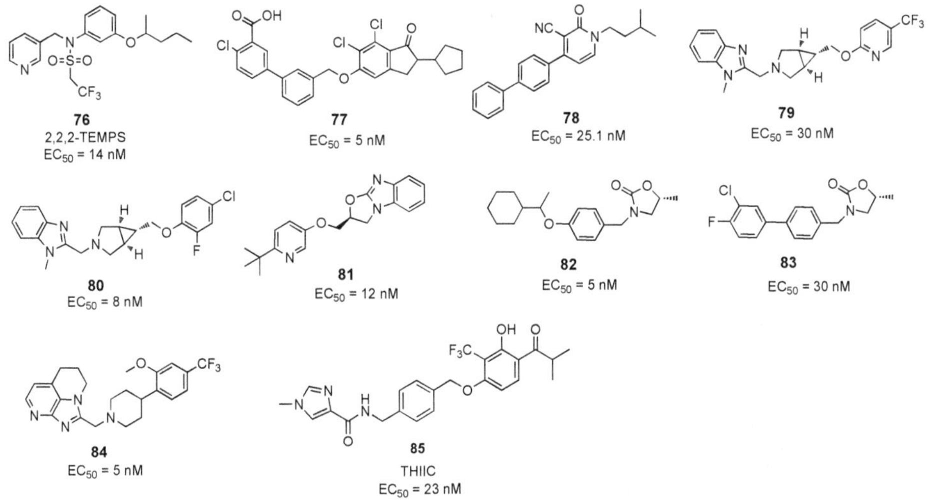

76
2,2,2-TEMPS
EC_{50} = 14 nM

77
EC_{50} = 5 nM

78
EC_{50} = 25.1 nM

79
EC_{50} = 30 nM

80
EC_{50} = 8 nM

81
EC_{50} = 12 nM

82
EC_{50} = 5 nM

83
EC_{50} = 30 nM

84
EC_{50} = 5 nM

85
THIIC
EC_{50} = 23 nM

Fig. 8. Chemical structures of mGluR2 positive allosteric modulators

Many series of selective mGluR2 positive allosteric modulators have been reported to date. Figure 8 shows the compounds that were reported to have an EC_{50} value of less than 30 nM. They are N-aryl-N-(pyridylmethyl)ethanesulfonamides (**76**) (Barda et al., 2004; Johnson et al., 2003), biphenyl-indanones (**77**) (Bonnefous et al., 2005), 1,4-disubstituted 3-cyano-pyridone derivatives (**78**) (Imogai et al., 2007), 3-(Imidazolyl methyl)-3-aza-bicyclo[3.1.0]hexan-6-yl)methyl ethers (**79** and **80**) (Zhang et al., 2008), oxazolobenzimidazoles (**81**) (Garbaccio et al., 2010), 3-Benzyl-1,3-oxazolidin-2-ones (**82** and **83**) (Duplantier et al., 2009), 2-((4-(2-methoxy-4-(trifluoromethyl)phenyl)piperidin-1-yl)methyl)-5,6-dihydro-4H-imidazo[4,5,1-ij][1,7]naphthyridine (**84**) (Efremov et al., 2008) and THIIC (**85**) (Fell et al., 2011).

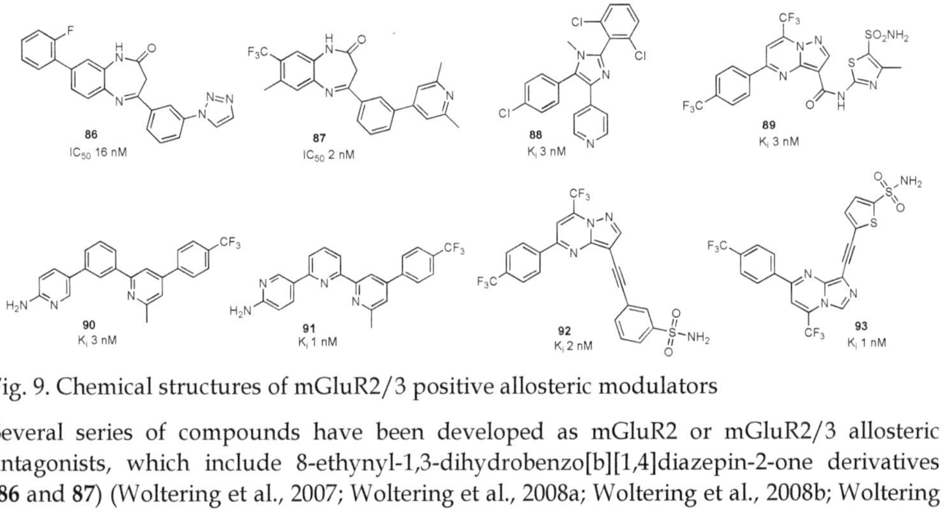

86
IC_{50} 16 nM

87
IC_{50} 2 nM

88
K_i 3 nM

89
K_i 3 nM

90
K_i 3 nM

91
K_i 1 nM

92
K_i 2 nM

93
K_i 1 nM

Fig. 9. Chemical structures of mGluR2/3 positive allosteric modulators

Several series of compounds have been developed as mGluR2 or mGluR2/3 allosteric antagonists, which include 8-ethynyl-1,3-dihydrobenzo[b][1,4]diazepin-2-one derivatives (**86** and **87**) (Woltering et al., 2007; Woltering et al., 2008a; Woltering et al., 2008b; Woltering et al., 2010), imidazole derivatives (**88**) (Gatti McArthur et al., 2006b), pyrazolopyrimidines

(89) (Gatti McArthur et al., 2006c), Pyridine and pyrimidine derivatives (90 and 91) (Gatti Mcarthur et al., 2007), acetylenyl-pyrazolo-pyrimidine derivatives (92 and 93) (Gatti McArthur et al., 2006a). Representative compounds listed in Fig. 9 exhibit high binding affinity towards mGluR2, however, their binding selectivity over mGluR3 is either very low or is not disclosed.

Currently, no positron emitting radioligand has been developed for imaging mGluR2.

3.2.2 PET imaging studies of mGluR2/3 expression

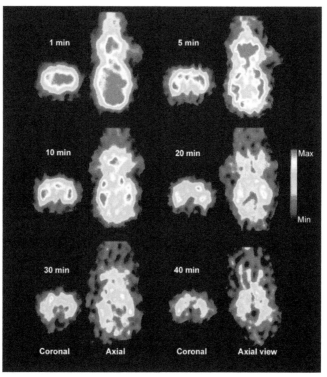

Fig. 10. To investigate preliminary imaging characteristics of (S,S,S)-2-(2-carboxycyclopropyl)-2-(3-[^{11}C]methoxyphenethyl) glycine dimethyl ester ([^{11}C]CMG) 0.4-0.5 mCi of [^{11}C]CMG was administered iv. into the anesthetized (isoflurane 1.5% with O2 flow of 1L/min) rats (male Spraque Dawley) in a microPET scanner (P4, Concord Microsystems). Dynamic volumetric data were acquired in 6 rats for 60 min. Fast reversible binding was observed in several cortical areas, hippocampus, striatum and olfactory bulb, the sites which are known to express group II mGluRs. The maximum binding (1.1-1.6% of the injected dose per cm3) was observed 2 min after administration. These data provide a foundation for future development of specific PET imaging ligands for group II mGluRs. Coronal and axial slices of [^{11}C]CMG distribution in the rat brain from 1 min till 40 min after administration of the radioligand are illustrated. Color coded images are normalized to each other and correspond the acquisition time of 1 min at the same midbrain level (coronal slice at bregma -1.6 mm; axial slice at bregma -5.4 mm).

3.2.3 Allosteric modulators for mGluR3

Eli Lilly and Company reported the first series of compounds, 1-(heteroaryl)-3-(2,4-dichlorobenzyl)amino-pyrolidine, acting as mGluR3 negative allosteric modulators (Britton et al., 2006). Figure 11 shows the chemical structures of two most potent ligands reported in the patent. Compounds, **94** and **95**, have an IC_{50} value of 77 nM, which is insufficient for *in vivo* detection of the receptors. Further SAR studies are needed to find more potent ligands. No PET radioligands have been identified for mGluR3 so far.

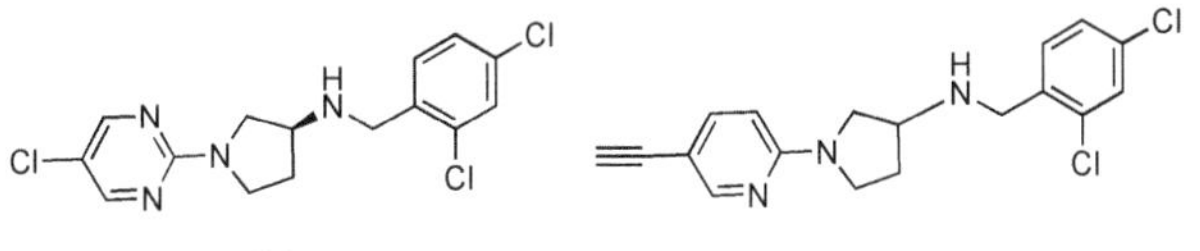

94
IC_{50} = 77 nM

95
IC_{50} = 77 nM

Fig. 11. Chemical structures of mGluR3 negative allosteric modulators

3.3 Allosteric modulators and radiotracers for Group III mGluRs

Group III metabotropic glutamate receptors are mGluR4, mGluR6, mGluR7 and mGluR8. There is no publication reporting mGluR6 allosteric ligands.

3.3.1 Allosteric modulators for mGluR4

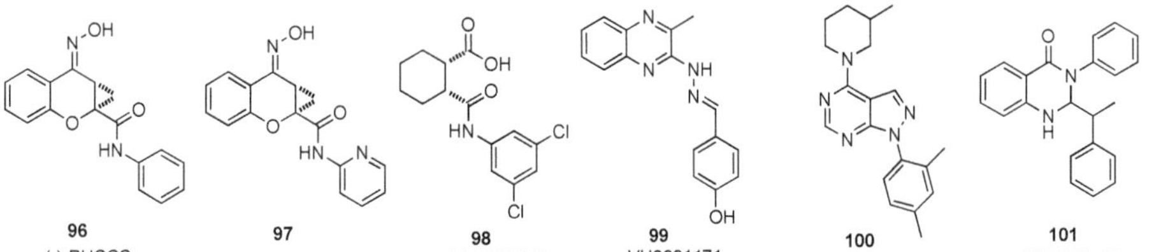

96
(-)-PHCCC
EC_{50}: 4.7 mM

97
VU0359516
EC_{50}: 380 nM

98
VU0155041
EC_{50}: 0.75 mM

99
VU0001171
EC_{50}: 0.65 mM

100
VU0080241
EC_{50}: 5.0 mM

101
VU0092145
EC_{50}: 3.0 mM

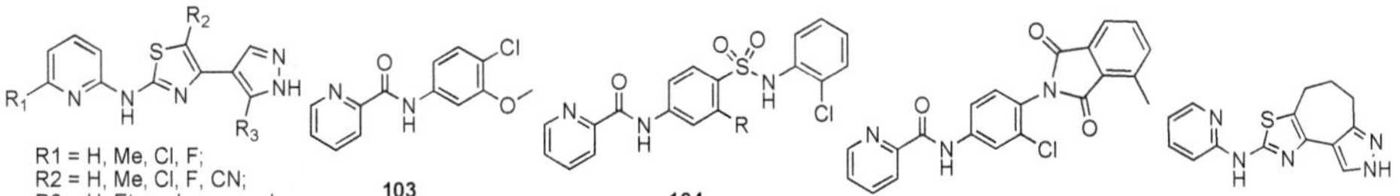

R1 = H, Me, Cl, F;
R2 = H, Me, Cl, F, CN;
R3 = H, Et, cyclopropanyl.

102
Addex compounds
EC_{50} < 0.5 µM

103
VU0361737
EC_{50}: 110 nM

104
A: R = H
EC_{50}: 160 nM
B: R = Cl (VU0364439)
EC_{50}: 20 nM

105
EC_{50}: 45 nM

106
EC_{50}: 9 nM

Fig. 12. Chemical structures of mGluR4 positive allosteric modulators

MGluR4 has received much attention lately due to its implication in several diseases, such as PD, epilepsy, and anxiety. There has been substantial progress in identifying positive allosteric modulators for mGluR4. The compound PHCCC (**96**, Fig. 12), a partial selective mGluR4 potentiator, has been studied for many years. Unfortunately PHCCC and other early disclosed mGluR4 PAMs such as **98–101** (Fig.12) are deficient in their BBB penetration (Engers et al., 2009). The potencies of these compounds are also relatively low (EC_{50}: 0.65 –

5.0 µM) and SAR studies around these structures have given 'flat' results. Addex Pharma disclosed a series of heteroaromatic compounds (**102** in Fig. 12) as positive allosteric modulators for mGluR4, with many compounds having $EC_{50} < 0.5$ µM (Bolea & Celanire, 2009). However, no other information was reported about these compounds.

Two research groups; Addex Pharma (Bolea, 2009) and Vanderbilt University (Engers et al., 2009), have independently disclosed a series of small arylamide compounds as a new class of mGluR4 PAMs. Engers et al (Vanderbilt University) found from a high-throughput screening that there were a number of small arylamide compounds having mGluR4 PAM activity (Engers et al., 2009). They reported studies on SAR and *in vitro* and *in vivo* pharmacokinetic parameters in rat. The most potent compound in this series was **103** shown in Fig. 12. Researchers at Merck presented two new compounds, **104A** and **105**, with improved activity (Reynolds, 2008). Engers et al. further studied SAR of 4-(phenylsulfamoyl)phenylacetamide derivatives and found that **104B** was the most potent (19.8 nM) mGluR4 positive allosteric modulator reported to date (Engers et al., 2010). Doller and co-workers (Lundbeck Research USA) have recently reported on a series of tricyclic thiazolopyrazole derivatives including compound **106**, which was identified as a very potent and orally available compound with excellent brain penetration and good physicochemical properties (Hong et al., 2011).

3.3.2 PET imaging studies of mGluR4 expression

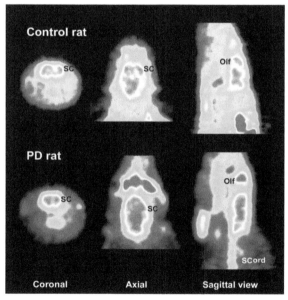

Fig. 13. Distribution of [¹¹C]methyl-PHCCC between 10-20 min after administration of radioligand in a control (1.2 mCi iv.) and PD (1.1 mCi iv.) rat brain. Coronal and axial views localize cortex at the level of S1 and S2 areas. It is noticeable that the accumulation of [¹¹C]methyl-PHCCC is enhanced in PD rat in the areas of subthalamic nucleus and spinal cord. The motor neurons in the ventral horn in the spinal cord express mGluR4 and the observed enhanced accumulation of mGluR4 ligand, [¹¹C]methyl-PHCCC is an indication of excess glutamate. This is the first time, when this aspect has been demonstrated *in vivo* in a PD model.

3.3.3 Allosteric modulators for mGluR7

It is reported that mGluR7 is widely expressed in the central nervous system and is primarily located on presynaptic terminals in brain regions such as the hippocampus, amygdala, and locus coeruleus. Mitsukawa et al. developed the first selective allosteric agonist of mGluR7, AMN082 (107), which has an EC_{50} value of 64-290 nM and it is brain penetrating (Mitsukawa, 2005). However, converting it to a PET tracer is not straightforward. Researchers of Banyu Pharmaceutical Co reported a series of isoxazolopyridone derivatives as allosteric mGluR7 antagonists (Suzuki et al., 2007b). Compound MDIP (108) that was identified by random screening displayed mGluR7 antagonistic activity (IC_{50} = 20 nM) and had no detectable activity on other mGluRs at 1000 nM. However, MDIP showed poor metabolic stability (predicted F_H: 34%) on rat hepatocyte assay and low aqueous solubility (0.17 µg/mL, pH 7.4). It is assumed that poor metabolic stability and low aqueous solubility may be due to its high lipophilicity (clog$D_{7.4}$: 3.5). Recently, Nakamura et al. have identified some isoxazolopyridone derivatives with potent mGluR7 antagonistic activity and metabolic stability, in which MMPIP (109) with improved physicochemical properties and metabolic stability showed good oral bioavailability and brain penetrability in rats (Nakamura et al., 2010).

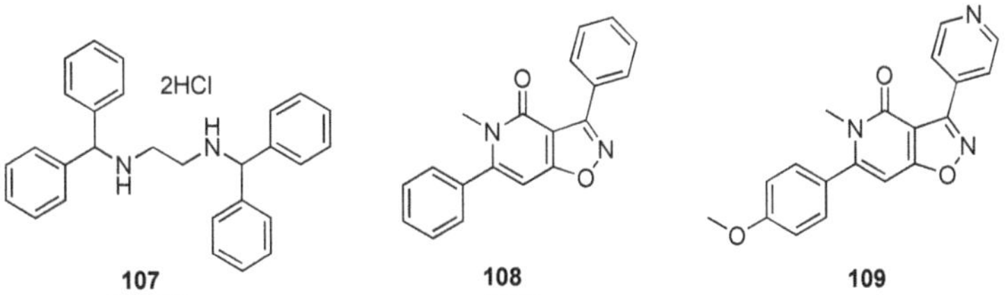

Fig. 14. Chemical structures of mGluR7 modulators

3.3.4 Allosteric modulators for mGluR8

Recently, AstraZeneca developed a positive allosteric modulator for mGluR8 (Duvoisin et al., 2010; Duvoisin et al., 2011). The compound AZ12216052 as injected into the amygdale, reduced measures of anxiety. There is no PET ligand available and AZ12216052 does not cross blood brain barrier.

4. Conclusion

Glutamate is an interesting transmitter since it can participate also on glutamate metabolism to be converted to glutamine and its function as a neurotransmitter can be investigated based on its receptor functions. To understand the diverse physiological effects of glutamate it is important to know molecular identity of mGluRs expressed in distinct subpopulations of neurons. For instance, group I mGluRs are coupled to phospholipase C and subsequent production of inositol triphosphates and induces intracellular calcium release in Purkinje cells and hippocampal CA1 neurons, but the same receptor types are also coupled to inhibition of voltage-dependent calcium channel in hippocampal neurons without intracellular diffusible messengers (Choi & Lovinger, 1996). Group II mGluRs can be coupled to inhibition of cyclic AMP cascade in neural and glial cells while they are also linked to rapid-onset regulation of various channels including calcium channels and G-protein. The group III mGluRs-mediated effect is inhibition of neurotransmission through suppression of presynaptic voltage-dependent calcium channels (Pekhletski et al., 1996). This basic functional information of mGluRs has been obtained with *in situ* hybridization, immunohistochemistry and *ex vivo* studies with tritium labeled antibodies. While *ex vivo* studies can provide accurate endpoint information in steady state, they cannot provide information of the active inhibitory or stimulating effects in the system or interplay with other systems. To obtain functional information in real time, the investigation has to be done by using *in vivo* imaging methods. However, a lack of specific agonists and antagonists has limited the precise characterization of the role of individual metabotropic glutamate receptors in glutamatergic neurotransmission and hampered progress in identifying the physiological and pathological roles of mGluRs *in vivo*.

Recently, the modern computational chemistry has opened a wide range of technical approaches to design and construct molecules for imaging and to simulate their molecular targets. This technology has been used to design molecules for tracking different mGluRs. Especially, approach of allosteric compounds relies on sophisticated design of three-dimensional arrangement of the tracer molecules responsible for the biological activity. Pharmacophore models can be constructed based on known biological activity. Design of novel allosteric modulators is an iterative process where structure-activity relationship information generated in the biological assays guides how to make structural alternations towards the optimal compound. Recently several non-competitive structurally diverse mGluR ligands have been published. These ligands, positive, negative and neutral modulators, bind to the allosteric binding sites located in the seven strand transmembrane domain. Based on these modulators, a number of radiotracers useful for imaging specific metabotropic glutamate receptors have been developed and their *in vivo* biological properties have been characterized.

Development of metabotropic glutamate receptor ligands will open a new perspective for molecular imaging. Modulation of receptor functions might be used as diagnostic tools as well as to follow progression/regression of neural diseases. Presently, three mGluR ligands have been used in human studies. They are developed as negative allosteric modulators for mGluR5. For example, concerning PD, the death of dopamine neurons in the substantia nigra pars compacta causes a loss of dopamine in the basal ganglia. Dopamine modulation of neurotransmission in the striatum and other basal ganglia structures is crucial to gate cortical and thalamic excitatory input through the direct and indirect pathways. By using *in vivo* PET imaging studies and [18F]FPEB we have found an upregulation of mGluR5 expression following dopamine denervation in animal models of PD (Figures 7 & 13), which probably represents a local compensatory mechanism, directed to dampen an excessive excitability of striatopallidal neurons. Drugs targeting the mGluR5 might provide new approaches by selectively reducing glutamate transmission in the areas where it is abnormally enhanced. In addition, we and others have found enhanced mGluR5 expression in several brain areas related to the indirect pathway in models of L-DOPA induced dyskinesias and some studies have shown promising therapeutic results after using mGluR5 antagonists. In gut glutamate is the main energy source and its neurotransmission is conducted by vagal afferents. The gut expresses also mGlu5 receptors and we have localized them with [18F]FPEB. This phenomenon has raised a hypothesis that gut-brain axis as well as interplay with dopamine transmission might contribute to obesity.

Even mGlu2 receptors had the earliest interest as targets for drug development and Eli Lilly developed several potent ligands targeted to mGluR2 there is not yet any specific allosteric modulators available for imaging purposes of mGluR2 function. The earlier compounds were missing receptor selectivity and sensitivity for imaging purposes since sequence similarity at the orthosteric binding site to which endogenous agonists bind.

Present application of glutamate transmission has evoked an active drug development especially to develop allosteric modulators for neurodegenerative disorders, pain and schizophrenia. It should be noted that these disorders are affected also by modulation of dopaminergic system supporting hypothesis of interplay of these powerful transmitter systems. Future pharmacological and imaging studies will show which specific ligands acting at individual receptor subtypes could be used as sensitive indicators for diagnostic imaging. Therefore, there is an urgent need for development of allosteric modulators as imaging ligands for different of mGluRs for human use.

5. Acknowledgement

This work was supported by the NIH grant NIBIB-EB12864 to A-LB.

6. References

Aguirre, J. A., Andbjer, B., Gonzalez-Baron, S., Hansson, A., Stromberg, I., et al. (2001). Group I mGluR antagonist AIDA protects nigral DA cells from MPTP-induced injury. *NeuroReport*, Vol. 12, pp. 2615-7

Ametamey, S. M., Kessler, L., Honer, M., Auberson, Y., Gasparini, F., Schubiger, P. A. (2003). Synthesis and evaluation of [^{11}C]MFPEP as a PET ligand for imaging the metabotropic glutamate receptor subtype 5 (mGluR5). *J. Label. Compd. Radiopharm.*, Vol. 46, pp. S188

Ametamey, S. M., Kessler, L. J., Honer, M., Wyss, M. T., Buck, A., et al. (2006). Radiosynthesis and preclinical evaluation of ^{11}C-ABP688 as a probe for imaging the metabotropic glutamate receptor subtype 5. *J. Nucl. Med.*, Vol. 47, pp. 698-705

Annoura, H., Fukunaga, A., Uesugi, M., Tatsuoka, T., Horikawa, Y. (1996). A novel class of antagonists for metabotropic glutamate receptors, 7-(hydroxyimino) cyclopropa[b]chromen-1a-carboxylates. *Bioorg Med chem Lett*, Vol. 6, pp.763-6

Bach, P., Nilsson, K., Svensson, T., Bauer, U., Hammerland, L., et al. (2006). Structure-activity relationships for the linker in a series of pyridinyl-alkynes that are antagonists of the metabotropic glutamate receptor 5 (mGluR5). *Bioorg. Med. Chem. Lett.*, Vol. 16, pp. 4788-91

Barda, D A., Wang, Z-Q., Britton, T. C., Henry, S. S., Jagdmann, G. E., et al. (2004). SAR study of a subtype selective allosteric potentiator of metabotropic glutamate 2 receptor, N-(4-phenoxyphenyl)-N-(3-pyridinylmethyl)ethanesulfonamide. *Bioorg. Med. Chem. Lett.*, Vol. 14, pp. 3099-102

Baumann, C., Mu, L., Johannsen, S., Honer, M., Schubiger, P., Ametamey, S. (2010a). Structure-activity relationships of fluorinated (E)-3-((6-methylpyridin-2-yl)ethynyl) cyclohex-2-enone-O-methyloxime (ABP688) derivatives and the discovery of a high affinity analogue as a potential candidate for imaging metabotropic glutamate recepors subtype 5 (mGluR5) with positron emission tomography (PET). *J. Med. Chem.*, Vol. 53, pp. 4009-17

Baumann, C., Mu, L., Wertli, N., Krämer, S., Honer, M, et al. (2010b). Syntheses and pharmacological characterization of novel thiazole derivatives as potential mGluR5 PET ligands. *Bioorg. Med. Chem.*, Vol. 18, pp. 6044-54

Berry-Kravis, E., Hessl, D., Coffey, S., Hervey, C., Schneider, A., et al. (2009). A pilot open label, single dose trial of fenobam in adults with fragile X syndrome. *J. Med. Genet.*, Vol 46, pp. 266-71

Bessis, A-S., Bonnet, B., Le Poul, E., Rocher, J-P., Epping-Jordan, M. (2005). *Application: WO Patent No. 2004-IB3822 2005044797*

Bhave, G., Karim, F., Carlton, S., Gereau, R. (2001). Peripheral group I metabotropic glutamate receptors modulate nociception in mice. *Nat. Neurosci.*, Vol. 4, pp. 417-23

Black, Y., Xiao, D., Pellegrino, D., Kachroo, A., Brownell, A., Schwarzschild, M. (2010). Protective effect of metabotroic glutamate mGluR5 receptor elimination in a 6-hydroxydopamine model of Parkinson's disease. *Neurosci. Lett.*, Vol. 486, pp. 161-5

Blakely, R. (2001). Neurobiology. Dopamine's reversal of fortune. *Science*, Vol 293, pp. 2407-9

Bliss, T., Collingridge, G. (1993). A synaptic model of memory: long-term potentiation in the hippocampus. *Nature*, Vol 361, pp. 31-9

Bolea, C. (2009). *Application: WO Patent No. 2008-EP59043 2009010454*

Bolea, C., Celanire, S. (2009). *WO Patent No. 2009/010455*

Bonnefous, C., Vernier, J-M., Hutchinson, J. H., Gardner, M. F., Cramer, M., et al. (2005). Biphenyl-indanones: Allosteric potentiators of the metabotropic glutamate subtype 2 receptor. *Bioorg. Med. Chem. Lett.*, Vol. 15, pp. 4354-8

Britton, T., Dehlinger, V., Dell, C., Dressman, B., Myers, J., Nisenbaum, S. (2006). *PCT Int Appl 2006; WO 2006/044454.*

Burdi, D., Hunt, R., Fan, L., Hu, T., Wang, J., et al. (2010). Design, synthesis, and structure-activity relationships of novel bicyclic azole-amines as negative allosteric modulators of metabotropic glutamate receptor 5. *J. Med. Chem.*, Vol. 53, pp. 7107-18

Cai, L., Lu, S., Pike, V. (2008). Chemistry with [18F]fluoride ion. *Eur. J. Org. Chem.*, Vol. 73, pp. 2853-73

Calabresi, P., Centonze, D., Pisani, A., Bernardi, G. (1999). Metabotropic glutamate receptors and cell-type-specific vulnerability in the striatum: implication for ischemia and Huntington's disease. *Exp Neurol*, Vol. 158, pp. 97-108

Carcache, D., Vranesic, I., Blanz, J., Desrayaud, S., Fendt, M., Glatthar, R. (2011). Benzimidazoles as potent and orally active mGlu5 receptor antagonists with an improved PK profile. *ACS Med. Chem. Lett.*, Vol. 2, pp. 58-62

Carroll, F. Y., Stolle, A., Beart, P. M., Voerste, A., Brabet, I., et al. (2001). BAY 36-7620: a potent non-competitive mGlu1 receptor antagonist with inverse agonist activity. *Mol. Pharmacol.*, Vol. 59, pp. 965-73

Chen, H., Shockcor, J., Chen, W., Espina, R., Gan, L-S., Mutlib, A. E. (2002). Delineating novel metabolic pathways of DPC 963, a non-nucleoside reverse transcriptase inhibitor, in rats. Characterization of glutathione conjugates of postulated oxirene and benzoquinone imine intermediates by LC/MS and LC/NMR. *Chem. Res. Toxicol*, Vol. 15, pp. 388-99

Choi, S., Lovinger, D. M. (1996). Metabotropic glutamate receptor modulation of voltage-gated Ca^{2+} channels involves multiple receptor subtypes in cortical neurons. *J Neurosci*, Vol. 16, pp. 36-45

Conn, J., Pin, J. (1997). Pharmacology and functions of metabotropic glutamate receptors. *Annu Rev Pharmacol Toxicol*, Vol. 37, pp. 205-37

Cosford, N., Roppe, J., Tehrani, L., Schweiger, E. J., Seiders, T. J., Chaudary, A., Rao, S., Varney, M. A. (2003). [^{3}H]-Methoxymethyl-MTEP and [3H]-methoxy-PEPy: potent and selective radioligands for the metabotropic glutamate subtype 5 (mGlu5) receptor. *Bioorg. Med. Chem. Lett.*, Vol. 13, pp. 351-4

Cosford, N., Tehrani, L., Roppe, J., Schweiger, E., Smith, N., et al. (2003). 3-[(2-Methyl-1,3-thiazol-4-yl)ethynyl]-pyridine: A potent and highly selective metabotropic glutamate subtype 5 receptor antagonist with anxiolytic activity. *J. Med. Chem.*, Vol. 46, pp. 204-6

De Paulis, T., Hemstapat, K., Chen, Y., Zhang, Y., Saleh, S., et al. (2006). Substituent effects of N-(1,3-diphenyl-1H-pyrazol-5-yl)benzamides on positive allosteric modulation of the metabotropic glutamate-5 receptor in rat cortical astrocytes. *J. Med. Chem.*, Vol. 49, pp. 3332-44

Dominguez, C., Prieto, L., Valli, M. J., Massey, S. M., Bures, M., et al. (2005). Methyl Substitution of 2-Aminobicyclo[3.1.0]hexane 2,6-Dicarboxylate (LY354740) Determines Functional Activity at Metabotropic Glutamate Receptors: Identification of a Subtype Selective mGlu2 Receptor Agonist. *J. Med. Chem.*, Vol. 48, pp. 3605-12

Duplantier, A. J., Efremov, I., Candler, J., Doran, A. C., Ganong, A. H., et al. (2009). 3-Benzyl-1,3-oxazolidin-2-ones as mGluR2 positive allosteric modulators: Hit-to lead and lead optimization. *Bioorg. Med. Chem. Lett.*, Vol. 19, pp. 2524-9

Duvoisin, R. M., Pfankuch, T., Wilson, J. M., Grabell, J., Chhajlani, V., et al. (2010). Acute pharmacological modulation of mGluR8 reduces measures of anxiety. *Behav. Brain Res.*, Vol. 212, pp. 168-73

Duvoisin, R. M., Villasana, L., Davis, M. J., Winder, D. G., Raber, J. (2011). Opposing roles of mGluR8 in measures of anxiety involving non-social and social challenges. *Behav. Brain Res.*, Vol. 221, pp. 50-4

Efremov, I., Rogers, B., Duplantier, A., Zhang, L., Maklad, N. (2008). *WO Patent No. 2008/012622*

Emmitte, K. A. (2011). Recent advances in the design and development of novel negative allosteric modulators of mGlu5. *ACS Chem. Neurosci.*, ACS ASAP

Engers, D., Gentry, P., Williams, R., Bolinger, J., Weaver, D., et al. (2010). Synthesis and SAR of novel, 4-(phenylsulfamoyl)phenylacetamide mGlu4 positive allosteric modulators (PAMs) identified by functional high-throughput screening (HTS). *Bioorg. Med. Chem. Lett.*, Vol. 20, pp. 5175-8

Engers, D., Niswender, C., Weaver, C., Jadhav, S., Menon, U., et al. (2009). Synthesis and evaluation of a series of heterobiarylamides that are centrally penetrant metabotropic glutamate receptor 4 (mGluR4) positive allosteric modulators (PAMs). *J. Med. Chem.*, Vol. 52, pp. 4115-8

Fell, M. J., Witkin, J. M., Falcone, J. F., Katner, J. S., Perry, K. W., et al. (2011). N-(4-((2-(trifluoromethyl)-3-hydroxy-4-(isobutyryl)phenoxy)methyl)benzyl)-1-methyl-1H-imidazole-4-carboxamide (THIIC), a novel metabotropic glutamate 2 potentiator with potential anxiolytic/antidepressant properties: in vivo profiling suggests a link between behavioral and central nervous system neurochemical changes. *J. Pharmacol. Exp. Ther.*, Vol. 336, pp. 165-77

Fontana, E., Dansette, P., Poli, S. (2005). Cytochrome P450 Enzymes Mechanism Based Inhibitors: Common Sub-Structures and Reactivity. *Curr. Drug. Metab.*, Vol. 6, pp. 413-54

Foroozesh, M., Primrose, G., Guo, Z., Bell, L., Alworth, W., Guengerich, F. (1997). Aryl acetylenes as mechanism-based inhibitors of cytochrome P450-dependent monooxygenase enzymes. *Chem. Res. Toxicol.*, Vol. 10, pp. 91-102

Fujinaga, M., Yamasaki, T., Kawamura, K., Kumata, K., Hatori, A., et al. (2011). Synthesis and evaluation of 6-[1-(2-[18F]fluoro-3-pyridyl)-5-methyl-1H-1,2,3-triazol-4-yl]quinoline for positron emission tomography imaging of the metabotropic glutamate receptor type 1 in brain. *Bioorg. Med. Chem.*, Vol. 19, pp. 102-10

Galambos, J., Wágner, G., Nógrádi, K., Bielik, A., Molnár, L., et al. (2010). Carbamoyloximes as novel non-competitive mGlu5 receptor antagonists. *Bioorg. Med. Chem. Lett.*, Vol. 20, pp. 4371-5

Garbaccio, R. M., Brnardic, E. J., Fraley, M. E., Hartman, G. D., Hutson, P. H., et al. (2010). Discovery of oxazolobenzimidazoles as positive allosteric modulators for the mGluR2 receptor. *ACS Med. Chem. Lett.*, Vol. 1, pp. 406-10

Gasparini, F., Andres, H., Flor, P. J., Heinrich, M., Inderbitzin, W., et al. (2002). [^{3}H]-M-MPEP, a potent, subtype-selective radioligand for the metabotropic glutamate receptor subtype 5. *Bioorg. Med. Chem. Lett.*, Vol. 12, pp. 407-9

Gasparini, F., Lingenhohl, K., Stoehr, N., Flor, P. J., Heinrich, M., et al. (1999). 2-Methyl-6-(phenylethynyl)-pyridine (MPEP), a potent, selective and systemically active mGlu5 receptor antagonist. *Neuropharmacology*, Vol. 38, pp. 1493-503

Gatti McArthur, S., Goetschi, E. Palmer, W. S., Wichmann, J., Woltering, T. J. (2006a). *Application: WO Patent No. 2006-EP2334 2006099972*

Gatti McArthur, S., Goetschi, E., Wichmann, J. (2006b). *WO Patent No. 2006/082002*

Gatti McArthur, S., Goetschi ,E., Wichmann, J., Woltering, T. J. (2006c). *Application: WO Patent No. 2006-EP940 2006084634*

Gatti Mcarthur, S., Goetschi, E., Wichmann, J., Woltering, T. J. (2007). *Application: WO Patent No. 2007-EP52560 2007110337*

Granberg, K., Holm, B. (2009). *Application: WO Patent No. 2008-SE51195 2009054792*

Granberg, K., Holm, B. (2010). *Application: WO Patent No. 2010-SE50440 2010123451*

Guitart, X., Khurdayan, V. (2005). Metabotropic glutamate receptors as therapeutic targets. *Drug News Perspect*, Vol. 18, pp. 587-93

Hamill, T. G., Krause, S., Ryan, C., Bonnefous, C., Govek, S., et al. (2005). Synthesis, characterization, and first successful monkey imaging studies of metabotropic glutamate receptor subtype 5 (mGluR5) PET radiotracers. *Synapse (Hoboken, NJ, U. S.)*, Vol. 56, pp. 205-16

Henrich, M., Weil, T., Mueller, S., Nagel, J., Gravius, A., et al. (2009). *Application: WO Patent No. 2009-EP616 2009095254*

Honer, M., Stoffel, A., Kessler, L., Schubiger, P., Ametamey, S. (2007). Radiolabeling and in vitro and in vivo evaluation of [(18)F]-FE-DABP688 as a PET radioligand for the metabotropic glutamate receptor subtype 5. *Nucl. Med. Biol.*, Vol. 34, pp. 973-80

Hong, S.-P., Liu, K. G., Ma, G., Sabio, M., Uberti, M. A., Bacolod, M. D., Peterson, , J., Zou, Z. Z., Robichaud, A. J., and Doller, D. (2011) Tricyclic thiazolopyrazole derivatives as novel, potent, selective, and orally available metabotropic glutamate receptor 4 positive allosteric modulators. *J. Med. Chem.* Vol 54, pp. 5070-81

Hostetler, E. D., Eng, W., Joshi, A. D., Sanabria-Bohorquez, S., Kawamoto, H., et al. (2011). Synthesis, characterization, and monkey PET studies of [18F]MK-1312, a PET tracer for quantification of mGluR1 receptor occupancy by MK-5435. *Synapse (Hoboken, NJ, U. S.)*, Vol. 65, pp. 125-35

Huang, Y., Narendran, R., Bischoff, F., Guo, N., Zhu, Z., et al. (2005). A positron emission tomography radioligand for the in vivo labeling of metabotropic glutamate 1 receptor: (3-ethyl-2-[11C]methyl-6-quinolinyl)(cis-   4-methoxycyclohexyl)methanone. *J. Med. Chem.*, Vol. 48, pp. 5096-9

Hwang, D-R., Narendran, R., Huang, Y., Slifstein, M., Talbot, P. S., et al. (2004). Quantitative analysis of (-)-N-11C-propyl-norapomorphine in vivo binding in nonhuman primates. *J. Nucl. Med.*, Vol. 45, pp. 338-46

Imogai, H. J., Cid-Nunez, J. M., Andres-Gil, J. I., Trabanco-Suarez, A. A., Oyarzabal-Santamarina J., et al. (2007). *Application: WO Patent No. 2007-EP52442 2007104783*

Isaac, M., Waallberg, A. (2009). *Application: WO Patent No. 2008-SE51197 2009054794*

Iso, Y., Grajkowska, E., Wroblewski, J. T., Davis, J., Goeders, N. E., et al. (2006). Synthesis and structure-activity relationships of 3-[(2-Methyl-1,3-thiazol-4-yl)ethynyl]pyridine analogues as potent, noncompetitive metabotropic glutamate receptor subtype 5 antagonists; Search for cocaine medications. *J. Med. Chem.*, Vol. 49, pp. 1080-100

Jimenez, H. N., Li, G., Doller, D., Grenon, M., White, A. D., et al. (2010). *Application: WO Patent No. 2009-US50934 2010011570*

Johnson, M. P., Baez, M., Jagdmann, G. E., Jr., Britton, T. C., Large, T. H., et al. (2003). Discovery of allosteric potentiators for the metabotropic glutamate 2 receptor: synthesis and subtype selectivity of N-(4-(2-Methoxyphenoxy)phenyl)-N-(2,2,2-trifluoroethylsulfonyl)pyrid-3-ylmethylamine. *J. Med. Chem.*, Vol. 46, pp. 3189-92

Karakossian, M., Otis, T. (2004). Excitation oof cerebellar interneurons by group I metabotropic glutamate receptors. *J. Neurophysiol.*, Vol. 92, pp. 1558-65

Kew, J. (2004). Positive and negative allosteric modulation of metabotropic glutamate receptors: emerging therapeutic potential. *Pharmacol Ther*, Vol. 104, pp. 233-44

Kew, J., Kemp, J. (2005). Ionotropic and metabotropic glutamate receptor structure and pharmacology. *Psychopharmacology*, Vol. 179, pp. 4-29

Keyvani, K., Bosse, F., Reinecke, S., Paulus, W., Witte, O. (2001). Postlesional transcriptional regulation of metabotropic glutamate receptors: implications for plasticity and excitotoxicity. *Acta Neuropathol*, Vol. 101, pp. 79-84

Keywood, C., Wakefield, M., Tack, J. (2009). A proof-of-concept study evaluating the effect of ADX 10059, a metabotropic glutamate receptor-5 negative allosteric modulator, on acid exposure and symptoms in gastro-oesophageal reflux disease. *Gut*, Vol. 58, pp. 1192-9

Kinney, G. G., O'Brien, J. A., Lemaire, W., Burno, M., Bickel, D. J., et al. (2005). A novel selective positive allosteric modulator of metabotropic glutamate receptor subtype 5 has in vivo activity and antipsychotic-like effects in rat behavioral models. *J. Pharmacol. Exp. Ther.*, Vol. 313, pp. 199-206

Knoflach, F., Mutel, V., Jolidon, S., Kew, J. N. C., Malherbe, P., et al. (2001). Positive allosteric modulators of metabotropic glutamate 1 receptor: characterization, mechanism of action, and binding site. *Proc. Natl. Acad. Sci. U. S. A.*, Vol. 98, pp. 13402-7

Kohara, A., Takahashi, M., Yatsugi, S-i., Tamura, S., Shitaka, Y., et al. (2008). Neuroprotective effects of the selective type 1 metabotropic glutamate receptor antagonist YM-202074 in rat stroke models. *Brain Res.*, Vol. 1191, pp. 168-79

Kornhuber, J., Weller, M. (1997). Psychotogenicity and N-methyl-D-aspartate receptor antagonism: implications for neuroprotective pharmacotherapy. *Biol Psychiatry*, Vol. 41, pp. 135-44

Kozikowski, A. P., Steensma, D., Araldi, G. L., Tueckmantel, W., Wang, S., et al. (1998). Synthesis and biology of the conformationally restricted ACPD analog, 2-aminobicyclo[2.1.1]hexane-2,5-dicarboxylic acid-I, a potent mGluR agonist. *J. Med. Chem.*, Vol. 41, pp. 1641-50

Krause, S., Hamill, T., Seiders, T., et al. (2003). In vivo characterizations of PET ligands for the mGluR5 receptor in rhesus monkey. *Mol. Imaging Biol.*, Vol. 5, pp. 166

Kulkarni, S., Zou, M-F., Cao, J., Deschamps, J., Rodriguez, A., et al. (2009). Structure-activity relationships comparing N-(6-Methylpyridin-yl)-substituted aryl amides to 2-methyl-6-(substituted-arylethynyl)pyridines or 2-methyl-4-(substituted-arylethynyl thiazoles as novel metabotropic glutamate receptor subtype 5 antagonists. *J. Med. Chem.*, Vol. 52, pp. 3563-75

Kumar, J. S. D., Majo, V. J., Hsiung, S-C., Millak, M. S., Liu, K-P., et al. (2006). Synthesis and in vivo validation of [O-methyl-^{11}C]-2-[4-[4-(7-methoxy-1-naphthalenyl)-1-piperazinyl]butyl]-4-methyl-2H-[1,2,4]triazine-3,5-dione: A novel 5-HT1A receptor agonist positron emission tomography ligand. *J. Med. Chem.*, Vol. 49, pp. 125-34

Lavreysen, H., Janssen, C., Bischoff, F., Langlois, X., Leysen, J., Lesage, A. (2003). [3H]R214127: a novel high-affinity radioligand for the mGlu1 receptor reveals a common binding site shared by multiple allosteric antagonists. *Mol. Pharmacol.*, Vol. 63, pp. 1082-93

Lavreysen, H., Pereira, S., Leysen, J., Langlois, X., Lesage, A. (2004a). Metabotropic glutamate 1 receptor distribution and occupancy in the rat brain: a quantitative autoradiographic study using [3H]R214127. *Neuropharmacology*, Vol. 46, pp. 609-19

Lavreysen, H., Wouters, R., Bischoff, F., Nobrega Pereira, S., Langlois, X., et al. (2004b). JNJ16259685, a highly potent, selective and systemically active mGlu1 receptor antagonist. *Neuropharmacology*, Vol. 47, pp. 961-72

Layton, M. (2005). Subtype-selective noncompetitive modulators of metabotropic glutamate receptor subtype 1 (mGluR1). . *Curr Top Med Chem*, Vol. 5, pp. 859-67

Lesage, A. (2004). Role of group I metabotropic glutamate receptors mGlu1 and mGlu5 in Nociceptive signalling. *Curr. Neuropharmacology*, Vol. 2, pp. 363-93

Lindsley, C., Bates, B., Menon, U., Jadhav, S., Kane, A., et al. (2011). (3-Cyano-5-fluorophenyl)biaryl negative allosteric modulators of mGlu5: Discovery of a new tool compound with activity in the OSS mouse model of addiction. *ACS Chem. Neurosci.*, Vol. 2, ASAP

Lindsley, C. W., Wisnoski, D. D., Leister, W. H., O'Brien, J. A., Lemaire, W., et al. (2004). Discovery of positive allosteric modulators for the metabotropic glutamate receptor subtype 5 from a series of N-(1,3-Diphenyl-1H- pyrazol-5-yl)benzamides that potentiate receptor function in vivo. *J. Med. Chem.*, Vol. 47, pp. 5825-8

Litschig, S., Gasparini, F., Rueegg, D., Stoehr, N., Flor, P. J., et al. (1999). CPCCOEt, a noncompetitive metabotropic glutamate receptor 1 antagonist, inhibits receptor signaling without affecting glutamate binding. *Mol. Pharmacol.*, Vol. 55, pp. 453-61

Lucas, D., Newhouse, J. (1957). The toxic effect of sodium L-glutamate on the inner layers of the retina. *AMA Arch Opthalmol*, Vol. 58, pp. 193-201

Lucatelli, C., Honer, M., Salazar, J-F., Ross, T. L., Schubiger, P., Ametamey, S. (2009). Synthesis, radiolabeling, in vitro and in vivo evaluation of [18F]-FPECMO as a positron emission tomography radioligand for imaging the metabotropic glutamate receptor subtype 5. *Nuclear Medicine and Biology*, Vol. 36, pp. 613-22

Mabire, D., Coupa, S., Adelinet, C., Poncelet, A., Simonnet, Y., et al. (2005). Synthesis, structure-activity relationship, and receptor pharmacology of a new series of quinoline derivatives acting as selective, noncompetitive mGlu1 antagonists. *J. Med. Chem.*, Vol. 48, pp. 2134-53

Malherbe, P., Kratochwil, N., Knoflach, F., Zenner, M-T., Kew, J. N. C., et al. (2003). Mutational analysis and molecular modeling of the allosteric binding site of a novel, selective, noncompetitive antagonist of the metabotropic glutamate 1 receptor. *J. Biol. Chem.*, Vol. 278, pp. 8340-7

Mantell, S. J., Gibson, K. R., Osborne, S. A., Maw, G. N., Rees, H., et al. (2009). In vitro and in vivo SAR of pyrido[3,4-d]pyramid-4-ylamine based mGluR1 antagonists. *Bioorg. Med. Chem. Lett.*, Vol. 19, pp. 2190-4

Marin, JC. A., Goadsby, P. J. (2010). Glutamatergic fine tuning with ADX-10059: a novel therapeutic approach for migraine? *Expert Opin. Invest. Drugs*, Vol. 19, pp. 555-61

Marino, M., Hess, J., Liverton, N. (2005). Targeting the metabotropic glutamate receptor mGluR4 for the treatment of diseases of the central nervous system. . *Curr Top Med Chem*, Vol. 5, pp. 885-95

Marino, M., Wittmann, M., Bradley, S., Hubert, G., Smith, Y., Conn, P. (2001). Activation of group I metabotropic glutamate receptors produces a direct excitation and disinhibition of GABAergic projection neurons in the substantia nigra pars reticulata. *J Neurosci*, Vol. 21, pp. 7001-12

Micheli, F., Di Fabio, R., Bordi, F., Cavallini, P., Cavanni, P., et al. (2003a). 2,4-Dicarboxypyrroles as selective non-competitive mGLUR1 antagonists: further characterization of 3,5-dimethylpyrrole-2,4-dicarboxylic acid 2-propyl ester 4-(1,2,2-trimethylpropyl) ester and structure-activity relationships. *Bioorg. Med. Chem. Lett.*, Vol. 13, pp. 2113-8

Micheli, F., Di Fabio, R., Cavanni, P., Rimland, J.M., Capelli, A. M., et al. (2003b). Synthesis and pharmacological characterization of 2,4-dicarboxy-pyrroles as selective non-competitive mGluR1 antagonists. *Bioorg. Med. Chem.*, Vol. 11, pp. 171-83

Milbank, J., Knauer, C., Augelli-Szafran, C., Sakkab-Tan, A., Lin, K., et al. (2007). Rational design of 7-arylquinolines as non-competitive metabotropic glutamate receptor subtype 5 antagonists. *Bioorg. Med. Chem. Lett.*, Vol. 17, pp. 4415-8

Miller, P., Long, N., Vilar, R., Gee, A. (2008). Synthesis of 11C, 18F, 15O, and 13N radiolabels for positron emission tomography. *Angew. Chem. int. ed*, Vol. 47, pp. 8998-9033

Mitsukawa, K,. Yamamoto, R., Ofner, S., Nozulak, J., Pescott, O., et al. (2005). A selective metabotropic glutamate receptor 7 agonist: activation of receptor signaling via an allosteric site modulates stress parameters in vivo. *Proc Natl Acad Sci U S A*, Vol. 102, pp. 18712-7

Musachio, J., Ghose, S., Toyama, H., et al. (2003). Two potential mGluR5 PET radioligands, [11C]M-MPEP and [11C]Methoxy-PEPy – synthesis and initial PET evaluation in rats and monkeys in vivo. *Mol. Imaging Biol.*, Vol. 5, pp. 168

Mutlib, A., Lam, W., Atherton, J., Chen, H., Galatsis, P., Stolle, W. (2005). Application of stable isotope labeled glutathione and rapid scanning mass spectrometers in detecting and characterizing reactive metabolites. *Rapid Commun. Mass Spectrom.*, Vol. 19, pp. 3482-92

Mutlib, A. E., Chen, H., Nemeth, G. A., Markwalder, J. A., Seitz, S. P., et al. (1999). Identification and characterization of efavirenz metabolites by liquid chromatography/mass spectrometry and high field NMR: species differences in the metabolism of efavirenz. *Drug Metab. Dispos.*, Vol. 27, pp. 1319-33

Nakamura, M., Kurihara, H., Suzuki, G., Mitsuya, M., Ohkubo, M., Ohta, H. (2010). Isoxazolopyridone derivatives as allosteric metabotropic glutamate receptor 7 antagonists. *Bioorganic & Medicinal Chemistry Letters*, Vol. 20, pp. 726-9

Niswender, C., Jones, C., Conn, P. (2005). New therapeutic frontiers for metabotropic glutamate receptors. *Curr Top Med Chem*, Vol. 5, pp. 847-57

O'Brien, J. A., Lemaire, W., Chen, T-B., Chang, R. S. L., Jacobson, M. A., et al. (2003). A family of highly selective allosteric modulators of the metabotropic glutamate receptor subtype 5. *Mol. Pharmacol.*, Vol. 64, pp. 731-40

O'Brien, J., Lemaire, W., Wittmann, M. (2004). A novel selective allosteric modulator potentiates the activity of native metabotropic glutamate receptor subtype 5 in rat forebrain. *J Pharmacol Exp Ther*, Vol. 309, pp. 568-77

O'Neill, M. (2001). Pharmacology and neuroprotective actions of mGlu receptor ligands. . *Dev Med Child Neurol Suppl*, Vol. 86, pp. 13-5

Ohgami, M., Haradahira, T., Takai, N., Zhang, M-R. (2009). *Eur. J. Nucl. Med. Mol. Imag.*, Vol. 36, pp. S310

Olive, M. F. (2009). Metabotropic glutamate receptor ligands as potential therapeutics for addiction. *Curr. Drug Abuse Rev.*, Vol. 2, pp. 83-98

Oney, J. (1978). *Neurotoxicity of excitatory amino acids*. New York: Raven Press. 27 pp.

Ott, D., Floersheim, P., Inderbitzin, W., Stoehr, N., Francotte, E., et al. (2000). Chiral resolution, pharmacological characterization, and receptor docking of the noncompetitive mGlu1 receptor antagonist (+-)-2-hydroxyimino- 1a,2-dihydro-1H-7-oxacyclopropa[b]naphthalene-7a-carboxylic acid ethyl ester. *J. Med. Chem.*, Vol. 43, pp. 4428-36

Owen, D. R., Dodd, P. G., Gayton, S., Greener, B. S., Harbottle, G. W., et al. (2007). Structure-activity relationships of novel non-competitive mGluR1 antagonists: A potential treatment for chronic pain. *Bioorg. Med. Chem. Lett.*, Vol. 17, pp. 486-90

Passchier, J., Gee, A., Willemsen, A., Vaalburg, W., Waarde, Av. (2002). Measuring drug related-receptor occupancy with positron emission tomography. *Methods*, Vol. 27, pp. 278-86

Patel, S., Hamill, T., Connolly, B., Jagoda, E., Li, W., Gibson, R. (2007). Species differences in mGluR5 binding sites in mammalian central nervous system determined using in vitro binding with [18F]F-PEB. *Nuclear Medicine and Biology*, Vol. 34, pp. 1009-17

Patel, S., Ndubizu, O., Hamill, T., Chaudhary, A., Burns, H. D., et al. (2005). Screening cascade and development of potential positron emission tomography radiotracers for mGluR5: in vitro and in vivo characterization. *Mol Imaging Biol*, Vol. 7, pp. 314-23

Pekhletski, R., Gerlai, R., Overstreet, L. S., et al. (1996). Impaired cerebellar synaptic plasticity and motor performance in mice lacking the mGluR4 subtype of metabotropic glutamate receptor. *J Neurosci*, Vol. 16, pp. 6364-73.

Pin, J., Duvoisin, R. (1995). Review: neurotransmitter receptors I. The metabotropic glutamate receptors: structure and functions. *Neuropharmacology*, Vol. 34, pp. 1-26

Pin, J-P., Galvez, T., Prezeau, L. (2003). Evolution, structure, and activation mechanism of family 3/C G-protein-coupled receptors. . *Pharmacol Ther*, Vol. 98, pp. 325-54

Popoli, P., Pezzola, A., Torvinen, M., et al. 2001. The selective mGlu(5) receptor agonist CHPG inhibits quinpirole-induced turning in 6-hydroxydopamine-lesioned rats and modulates the binding characteristics of dopamine D(2) receptors in the rat striatum: interactions with adenosine A(2a) receptors. *Neuropsychopharmacology*. Vol. 25, pp. 505-13

Porter, R. H. P., Jaeschke, G., Spooren, W., Ballard, T. M., Buttelmann, B., et al. (2005). Fenobam: A clinically validated nonbenzodiazepine anxiolytic is a potent, selective, and noncompetitive mGlu5 receptor antagonist with inverse agonist activity. *J. Pharmacol. Exp. Ther.*, Vol. 315, pp. 711-21

Prabhakaran, J., Majo, V. J., Milak, M. S., Kassir, S. A., Palner, M., et al. (2010). Synthesis, in vitro and in vivo evaluation of [^{11}C]MMTP: A potential PET ligand for mGluR1 receptors. *Bioorg. Med. Chem. Lett.*, Vol. 20, pp. 3499-501

Prabhakaran, J., Parsey, R. V., Majo, V. J., Hsiung, S-C., Milak, M. S., et al. (2006). Synthesis, in vitro and in vivo evaluation of [O-methyl-11C] 2-{4-[4-(3-methoxyphenyl)piperazin-1-yl]-butyl}-4-methyl-2H-[1,2,4]-triazine-3,5-dione: A novel agonist 5-HT1A receptor PET ligand. *Bioorg. Med. Chem. Lett.*, Vol. 16, pp. 2101-4

Rao, A., Hatcher, J., Dempsey, R. (2000). Neuroprotection by group I metabotropic glutamate receptor antagonist in forebrain ischemia of gerbil. *Neurosci Lett*, Vol. 293, pp. 1-4

Reynolds, I. J. (2008). Metabotropic glutamate receptors as therapeutic targets in Parkinson's disease. *6th international meeting on metabotropic glutamate receptors*. Taoromino, Sicily, Italy

Ritzen, A., Mathiesen, J., Thomsen, C. (2005). Molecular pharmacology and therapeutic prospects of metabotropic glutamate receptor allosteric modulators. *Basic Clin Pharmacol Toxicol*, Vol. 97, pp. 202-13

Rouse, S., Marino, M., Bradley, S., Award, H., Wittmann, M., Conn, P. (2000). Distribution and roles of metabotropic glutamate receptors in the basal ganglia motor circuit: implications for treatment of Parkinson's disease and related disorders. *Pharmacol Ther*, Vol. 88, pp. 427-35

Rudd, M., McCauley, J. (2005). Positive allosteric modulators of the metabotropic glutamate receptor subtype 2 (mGluR2). . *Curr Top Med Chem*, Vol. 5, pp. 869-84

Sanchez-Pernaute, R., Wang, J. Q., Kuruppu, D., Cao, L., Tueckmantel, W., et al. (2008). Enhanced binding of metabotropic glutamate receptor type 5 (mGluR5) PET tracers in the brain of parkinsonian primates. *Neuroimage*, Vol. 42, pp. 248-51

Sasikumar, T. K., Qiang, L., Burnett, D. A., Greenlee, W. J., Li, C., et al. (2010). A-ring modifications on the triazafluorenone core structure and their mGluR1 antagonist properties. *Bioorg. Med. Chem. Lett.*, Vol. 20, pp. 2474-7

Satoh, A., Nagatomi, Y., Hirata, Y., Ito, S., Suzuki, G., et al. (2009). Discovery and in vitro and in vivo profiles of 4-fluoro-N-[4-[6-(isopropylamino)pyrimidin-4-yl]-1,3-thiazol-2-yl]-N-methylbenzamide as novel class of an orally active metabotropic glutamate receptor 1 (mGluR1) antagonist. *Bioorg. Med. Chem. Lett.*, Vol. 19, pp. 5464-8

Schoepp, D., Goldsworthy, J., Johnson, B., Salhoff, C., Baker, S. (1994). 3,5-dihydroxyphenylglycine is a highly selective agonist for phosphorinositide-linked metabotropic glutamate receptors in the rat hippocampus. *J Neurochem*, Vol. 1994, pp. 769-72

Schoepp, D. D., Jane, D. E., Monn, J. A. (1999). Pharmacological agents acting at subtypes of metabotropic glutamate receptors. *Neuropharmacology*, Vol. 38, pp. 1431-76

Sharma, S., Lindsley, C. (2007). A new high affinity PET tracer for the metabotropic glutamate receptor subtype 5 (mGluR5). *Curr. Top. Med. Chem.*, Vol. 7, pp. 1541-2

Shigemoto, R., Mizuno, N. (2000). Metabotropic glutamate receptors - immunocytochemical and in situ hybridization analyses. *Handbook Chemical Neuroanat.*, Vol. 18, pp. 63-98

Shimada, T., Murayama, N., Okada, K., Funae, Y., Yamazaki, H., Guengerich, F. P. (2007). Different mechanisms for inhibition of human cytochromes P450 1A1, 1A2, and 1B1 by polycyclic aromatic inhibitors. *Chem. Res. Toxicol.*, Vol. 20, pp. 489-96

Sime´on, F., Brown, A., Zoghbi, S., Patterson, V., Innis, R., Pike, V. (2007). Synthesis and simple ^{18}F-labeling of 3-fluoro-5-(2-(2-(fluoromethyl)thiazol-4-yl)ethynyl benzonitrile as a high affinity radioligand for imaging monkey brain metabotropic glutamate subtype-5 receptors with positron emission tomography. *J. Med. Chem.*, Vol. 50, pp. 3256-66

Simonyi, A., Ngomba, R. T., Storto, M., Catania, M. V., Miller, L. A., et al. (2005). Expression of groups I and II metabotropic glutamate receptors in the rat brain during aging. *Brain Res.*, Vol. 1043, pp. 95-106

Skerry, T., Genever, P. (2001). Glutamate signaling in non-neuronal tissues. *Trends Pharmacol. Sci.*, Vol. 22, pp. 174-81

Slassi, A., Isaac, M., Edwards, L., Minidis, A., Wensbo, D., et al. (2005). Recent advances in non-competitive mGlu5 receptor antagonists and their potential therapeutic applications. *Curr. Top. Med. Chem. (Sharjah, United Arab Emirates)*, Vol. 5, pp. 897-911

Spanka, C., Glatthar, R., Desrayaud, S., Fendt, M., Orain, D., et al. (2010). Piperidyl amides as novel, potent and orally active mGlu5 receptor antagonists with anxiolytic-like activity. *Bioorganic & Medicinal Chemistry Letters*, Vol. 20, pp. 184-8

Spooren, W., Ballard, T., Gasparini, F., Amalric, M., Mutel, V., Schreiber, R. (2003). Insight into the function of group I and group II metabotropic glutamate (mGlu) receptors: behavioural characterization and implications for the treatment of CNS disorders. *Behav. Pharmacol.*, Vol. 14, pp. 257-77

Suzuki, G., Kawagoe-Takaki, H., Inoue, T., Kimura, T., Hikichi, H., et al. (2009). Correlation of receptor occupancy of metabotropic glutamate receptor subtype 1 (mGluR1) in mouse brain with in vivo activity of allosteric mGluR1 antagonists. *J. Pharmacol. Sci. (Tokyo, Jpn.)*, Vol. 110, pp. 315-25

Suzuki, G., Kimura, T., Satow, A., Kaneko, N., Fukuda, J., et al. (2007a). Pharmacological characterization of a new, orally active and potent allosteric metabotropic glutamate receptor 1 antagonist, 4-[1-(2-fluoropyridin-3-yl)-5-methyl-1H-1,2,3-

triazol-4-yl]-N-isopropyl-N-methyl-3,6-dihydropyridine-1(2H)-carboxamide
(FTIDC). *J. Pharmacol. Exp. Ther.*, Vol. 321, pp. 1144-53

Suzuki, G., Tsukamoto, N., Fushiki, H., Kawagishi, A., Nakamura, M., et al. (2007b). In vitro
pharmacological characterization of novel isoxazolopyridone derivatives as
allosteric metabotropic glutamate receptor 7 antagonists. *J. Pharmacol. Exp. Ther.*,
Vol. 323, pp. 147-56

Tanabe, Y., Nomura, A., Masu, M., Shigemoto, R., Mizuno, N., Nakanishi, S. (1997). Signal
transduction, pharmacological properties, and expression patterns of two
metabotropic glutamate receptors, mGluR3 and mGluR4. *J Neurosci*, Vol. 13, pp.
1372-8

Testa, B., Jenner, p. (1981). Inhibitors of Cytochrome P-450s and Their Mechanism of Action.
Drug Metab. Rev., Vol. 12, pp. 1-117

Varnes, J., Marcus, A., Mauger, R., Throner, S., Hoesch, V., et al. (2011). Discovery of novel
positive allosteric modulators of the metabotropic glutamate receptor 5 (mGlu5).
Bioorganic & Medicinal Chemistry Letters, Vol. 21, pp. 1402-6

Varney, M. A., Cosford, N. D., Jachec, C., Rao, S. P., Sacaan, A., et al. (1999). SIB-1757 and
SIB-1893: selective, noncompetitive antagonists of metabotropic glutamate receptor
type 5. *J Pharmacol Exp Ther*, Vol. 290, pp. 170-81

Wang, J-Q., Tueckmantel, W., Zhu, A., Pellegrino, D., Brownell, A-L. (2007a). Synthesis and
preliminary biological evaluation of 3-[18F]fluoro-5-(2-
pyridinylethynyl)benzonitrile as a PET radiotracer for imaging metabotropic
glutamate receptor subtype 5. *Synapse (Hoboken, NJ, U. S.)*, Vol. 61, pp. 951-61

Wang, X., Kolasa, T., El Kouhen, O. F., Chovan, L. E., Black-Shaefer, C. L., et al. (2007b).
Rapid hit to lead evaluation of pyrazolo[3,4-d]pyrimidin-4-one as selective and
orally bioavailable mGluR1 antagonists. *Bioorg. Med. Chem. Lett.*, Vol. 17, pp. 4303-7

Wichmann, J., Bleicher, K., Vieira, E., Woltering, T., Knoflach, F., Mutel, V. (2002). Alkyl
diphenylacetyl, 9H-xanthene- and 9H-thioxanthene-carbonyl carbamates as
positive allosteric modulators of mGlu1 receptors. *Farmaco*, Vol. 57, pp. 989-92

Williams, D. J., Lindsley, C. (2005). Discovery of positive allosteric modulators of
metabotropic glutamate receptor subtype 5 (mGluR5). *Curr Top Med Chem*, Vol. 5,
pp. 825-46

Williams, R., Manka, J., Rodriguez, A., Vinson, P., Niswender, C., et al. (2011). Synthesis and
SAR of centrally active mGlu5 positive allosteric modulators based on an aryl
acetylenic bicyclic lactam scaffold. *Bioorg. Med. Chem. Lett.*, Vol. 21, pp. 1350-3

Wilson. A. A., McCormick, P., Kapur, S., Willeit, M., Garcia, A., et al. (2005). Radiosynthesis
and evaluation of [11C]-(+)-4-propyl-3,4,4a,5,6,10b-hexahydro-2H-naphtho[1,2-
b][1,4]oxazin-9-ol as a potential radiotracer for in vivo imaging of the dopamine D2
high-affinity state with positron emission tomography. *J. Med. Chem.*, Vol. 48, pp.
4153-60

Woltering, T. J., Adam, G., Alanine, A., Wichmann, J., Knoflach, F., et al. 2007. Synthesis and
characterization of 8-ethynyl-1,3-dihydro-benzo[b][1,4]diazepin-2-one derivatives:
New potent non-competitive metabotropic glutamate receptor 2/3 antagonists. Part
1. *Bioorg. Med. Chem. Lett.*, Vol. 17, pp. 6811-5

Woltering, T. J., Adam, G., Wichmann, J., Goetschi, E, Kew, J. N. C., et al. (2008a). Synthesis
and characterization of 8-ethynyl-1,3-dihydro-benzo[b][1,4]diazepin-2-one

derivatives: Part 2. New potent non-competitive metabotropic glutamate receptor 2/3 antagonists. *Bioorg. Med. Chem. Lett.*, Vol. 18, pp. 1091-5

Woltering, T. J., Wichmann, J., Goetschi, E., Adam, G., Kew, J. N. C., et al. (2008b). Synthesis and characterization of 1,3-dihydro-benzo[b][1,4]diazepin-2-one derivatives: Part 3. New potent non-competitive metabotropic glutamate receptor 2/3 antagonists. *Bioorg. Med. Chem. Lett.*, Vol. 18, pp. 2725-9

Woltering, T. J., Wichmann, J., Goetschi, E., Knoflach, F., Ballard, T. M., et al. (2010). Synthesis and characterization of 1,3-dihydro-benzo[b][1,4]diazepin-2-one derivatives: Part 4. In vivo active potent and selective non-competitive metabotropic glutamate receptor 2/3 antagonists. *Bioorg. Med. Chem. Lett.*, Vol. 20, pp. 6969-74

Wu, W-L., Burnett, D. A., Domalski, M., Greenlee, W. J., Li, C., et al. (2007). Discovery of orally efficacious tetracyclic metabotropic glutamate receptor 1 (mGluR1) antagonists for the treatment of chronic pain. *J. Med. Chem.*, Vol. 50, pp. 5550-3

Yanamoto, K., Konno, F., Odawara, C., Yamasaki, T., Kawamura, K., et al. (2010). Radiosynthesis and evaluation of [^{11}C]YM-202074 as a PET ligand for imaging the metabotropic glutamate receptor type 1. *Nuclear Medicine and Biology*, Vol. 37, pp. 615-24

Yang, Z-Q. (2005). Agonists and antagonists for group III metabotropic glutamate receptors 6, 7, and 8. *Curr Top Med Chem*, Vol. 5, pp. 913-8

Yasuhara, A., Sakagami, K., Yoshikawa, R., Chaki, S., Nakamura, M., Nakazato, A. (2006). Synthesis, in vitro pharmacology, and structure-activity relationships of 2-aminobicyclo[3.1.0]hexane-2,6-dicarboxylic acid derivatives as mGluR2 antagonists. *Bioorg. Med. Chem.*, 14, pp. 3405-20

Yu, M., Brownell, A-L. (2002). Synthesis of C-11 CPCCOMe, a potent PET ligand for imaging mGluR1 in vivo. *Molecular Imaging*, Vol. 1, pp. 230

Yu, M., Tueckmantel, W., Wang, X., Zhu, A., Kozikowski, A., Brownell, A-L. (2005). Methoxyphenylethynyl, methoxypyridylethynyl and phenylethynylderivatives of pyridine: synthesis, radiolabeling and evaluation of new PET ligands for metabotropic glutamate subtype 5 receptors. . *Nucl. Med. Biol.*, Vol. 32, pp. 631-40

Yu, M., Tueckmantel, W., Wang, X., Zhu, A., Kozikowski, A. P., Brownell, A-L. (2005). Methoxyphenylethynyl, methoxypyridylethynyl and phenylethynyl derivatives of pyridine: synthesis, radiolabeling and evaluation of new PET ligands for metabotropic glutamate subtype 5 receptors. *Nucl Med Biol*, Vol. 32, pp. 631-40

Zhang, L., Rogers, B. N., Duplantier, A. J., McHardy, S. F., Efremov, I., et al. (2008). 3-(Imidazolylmethyl)-3-aza-bicyclo[3.1.0]hexan-6-yl)methyl ethers: A novel series of mGluR2 positive allosteric modulators. *Bioorg. Med. Chem. Lett.*, Vol. 18, pp. 5493-6

Zheng, G. Z., Bhatia, P., Daanen, J., Kolasa, T., Patel, M., et al. (2005). Structure-activity relationship of triazafluorenone derivatives as potent and selective mGluR1 antagonists. *J. Med. Chem.*, Vol. 48, pp. 7374-88

Zhu, A., Wang, X., Yu, M., Wang, J-Q., Brownell, A-L. (2007). Evaluation of four pyridine analogs to characterize 6-OHDA induced modulation of mGluR5 function in rat brain using microPET studies. *J. Cereb. Blood. Flow. Metab.*, Vol. 27, pp. 1623-31

7

Advances in MR Imaging of Leukodystrophies

Eva-Maria Ratai[1], Paul Caruso[1] and Florian Eichler[2]
[1]Department of Radiology,
[2]Department of Neurology,
Massachusetts General Hospital,
Harvard Medical School, Boston, MA,
USA

1. Introduction

Leukodystrophies are hereditary disorders of white matter that impair brain that is initially normally formed and developed (1, 2). They can affect brain myelin throughout life. The disorders are commonly progressive in nature and ultimately fatal. First manifestations are often cognitive deterioration and neuropsychological problems. Motor and balance difficulties occur, as do visual abnormalities. Classic leukodystrophies lead to a vegetative state or death within months to years. In general, the earlier the onset of symptoms, the more progressive the disease course.

Most leukodystrophies are monogenetic disorders. The mutant gene often encodes an enzyme or protein that maintains neuronal and/or glial health and is responsible for regulation of brain metabolism. Many enzymes involved play a role in lipid metabolism. The inability to degrade or synthesize substrate leads to an upstream excess or downstream lack of vital lipids. This can cause a wide range of pathology, from inflammatory demyelination to axonal degeneration and microglial activation. Hence, the often cited prominent demyelination is only one manifestation in leukodystrophies, and myelin-forming oligodendrocytes are not the only cells affected in these disorders.

Yet, there are some common characteristics that distinguish the pathology in leukodystrophies from that of other disorders. MRI has played a seminal role in visualization of the lesion pattern. (3). The demyelinating lesions are usually confluent and symmetric. Many of the classic disorders, such as X-linked adrenoleukodystrophy (X-ALD), metachromatic leukodystrophy (MLD) and Krabbe, show relative sparing of subcortical fibers. Yet again, other disorders have early involvement of the U fibers and other unique characteristics, such as cystic rarefaction and degeneration.

Hereditary disorders that do not show demyelination but rather hypomyelination have come to increasing attention (4). Common neurological features in hypomyelinating disorders are developmental delay, nystagmus, cerebellar ataxia and spasticity. One of the better characterized hypomyelinating disorders is Pelizaeus Merzbacher disease (PMD). Beyond this classic disorder, a multitude of other hypomyelinating disorders exist. Only about half of the patients with evidence of hypomyelination on MRI come to a definitive diagnosis. Yet, specific clinical and MRI features can be pathognomonic and lead to diagnosis.

The current review aims to present the diagnostic MRI lesion patterns of leukodystrophies, as well as the utility of advanced MR techniques. While some of these techniques are already established in clinical practice, others are still experimental in nature and require future validation.

2. Conventional brain MRI lesion patterns in LD

Overall, MR imaging has made an enormous contribution to the field of leukodystrophies due to the precise lesion pattern evident on MRI (5). Many leukodystophies classically show imaging features that, in some cases, are pathognomonic and, in some cases, highly suggestive of the diagnosis. Both demyelinating and hypomyelinating disorders carry distinct features and are listed in **Tables 1 and 2**. While the patterns of maturation of white matter are similar on T1 and T2 weighted images, white matter appears to mature at a later time on T2 weighted images. This is crucial, as it indicates that T1 weighted imaging may be more sensitive to immature myelin than T2 weighted imaging.

In its most severe form, X-ALD is a lethal neurodegenerative disorder with inflammatory demyelination. Defective peroxisomal beta-oxidation causes accumulation of very long-chain fatty acids (VLCFA) in tissues and plasma, particularly in the nervous system and adrenal glands. At least four clinical phenotypes have been delineated: childhood cerebral (CCALD), adult cerebral, adrenomyeloneuropathy (AMN), and female heterozygotes for X-ALD.

In CCALD, the posterior regions of the brain are involved in 80-90% and the frontal regions are involved in 5-10% (6, 7). The lesion evolves in a symmetric confluent fashion starting in the splenium or genu of the corpus callosum and spreading into the periventricular white matter (**Figure 1**). The arcuate fibers are most often spared. In the acute phase, a garland of contrast enhancement is present. In the final stages, white matter atrophy is seen. The systematic progression has given rise to a scoring system of 34 points (8, 9). This pattern is markedly different than that seen in the adult form of the disease, AMN, a non-inflammatory chronic axonopathy.

In Krabbe disease, the parieto-occipital lesions are also present, although a garland of contrast enhancement is never seen (10, 11). MLD shows more diffuse involvement of both frontal and posterior regions of the brain (12). Involvement of the corpus callosum is seen early, although not as striking as that seen in ALD or GLD. A tigroid pattern is often apparent in the centrum semiovale. In contrast to ALD, the outer subarachnoid spaces are not enlarged in MLD, even in the most advanced stages of disease.

Other disorders have characteristic early involvement of the subcortical fibers. Children with Canavan disease present with an enlarged head ("megalencephaly"), but show less behavioral changes than other leukodystrophies of infancy. (13, 14). Their MRI shows diffuse involvement of white matter including the subcortical U fibers (15). There is also involvement of basal ganglia and other gray matter structures. Alexander disease is another leukodystrophy that often manifests with megalencephaly (16). Imaging studies of the brain typically show cerebral white matter abnormalities, preferentially affecting the frontal region, although unusual variants are coming to increasing attention (17, 18).

The MRI of vanishing white matter disease (VWMD) also has a characteristic pattern. It shows progressive loss of white matter over time on proton density and FLAIR images (19-21). The findings on autopsy confirm the white matter rarefaction and cystic degeneration suggested by the MRI. Regions of relative sparing include the U-fibers, corpus callosum, internal capsule, and the anterior commissure. The cerebellar white matter and brainstem show variable degrees of involvement but do not undergo cystic degeneration.

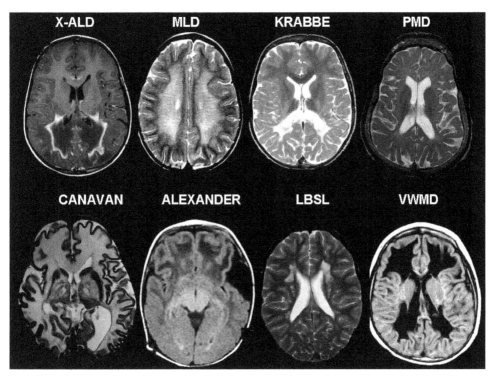

Fig. 1. Lesion Patterns on Conventional MRI in Leukodystrophies and Hypomyelinating Disorders

Brainstem lesion patterns can also often provide critical clues to the diagnosis. Leukoencephalopathy with Brainstem and Spinal Cord Involvement and Elevated White Matter Lactate (LBSL) has recently been described and shows distinct involvement of the pyramidal tracts, medial lemniscus, mesencephalic trigeminal tracts, corticobulbar tracts, and superior cerebellar peduncles. (22). Recognition of the distinct lesion pattern led to the identification of the responsible gene DARS2, which encodes mitochondrial aspartyl-tRNA synthetase.

In hypomyelinating disorders, the boundaries between gray and white matter often appear "blurred" (4). The T2 hypointensity of the white matter is milder in hypomyelination than in demyelination and other white matter pathology. Overall, the brain MRI in hypomyelination looks like that of a young child, with less well distinguished gray and white matter. As opposed to "delayed myelination," the pattern on brain MRI is unchanged, as in myelination is "stuck" on two MRIs 6-12 months apart in a child older than one year of age. While at first glance, hypomyelinating disorders may all have a similar MRI appearance, there are a group of disorders for which the MRI scan can provide clues to the diagnosis (see **Table 2**). In these individual disorders attention to the deep gray matter structures will often reveal a characteristic "signature" (4).

Leukodystrophy	Mutated genes	Characteristics on Brain MRI
Aicardi-Goutières syndrome (78, 79)	TREX1	Often with microcephaly and intracranial calcifications (CT)
Alexander Disease	GFAP	Macrocephaly with frequent frontal lesion predominance in childhood, variants with abnormalities in medulla and spinal cord, ventricular garlands
Canavan Disease	ASPA	Macrocephaly, subcortical U fibers and basal ganglia involved
Cerebral autosomal dominant arteriopathy with subcortical infarcts and leukoencephalopathy (CADASIL)	NOTCH3	Multiple small hemorrhages. Widened perivascular spaces in the centrum semiovale and basal ganglia
Cerebrotendineous Xanthomatosis	CYP27A1	Cerebellar lesions, calcifications visible on CT
Globoid Leukodystrophy (Krabbe Disease)	GALC	Posterior predominance, no contrast enhancement
Leukoencephalopathy with Brain Stem and Spinal Cord Involvement and Elevated Lactate	DARS2	Characteristic brainstem pattern: pyramidal tracts, cerebellar connections and intraparenchymal trajectories of trigeminal nerve
Megalencephalic Leukodystrophy with Cysts (80, 81)	MLC1, GLIALCAM	Macrocephaly with swelling of cerebral white matter and cystic lesions (bilateral anterior temporal lobes)
Metachromatic leukodystrophy	ARSA	Diffuse with initial subcortical sparing, "tigroid pattern" in centrum semiovale
Vanishing White Matter Disease	EIF2B1-5	Confluent cystic degeneration, white matter signal appears CSF-like
X-Linked Adrenoleukodystrophy	ABCD1	CCALD: posterior predominance with contrast enhancement in acute phase AMN: corticospinal tracts and dorsal columns, no contrast enhancement

Table 1. Characteristics on Brain MRI in Leukodystrophies

Hypomyelinating Disorder	Mutated genes	Characteristics on Brain MRI
Fucosidosis	FUCA1	T2 hypointensity globus pallidus
GM2 gangliosidoses	HEXA, HEXB	T2 hyperintensity in the basal ganglia
Hypomyelination with atrophy of the basal ganglia and cerebellum	unknown	Atrophy of the basal ganglia and cerebellum
Hypomyelination, Hypodontia, Hypogonadotropic Hypogonadism	unknown	Early cerebellar atrophy with absence of putamen
Pelizaeus-Merzbacher Disease	PLP1	Homogeneous T2 hyperintensity of cerebral white matter
Pelizaeus-Merzbacher-like Disease	GJC2, SLC16A2	Pontine T2 hyperintensity

Table 2. Characteristics on Brain MRI in Hypomyelinating Disorders

Advanced magnetic resonance (MR) imaging techniques, such as proton MR spectroscopic and diffusion tensor (DT) MR imaging, permit the investigation of changes in metabolite levels and water diffusion parameters in leukodystrophy patients. Both metabolite measures and water diffusion parameters offer an opportunity to assess the degree of axonal loss and demyelination in the leukodystrophies.

3. Proton MR spectroscopy

Magnetic resonance spectroscopy (MRS) offers the unique ability to measure metabolite levels in vivo in a non-invasive manner (23, 24, 25). These metabolite quantifications can be used to identify disease, measure the severity of an injury, or monitor a patient's response to treatment. Table 3 shows the most well characterized metabolite abnormalities detected by MRS in leukodystrophies.

The resonances seen in the brain by MRS are typically low weight molecules (see Figure 2). In the normal brain, the most prominent peak arises from N-acetylaspartate (NAA) at 2.0 ppm. The other major peaks include creatine (Cr) and phosphocreatine (phospho-Cr), which are observed at 3.0 and 3.3 ppm, respectively, as well as choline containing compounds. 1H MR spectra acquired with short echo times are characterized by additional resonances from myo-inositol (MI) at 3.5 ppm, and glutamate and glutamine, which overlap with each other so that they are often referred to as Glx, at ~2.5 ppm. Under normal conditions, the lactate concentration is very low in the adult brain. This resonance (observed as a doublet) occurs at 1.32 ppm.

NAA within the adult brain is found exclusively in neurons, serving as a marker of neuronal density and viability and reported to be decreased in a number of neurological disorders.

Leukodystrophy or Hypomyelinating Disorder	Systemic metabolites	Brain metabolites abnormalities on proton MR spectroscopy
Alexander Disease	Unknown	Infantile form: myoinositol elevations in white and gray matter, decreased N-acetylaspartate
Canavan Disease	Urine N-acetylaspartate	Highly elevated N-acetylaspartate
Cerebrotendineous Xanthomatosis	Plasma cholestanol	Lipid peaks seen in cerebellum
Globoid Leukodystrophy (Krabbe Disease)	Plasma glucocerebrosides, psychosine	Choline and myoinositol elevations, decreased N-acetylaspartate
GM2 gangliosidoses	GM2 gangliosides	Infantile: variable choline, myoinositol and N-acetylaspartate. Late onset: decreased N-acetylaspartate
Hypomyelination with atrophy of the basal ganglia and cerebellum	Unknown	Increased myoinositol and creatine
Leukoencephalopathy with Brain Stem and Spinal Cord Involvement and Elevated Lactate	Unknown	Decreased N-acetylaspartate and increased myo-inositol, choline and lactate
Leukoencephalopathy associated with a disturbance in the metabolism of polyols (83, 84)	Arabinitol and ribitol in urine, plasma and CSF	Elevated levels of arabinitol and ribitol (coupled resonances between 3.5 and 4ppm)
Megalencephalic Leukodystrophy with Cysts	Unknown	Decreased ratio of N-acetylaspartate to Creatine
Pelizaeus-Merzbacher Disease	Unknown	Variable reports on changes in N-acetylaspartate and choline
Vanishing White Matter Disease	Decreased ratio of asialotransferrin to transferrin in CSF	Within cystic white matter complete absence of all metabolites
X-Linked Adrenoleukodystrophy	Plasma very long chain fatty acids	CCALD: Choline elevations within normal appearing white matter, elevations of lactate within the lesion. AMN: decreased N-acetylaspartate in adrenomyeloneuropathy

Table 3. Brain Metabolites Abnormalities on Proton MR Spectroscopy

NAA is the source of acetyl in myelin membrane biosynthesis (26) and is coupled to lipid metabolism and energy generation (27). Creatine serves as a marker for energy-dependent systems in cells and it tends to be low in processes that have low metabolism, such as necrosis and infarction. As Cr and phospho-Cr are in equilibrium, the Cr peak is thought to remain stable in size, despite bioenergetic abnormalities that occur with multiple pathologies. Consequently, the Cr resonance is often used as an internal standard.

The choline (Cho) resonance arises from signals of several soluble components that resonate at 3.2 ppm. This resonance contains contributions primarily from glycerophosphocholine (GPC), phosphocholine (PCho), and Cho. Changes in this resonance are commonly seen with diseases that have alterations in membrane turnover and in inflammatory and gliotic processes (28, 29). The function of MI is not fully understood, although it is believed to be an essential requirement for cell growth, an osmolyte, and a storage form for glucose (30). MI is primarily located in glia, and an increase in MI is commonly thought to be a marker of gliosis (31). Lactate is produced by anaerobic metabolism, and increased lactate has been found during hypoxia (32), mitochondrial diseases (33, 34), seizures (35), and in the first hours after birth (36, 37).

In the developing brain, Cho and MI are the dominant peaks in the MR spectrum. Their levels are high compared to Cr. In contrast, NAA levels are low in newborns and increase with age, while Cho and MI decrease with age. During the first 6 months of life, these metabolic changes are most rapid, leveling off at about 30 months of age (50). These changes are crucial, as both hypomyelination and delayed myelination affect changes of these metabolites.

In X-ALD, proton MRS sometimes shows metabolite abnormalities beyond the margins of disease depicted by conventional MR imaging (38). The white matter lesion in children with X-ALD shows reduced NAA/Cr and increased Cho/Cr, MI/Cr and Glx/Cr (30). Spectroscopic changes in normal appearing white matter (NAWM) that precede disease progression in patients with X-ALD have been described (39). The changes are an increase in choline and a decrease in NAA. They occur in areas where subsequent lesion progression is observed, but not in the remainder of the brain. These areas may represent a zone of impending or beginning demyelination.

Adrenomyeloneuropathy (AMN) is the adult variant of X-ALD. The disease pathology is usually limited to spinal cord and peripheral nerves ("'pure AMN") but shows cerebral involvement on histopathology. MRS studies showed reduced global NAA/Cho and NAA/Cr compared to controls. These changes are most prominent in internal capsule and parieto-occipital white matter. Decreased ratios of NAA in the absence of Cho/Cr elevation suggest prominent axonal involvement (40). Furthermore, Dubey et al demonstrated that the Expanded Disability Status Scale (EDSS) score inversely correlated with global NAA/Cr, suggesting a potential role of axonal injury in clinical disability in pure AMN. (40). Brain involvement demonstrable by MRI is rare in female subjects heterozygous for X-ALD, including those who have clinical evidence of spinal cord involvement. Nevertheless, NAA levels are reduced in the corticospinal projection fibers in female subjects with normal results on MRI, suggesting axonal dysfunction (41).

Canavan disease is caused by a deficiency in aspartoacylase (ASPA), an enzyme involved in the process of degrading NAA to aspartate and acetate. Deficiency leads to the accumulation of NAA, which impairs normal myelination and results in spongiform degeneration of the brain (42, 43). The elevations in NAA can be detected by MR spectroscopy in vivo (**Figure 2**), a diagnostic clue that can then be confirmed by urine measurement of NAA. The distinctly higher NAA peak can even be detected in the newborn

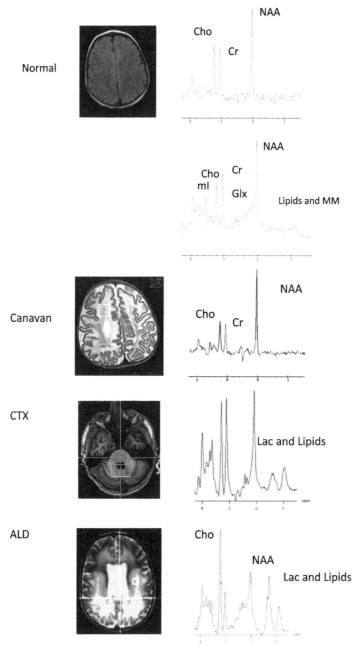

Fig. 2. The spectra of a normal brain are shown at both long echo time (top), TE = 250-280 ms, and short echo time (bottom), TE = 20-50 ms. The spectra for the disease states are as follows: the Canavan spectra are acquired at long echo time, and the ALD and CTX spectra are acquired at short echo time.

although a radiologist only familiar with MR spectra in adults may not recognize the elevation in the newborn as pathologic.

LBSL is a disorder clinically characterized by slowly progressive signs of pyramidal, cerebellar and dorsal column dysfunction. LBSL shows a very distinct MRI pattern, with selective involvement of cerebral and cerebellar white matter and brainstem and spinal tracks, while U-fibers are spared (44). In LBSL, MR spectroscopy characteristically reveals decreased NAA and increased lactate, Cho and MI in the white matter, suggesting axonal damage and gliosis (45). Lately, mutations in the DARS2 gene, which encodes mitochondrial aspartyl-tRNA synthetase, have been identified as the underlying defect.

Cerebrotendinous xanthomatosis (CTX) is a rare but treatable disorder characterized by a defect in the metabolic pathway of cholesterol (46). Symptoms in infancy include diarrhea, cataracts and psychomotor retardation. In adulthood, the spectrum of neurologic dysfunction includes mental retardation leading to dementia, psychiatric symptoms, premature retinal aging, and epileptic seizures. The most distinctive MR imaging abnormalities are bilateral T2 hyperintensities in the dentate nuclei and adjacent cerebellar white matter (47). An MRS study showed a reduction in NAA levels and the presence of a lactate peak (see Figure 2). NAA decreases are attributed to neuroaxonal damage due to neurotoxic deposition of cholesterol (48). A recent case report described the presence of abnormal lipid peaks at 0.9 and 1.3 ppm in the cerebellar hemisphere (49). These peaks can either be attributed to membrane breakdown or they may serve as surrogate markers of major lipid storage, with a potential role in monitoring therapeutic response. In addition, one patient had an increase in MI concentration, pointing to gliosis and astrocytic proliferation (50).

The MR spectra of patients with 4H-Syndrome, a rare form of hypomyelinating leukodystrophy, reveals low Cho/Cr and NAA/Cr, while a prominent MI peak can be observed (51, 52). Low Cho levels are indicative of hypomyelination due to decreased membrane synthesis and turnover. In a new syndrome characterized by Hypomyelination with Atrophy of the Basal Ganglia and Cerebellum (H-ABC), MI and Cr levels are found to be elevated in the cerebral white matter, while NAA and choline levels are normal (53). These findings suggest that neither axonal loss nor active demyelination occurs in the setting of gliosis. In Pelizaeus Merzbacher disease, another hypomyelinating disorder, there have been discrepant reports on metabolite abnormalities detected by MRS. In part, these findings may be explained by the concurrent pathophysiologic processes of hypomyelination, gliosis, and neuronal loss over time (54).

4. Diffusion tensor imaging

While conventional MRI and MR spectroscopy show greatest utility in the diagnoses of leukodystrophies, other techniques, such as diffusion tensor imaging, are starting to be applied to leukodystrophies as well. Diffusion tensor (DT) MRI measures diffusivity of free water molecules in the brain. From the diffusion tensor, one can calculate indices that describe features of the orientationally averaged water diffusivity (isotropic part) and the water molecule displacements affected by the orientation of a regularly ordered structure in the tissue (anisotropic diffusion). Compared to gray matter, in which diffusion shows less directional dependence, white matter apparent diffusion is very anisotropic. (55). This property, termed fractional anisotropy (FA), depends on the orientation of the white matter tracks and on the degree and integrity of myelination (56-59).

In X-ALD, DT imaging may reflect the different abnormal white matter (AWM) zones in patients with X-ALD (60). We and others have observed that FA decreases and the isotropic apparent diffusion coefficient (iADC) increases over the zones toward the center of the lesion. The decrease in mean FA indicates the loss of an ordered structure governing the directionality of water molecule displacement. The increase in mean iADC suggests an increase in free water and a decrease in structures that restrict water diffusion.

In X-ALD, a strong correlation exists between NAA levels and FA, reinforcing the concept that both reflect axonal integrity. However, proton MR spectroscopic imaging reveals a low NAA level in regions with normal MR and DT imaging findings (61). In contrast, DT imaging showed no abnormalities outside the lesion on T2-weighted images. Further, the membrane turnover and cell accumulation associated with beginning demyelination, recognized in the enhanced choline and creatine signal intensity on proton MR spectroscopic imaging, did not have an effect on diffusion parameters. This suggests that proton MR spectroscopic imaging may have a higher sensitivity than both conventional MR and DT imaging in the early detection of abnormalities related to demyelination or axonal loss in X-ALD patients.

However, in other instances, DTI has proven utility over proton MRSI. In pure AMN patients, DTI-based three-dimensional fiber tracking has shown occult tract-specific cerebral microstructural abnormalities in patients who had a normal conventional brain magnetic resonance image (62). This advance in MR imaging demonstrates that the corticospinal tract abnormalities in AMN reflect a centripetal extension of the spinal cord long-tract distal axonopathy.

DTI anisotropy has also proved useful in Krabbe disease (63, 64). In particular, measurements of white matter metabolites may help assess disease progression and determine optimal candidates for treatment options. Patients with Krabbe disease who underwent stem cell transplantation within the 1st month of life showed substantially smaller decreases in anisotropy ratios than those who were treated later. These findings correlate well with global assessments of disease progression as recognized by neurodevelopmental evaluations and conventional MR imaging.

DT MR imaging studies of cerebral white matter development in human premature and term infants demonstrated that, in general, the apparent diffusion coefficient decreases while relative anisotropy increases with brain maturation. The most prominent regional difference at term is the increased relative anisotropy in the internal capsule, indicative of high directionality of diffusion, which could in part be related to myelination. Axonal diameter increases before and during myelination. This diameter change could also contribute in an important way to the diminished water diffusion perpendicular to the orientation of the fiber and thereby contribute to the increase in relative anisotropy. As anisotropy precedes myelination changes seen on conventional imaging, it is expected that quantitative analysis of diffusion parameters would add to the field of hypomyelinating disorders. Yet, little or no data is currently available in this group of disorders. Clearly, more systematic research is needed in regards to hypomyelination and DTI.

5. Recent applications of advanced MR technology

One major technological advance has been imaging at higher field strength. Magnetic resonance imaging at 4 and 7T allows for better visualization of lesion architecture, white matter tracts, and gray-white matter distinction compared with 1.5T. The field of proton MR spectroscopy has also benefited from higher field strength (65, 66). Better spectral resolution results from improved signal-to-noise ratio and chemical-shift dispersion, and this in turn leads to more reliable detection of metabolites such as myoinositol and glutamine.

Using 7T MRSI, decreases in NAA in the cortex of X-ALD patients were detected, which appears greater in male hemizygotes than in female heterozygotes and most pronounced with the occurrence of white matter lesions in males. (66). Although the cytoarchitecture of the cerebral cortex generally appears normal in X-ALD, scattered neuronal loss can be seen in gray matter during a pathologic examination. Both ratios of myoinositol and choline to creatine were found to be higher in normal appearing white matter of adult ALD patients with brain lesions compared to those without lesions. Yet, the interpretation of 7T MRSI data also poses challenges. Voxels close to the scalp show poor water and lipid suppression. Also, the quantification of spectral data in the presence of substantial radiofrequency excitation field (B1) variations is difficult. Therefore, focus has shifted on using adiabatic pulses to compensate for radiofrequency inhomogeneity and reduce the chemical shift displacement error (67, 68).

Overcoming some of the shortcomings of DTI, novel methods now exist to map complex fiber architectures of white matter and other brain tissues. Diffusion spectrum imaging (DSI) allows resolution of regions of 3 way fiber crossings (69-71). On DTI this was not possible as fiber crossing led to decreases in FA, making it difficult to distinguish pathological changes from normal fiber crossings. The years ahead will likely bring more studies employing DSI in leukodystrophy patients.

Advances have also been in the development of ex vivo MRI and novel magnetic resonance contrast agents for imaging of autopsy specimen. In metachromatic leukodystrophy, postmortem studies have demonstrated the pathological correlate of the "tigroid stripes" characteristically seen on conventional imaging (72). Through direct correlation of postmortem MR imaging on 1 cm thick blocks with neuropathology staining, the authors were able to show that perivascular clusters of glial cells containing lipid material corresponded to the stripes on MRI.

Using contrast agents ex vivo, the corresponding substrate of imaging can be further elucidated. One such example is luxol fast blue that displays a binding affinity for myelinated constituents of the brain (73). The specificity of luxol fast blue for lipid constituents results in an increase in longitudinal and transverse relaxation rates of tissue dependent on myelination status. The relaxation rates of white matter increase sufficiently to permit T1-weighted images of ex vivo samples that are similar in contrast behavior to T1-weighted in vivo imaging. The contrast increases in MR images of LFB-stained ex vivo brain tissues enhancing delineation between upper lamina and the more myelinated lower lamina.

Other advances in MR technology have brought great practical benefits. Sedation and anesthesia represent risks in advanced brain disease of LD patients. Using new techniques, such as propeller MRI, it has become possible to oversample k space and, thereby, compensate for motion and allow follow-up MR imaging without sedation (74, 75). As an alternative to these retrospective motion-correction techniques, it is also possible to prospectively correct motion in structural imaging and single-voxel spectroscopy using image-based navigators (76-78). In patients with more advanced leukodystrophies, these advances may allow for imaging without sedation and thereby give insight into the more advanced stages of disease.

Overall, not one advanced imaging technology is expected to bring about a breakthrough in the leukodystrophies. Rather, the multimodal approach with coregistration of high resolution imaging with advanced spectroscopic and diffusion imaging will lead to new pathophysiological insights in the years to come. Different diseases, varying phenotypes, and stages within the disease will require varying imaging modalities.

6. Conclusions

MRI has allowed for much progress in the field of leukodystrophies. Prior to arrival of MRI, the specific vulnerability of brain white matter was not well understood. Today, MRI has helped define disorders through the recognition of specific lesion patterns and their evolution over time. This has also led to identification of novel leukodystrophies and the genes underlying these disorders. Even in previously well characterized disorders, MRI patterns have shed light on disease mechanisms.

The understanding of the pathology and molecular basis of leukodystrophies has in turn allowed for new insight into the significance of MRI changes and elucidated the capabilities of MR techniques. Brain MRI today is a valuable tool in monitoring disease progression and the success of therapeutic interventions in leukodystrophies. Advances in new techniques encourage a multimodal approach employing a variety of sequences sensitive to different brain tissue characteristics. Together, these techniques will be able to provide clues to the early stages of disease – insight not gained by pathology in the past.

7. References

[1] Costello DJ, Eichler AF, Eichler FS. Leukodystrophies: classification, diagnosis, and treatment. Neurologist 2009;15(6):319-28.
[2] Kohlschutter A, Bley A, Brockmann K, Gartner J, Krageloh-Mann I, Rolfs A, et al. Leukodystrophies and other genetic metabolic leukoencephalopathies in children and adults. Brain Dev;32(2):82-9.
[3] van Der Knaap MS. Magnetic Resonance of Myelination and Myelin Disorders, 3rd edition. 2005.
[4] Steenweg ME, Vanderver A, Blaser S, Bizzi A, de Koning TJ, Mancini GM, et al. Magnetic resonance imaging pattern recognition in hypomyelinating disorders. Brain;133(10):2971-82.
[5] Schiffmann R, van der Knaap MS. Invited article: an MRI-based approach to the diagnosis of white matter disorders. Neurology 2009;72(8):750-9.
[6] Moser H SK, Watkins P, Powers J, Moser A. X-linked adrenoleukodystrophy. 8th ed. New York: McGraw Hill; 2000.

[7] Melhem ER, Barker PB, Raymond GV, Moser HW. X-linked adrenoleukodystrophy in children: review of genetic, clinical, and MR imaging characteristics. AJR Am J Roentgenol 1999;173(6):1575-81.

[8] Loes DJ, Hite S, Moser H, Stillman AE, Shapiro E, Lockman L, et al. Adrenoleukodystrophy: a scoring method for brain MR observations. AJNR Am J Neuroradiol 1994;15(9):1761-6.

[9] Loes DJ, Fatemi A, Melhem ER, Gupte N, Bezman L, Moser HW, et al. Analysis of MRI patterns aids prediction of progression in X-linked adrenoleukodystrophy. Neurology 2003;61(3):369-74.

[10] Wenger DA SK, Suzuki Y, Suzuki K. Galactosylceramide lipidosis: globoid cell leukodystrophy (Krabbe disease). 2001:3669-94.

[11] Loes DJ, Peters C, Krivit W. Globoid cell leukodystrophy: distinguishing early-onset from late-onset disease using a brain MR imaging scoring method. AJNR Am J Neuroradiol 1999;20(2):316-23.

[12] Eichler F, Grodd W, Grant E, Sessa M, Biffi A, Bley A, et al. Metachromatic leukodystrophy: a scoring system for brain MR imaging observations. AJNR Am J Neuroradiol 2009;30(10):1893-7.

[13] Kumar S, Mattan NS, de Vellis J. Canavan disease: a white matter disorder. Ment Retard Dev Disabil Res Rev 2006;12(2):157-65.

[14] Surendran S, Matalon KM, Tyring SK, Matalon R. Molecular basis of Canavan's disease: from human to mouse. J Child Neurol 2003;18(9):604-10.

[15] Janson CG, McPhee SW, Francis J, Shera D, Assadi M, Freese A, et al. Natural history of Canavan disease revealed by proton magnetic resonance spectroscopy (1H-MRS) and diffusion-weighted MRI. Neuropediatrics 2006;37(4):209-21.

[16] van der Knaap MS, Naidu S, Breiter SN, Blaser S, Stroink H, Springer S, et al. Alexander disease: diagnosis with MR imaging. AJNR Am J Neuroradiol 2001;22(3):541-52.

[17] van der Knaap MS, Salomons GS, Li R, Franzoni E, Gutierrez-Solana LG, Smit LM, et al. Unusual variants of Alexander's disease. Ann Neurol 2005;57(3):327-38.

[18] van der Knaap MS, Ramesh V, Schiffmann R, Blaser S, Kyllerman M, Gholkar A, et al. Alexander disease: ventricular garlands and abnormalities of the medulla and spinal cord. Neurology 2006;66(4):494-8.

[19] van der Knaap MS, Barth PG, Gabreels FJ, Franzoni E, Begeer JH, Stroink H, et al. A new leukoencephalopathy with vanishing white matter. Neurology 1997;48(4):845-55.

[20] van der Knaap MS, Leegwater PA, Konst AA, Visser A, Naidu S, Oudejans CB, et al. Mutations in each of the five subunits of translation initiation factor eIF2B can cause leukoencephalopathy with vanishing white matter. Ann Neurol 2002;51(2):264-70.

[21] Leegwater PA, Vermeulen G, Konst AA, Naidu S, Mulders J, Visser A, et al. Subunits of the translation initiation factor eIF2B are mutant in leukoencephalopathy with vanishing white matter. Nat Genet 2001;29(4):383-8.

[22] Scheper GC, van der Klok T, van Andel RJ, van Berkel CG, Sissler M, Smet J, et al. Mitochondrial aspartyl-tRNA synthetase deficiency causes eukoencephalopathy

with brain stem and spinal cord involvement and lactate elevation. Nat Genet 2007;39(4):534-9.

[23] Barker PB, Horska A. Neuroimaging in leukodystrophies. J Child Neurol 2004;19(8):559-70.

[24] Barker PB BB, De Stefano N, Gullapalli R, Lin DDM Clinical MR Spectroscopy: Techniques and Applications. 2010.

[25] Lin A, Ross BD, Harris K, Wong W. Efficacy of proton magnetic resonance spectroscopy in neurological diagnosis and neurotherapeutic decision making. NeuroRx, 2(2), 197-214, review (2005).

[26] Chakraborty G, Mekala P, Yahya D, Wu G, Ledeen RW. Intraneuronal N-acetylaspartate supplies acetyl groups for myelin lipid synthesis: evidence for myelin-associated aspartoacylase. J Neurochem 2001;78(4):736-45.

[27] Moffett JR, Ross B, Arun P, Madhavarao CN, Namboodiri AM. N-Acetylaspartate in the CNS: from neurodiagnostics to neurobiology. Prog Neurobiol 2007;81(2): 89-131.

[28] Pouwels PJ, Kruse B, Korenke GC, Mao X, Hanefeld FA, Frahm J. Quantitative proton magnetic resonance spectroscopy of childhood adrenoleukodystrophy. Neuropediatrics 1998;29(5):254-64.

[29] Tzika AA, Ball WS, Jr., Vigneron DB, Dunn RS, Nelson SJ, Kirks DR. Childhood adrenoleukodystrophy: assessment with proton MR pectroscopy. Radiology 1993;189(2):467-80.

[30] Ross BD. Biochemical considerations in 1H spectroscopy. Glutamate and glutamine; myo-inositol and related metabolites. NMR Biomed 1991;4(2):59-63.

[31] Brand A, Richter-Landsberg C, Leibfritz D. Multinuclear NMR studies on the energy metabolism of glial and neuronal cells. Dev Neurosci 1993;15(3-5):289-98.

[32] Kreis R, Arcinue E, Ernst T, Shonk TK, Flores R, Ross BD. Hypoxic encephalopathy after near-drowning studied by quantitative 1H-magnetic resonance spectroscopy. J Clin Invest 1996;97(5):1142-54.

[33] Castillo M, Kwock L, Green C. MELAS syndrome: imaging and proton MR spectroscopic findings. AJNR Am J Neuroradiol 1995;16(2):233-9.

[34] Mathews PM, Andermann F, Silver K, Karpati G, Arnold DL. Proton MR spectroscopic characterization of differences in regional brain metabolic abnormalities in mitochondrial encephalomyopathies. Neurology 1993;43(12):2484-90.

[35] Breiter SN, Arroyo S, Mathews VP, Lesser RP, Bryan RN, Barker PB. Proton MR spectroscopy in patients with seizure disorders. AJNR Am J Neuroradiol 1994;15(2):373-84.

[36] Barkovich AJ, Miller SP, Bartha A, Newton N, Hamrick SE, Mukherjee P, et al. MR imaging, MR spectroscopy, and diffusion tensor imaging of sequential studies in neonates with encephalopathy. AJNR Am J Neuroradiol 2006;27(3):533-47.

[37] Barkovich AJ, Westmark KD, Bedi HS, Partridge JC, Ferriero DM, Vigneron DB. Proton spectroscopy and diffusion imaging on the first day of life after perinatal asphyxia: preliminary report. AJNR Am J Neuroradiol 2001;22(9):1786-94.

[38] Holshouser BA, Ashwal S, Luh GY, Shu S, Kahlon S, Auld KL, et al. Proton MR spectroscopy after acute central nervous system injury: outcome prediction in neonates, infants, and children. Radiology 1997;202(2):487-96.

[39] Kruse B, Barker PB, van Zijl PC, Duyn JH, Moonen CT, Moser HW. Multislice proton magnetic resonance spectroscopic imaging in X-linked adrenoleukodystrophy. Ann Neurol 1994;36(4):595-608.

[40] Eichler FS, Barker PB, Cox C, Edwin D, Ulug AM, Moser HW, et al. Proton MR spectroscopic imaging predicts lesion progression on MRI in X-linked adrenoleukodystrophy. Neurology 2002;58(6):901-7.

[41] Dubey P, Fatemi A, Barker PB, Degaonkar M, Troeger M, Zackowski K, et al. Spectroscopic evidence of cerebral axonopathy in patients with "pure" adrenomyeloneuropathy. Neurology 2005;64(2):304-10.

[42] Fatemi A, Barker PB, Ulug AM, Nagae-Poetscher LM, Beauchamp NJ, Moser AB, et al. MRI and proton MRSI in women heterozygous for X-linked adrenoleukodystrophy. Neurology 2003;60(8):1301-7.

[43] Tsai G, Coyle JT. N-acetylaspartate in neuropsychiatric disorders. Prog Neurobiol 1995;46(5):531-40.

[44] Grodd W, Krageloh-Mann I, Klose U, Sauter R. Metabolic and destructive brain disorders in children: findings with localized proton MR spectroscopy. Radiology 1991;181(1):173-81.

[45] van der Knaap MS, Scheper GC. Leukoencephalopathy with Brain Stem and Spinal Cord Involvement and Lactate Elevation. 1993.

[46] Uluc K, Baskan O, Yildirim KA, Ozsahin S, Koseoglu M, Isak B, et al. Leukoencephalopathy with brain stem and spinal cord involvement and high lactate: a genetically proven case with distinct MRI findings. J Neurol Sci 2008;273(1-2):118-22.

[47] Salen G, Berginer V, Shore V, Horak I, Horak E, Tint GS, et al. Increased concentrations of cholestanol and apolipoprotein B in the cerebrospinal fluid of patients with cerebrotendinous xanthomatosis. Effect of chenodeoxycholic acid. N Engl J Med 1987;316(20):1233-8.

[48] De Stefano N, Dotti MT, Mortilla M, Federico A. Magnetic resonance imaging and spectroscopic changes in brains of patients with cerebrotendinous xanthomatosis. Brain 2001;124(Pt 1):121-31.

[49] Pilo de la Fuente B, Ruiz I, Lopez de Munain A, Jimenez-Escrig A. Cerebrotendinous xanthomatosis: neuropathological findings. J Neurol 2008;255(6):839-42.

[50] Embirucu EK, Otaduy MC, Taneja AK, Leite CC, Kok F, Lucato LT. MR spectroscopy detects lipid peaks in cerebrotendinous xanthomatosis. AJNR Am J Neuroradiol;31(7):1347-9.

[51] Outteryck O, Devos D, Jissendi P, Boespflug-Tanguy O, Hopes L, Renard D, et al. 4H syndrome: a rare cause of leukodystrophy. J Neurol;257(10):1759-61.

[52] Wolf NI, Harting I, Boltshauser E, Wiegand G, Koch MJ, Schmitt-Mechelke T, et al. Leukoencephalopathy with ataxia, hypodontia, and hypomyelination. Neurology 2005;64(8):1461-4.

[53] van der Knaap MS, Linnankivi T, Paetau A, Feigenbaum A, Wakusawa K, Haginoya K, et al. Hypomyelination with atrophy of the basal ganglia and cerebellum: follow-up and pathology. Neurology 2007;69(2):166-71.

[54] Cecil KM. MR spectroscopy of metabolic disorders. Neuroimaging Clin N Am 2006;16(1):87-116, viii.

[55] Basser PJ, Mattiello J, LeBihan D. MR diffusion tensor spectroscopy and imaging. Biophys J 1994;66(1):259-67.

[56] Mori S, Crain BJ, Chacko VP, van Zijl PC. Three-dimensional tracking of axonal projections in the brain by magnetic resonance imaging. Ann Neurol 1999;45(2):265-9.

[57] Wakana S, Jiang H, Nagae-Poetscher LM, van Zijl PC, Mori S. Fiber tract-based atlas of human white matter anatomy. Radiology 2004;230(1):77-87.

[58] Mori S, Oishi K, Faria AV. White matter atlases based on diffusion tensor imaging. Curr Opin Neurol 2009;22(4):362-9.

[59] Wakana S, Caprihan A, Panzenboeck MM, Fallon JH, Perry M, Gollub RL, et al. Reproducibility of quantitative tractography methods applied to cerebral white matter. Neuroimage 2007;36(3):630-44.

[60] Ito R, Melhem ER, Mori S, Eichler FS, Raymond GV, Moser HW. Diffusion tensor brain MR imaging in X-linked cerebral adrenoleukodystrophy. Neurology 2001;56(4):544-7.

[61] Eichler FS, Itoh R, Barker PB, Mori S, Garrett ES, van Zijl PC, et al. Proton MR spectroscopic and diffusion tensor brain MR imaging in X-linked adrenoleukodystrophy: initial experience. Radiology 2002;225(1):245-52.

[62] Dubey P, Fatemi A, Huang H, Nagae-Poetscher L, Wakana S, Barker PB, et al. Diffusion tensor-based imaging reveals occult abnormalities in adrenomyeloneuropathy. Ann Neurol 2005;58(5):758-66.

[63] Escolar ML, Poe MD, Smith JK, Gilmore JH, Kurtzberg J, Lin W, et al. Diffusion tensor imaging detects abnormalities in the corticospinal tracts of neonates with infantile Krabbe disease. AJNR Am J Neuroradiol 2009;30(5):1017-21.

[64] Provenzale JM, Escolar M, Kurtzberg J. Quantitative analysis of diffusion tensor imaging data in serial assessment of Krabbe disease. Ann N Y Acad Sci 2005;1064:220-9.

[65] Oz G, Tkac I, Charnas LR, Choi IY, Bjoraker KJ, Shapiro EG, et al. Assessment of adrenoleukodystrophy lesions by high field MRS in non-sedated pediatric patients. Neurology 2005;64(3):434-41.

[66] Ratai E, Kok T, Wiggins C, Wiggins G, Grant E, Gagoski B, et al. Seven-Tesla proton magnetic resonance spectroscopic imaging in adult X-linked adrenoleukodystrophy. Arch Neurol 2008;65(11):1488-94.

[67] Tannus A, Garwood M. Adiabatic pulses. NMR Biomed 1997;10(8):423-34.

[68] Andronesi OC, Ramadan S, Ratai EM, Jennings D, Mountford CE, Sorensen AG. Spectroscopic imaging with improved gradient modulated constant adiabaticity pulses on high-field clinical scanners. J Magn Reson;203(2):283-93.

[69] Wedeen VJ, Wang RP, Schmahmann JD, Benner T, Tseng WY, Dai G, et al. Diffusion spectrum magnetic resonance imaging (DSI) tractography of crossing fibers. Neuroimage 2008;41(4):1267-77.

[70] Schmahmann JD, Pandya DN, Wang R, Dai G, D'Arceuil HE, de Crespigny AJ, et al. Association fibre pathways of the brain: parallel observations from diffusion spectrum imaging and autoradiography. Brain 2007;130(Pt 3):630- 53.

[71] Hagmann P, Sporns O, Madan N, Cammoun L, Pienaar R, Wedeen VJ, et al. White matter maturation reshapes structural connectivity in the late developing human brain. Proc Natl Acad Sci U S A;107(44):19067-72.

[72] van der Voorn JP, Pouwels PJ, Kamphorst W, Powers JM, Lammens M, Barkhof F, et al. Histopathologic correlates of radial stripes on MR images in lysosomal storage disorders. AJNR Am J Neuroradiol 2005;26(3):442-6.

[73] Blackwell ML, Farrar CT, Fischl B, Rosen BR. Target-specific contrast agents for magnetic resonance microscopy. Neuroimage 2009;46(2):382-93.

[74] Tamhane AA, Arfanakis K. Motion correction in periodically-rotated overlapping parallel lines with enhanced reconstruction (PROPELLER) and turboprop MRI. Magn Reson Med 2009;62(1):174-82.

[75] Forbes KP, Pipe JG, Karis JP, Farthing V, Heiserman JE. Brain imaging in the unsedated pediatric patient: comparison of periodically rotated overlapping parallel lines with enhanced reconstruction and single-shot fast spin-echo sequences. AJNR Am J Neuroradiol 2003;24(5):794-8.

[76] Hess AT TM, Andronesi OC, Meintjes EM, van der Kouwe AJW. Real-time Motion and B0 corrected single voxel spectroscopy using volumetric navigators. Magnetic Resonance in Medicine (in press) 2011.

[77] Tisdall MD HA, van der Kouwe AJW. Selective k-space Reacquisition in Anatomical Brain Sequences using EPI Navigators. 2010.

[78] White N, Roddey C, Shankaranarayanan A, Han E, Rettmann D, Santos J, et al. PROMO: Real-time prospective motion correction in MRI using image-based tracking. Magn Reson Med;63(1):91-105.

[79] Orcesi S, La Piana R, Fazzi E. Aicardi-Goutieres syndrome. Br Med Bull 2009;89:183-201.

[80] Uggetti C, La Piana R, Orcesi S, Egitto MG, Crow YJ, Fazzi E. Aicardi-Goutieres syndrome: neuroradiologic findings and follow-up. AJNR Am J Neuroradiol 2009;30(10):1971-6.

[81] Lopez-Hernandez T, Ridder MC, Montolio M, Capdevila-Nortes X, Polder E, Sirisi S, et al. Mutant GlialCAM causes megalencephalic leukoencephalopathy with subcortical cysts, benign familial macrocephaly, and macrocephaly with retardation and autism. Am J Hum Genet;88(4):422-32.

[82] Lopez-Hernandez T, Sirisi S, Capdevila-Nortes X, Montolio M, Fernandez-Duenas V, Scheper GC, et al. Molecular mechanisms of MLC1 and GLIALCAM mutations in megalencephalic leukoencephalopathy with subcortical cysts. Hum Mol Genet.

[83] van der Knaap MS, Wevers RA, Struys EA, Verhoeven NM, Pouwels PJ, Engelke UF, et al. Leukoencephalopathy associated with a disturbance in the metabolism of polyols. Ann Neurol 1999;46(6):925-8.
[84] Moolenaar SH, van der Knaap MS, Engelke UF, Pouwels PJ, Janssen-Zijlstra FS, Verhoeven NM, et al. In vivo and in vitro NMR spectroscopy reveal a putative novel inborn error involving polyol metabolism. NMR Biomed 2001;14(3):167-76.

8

Molecular Imaging of α7 Nicotinic Acetylcholine Receptors *In Vivo*: Current Status and Perspectives

Peter Brust and Winnie Deuther-Conrad
Helmholtz-Zentrum Dresden – Rossendorf
Research Site Leipzig
Germany

1. Introduction

Nicotine, named after the French diplomat Jean Nicot who brought the tobacco plant (Nicotiana tabacum) to France, isolated in 1828 as the major pharmacologically active compound in this plant (Posselt & Reimann, 1828), structurally identified between 1890 and 1893 (Pinner, 1893; Pinner & Wolffenstein, 1891), and first synthesized chemically in 1903 (Pictet, 1903), acts on various subtypes of nicotinic acetylcholine receptors (nAChRs) in the brain and in the periphery (Changeux, 2010; Langley, 1906).

Besides tobacco, nicotine is found in plants of the nightshade family (solanaceae) such as tomato, potato, peppers and aubergine (eggplant) but also in tea plants (Schep et al., 2009). Accordingly, it is regularly taken up by the great majority of the human population with a mean daily dietary intake of approximately 1.4 µg per day (Siegmund et al., 1999). The alkaloid is readily absorbed by the lung or intestinal tissue, distributed by the blood and transported across the blood-brain barrier (Allen & Lockman, 2003; Oldendorf et al., 1979). When inhaled it takes about seven seconds for nicotine to reach the brain (Rose et al., 2010), where it binds with high affinity to the heteromeric α4β2 and the homomeric α7 nAChRs, the two most abundant nAChR populations (Changeux, 2010). In the brain, nAChRs are involved in attention and cognition, locomotion, vigilance control, and rewarding mechanisms (Changeux, 2010; Graef et al., 2011), and they are suggested to play a major role in brain development (Hruska et al., 2009; Ross et al., 2010).

Notably, nicotinic receptors, and in particular α7 nAChR, are not only expressed on neurons but virtually on all cell types present in the brain including astrocytes (Sharma & Vijayaraghavan, 2001), microglia (De Simone et al., 2005; Suzuki et al., 2006), oligodendrocyte precursor cells (Sharma & Vijayaraghavan, 2002), and endothelial cells (Hawkins et al., 2005). Accordingly, neuronal and non-neuronal expression of α7 nAChR has also been found in peripheral organs (Albuquerque et al., 2009; Sharma & Vijayaraghavan, 2002).

Molecular imaging *in vivo* as considered in this review relates exclusively to the use of radiolabelled receptor ligands, although occasionally optical imaging has been used to investigate the cholinergic system (Prakash & Frostig, 2005). Molecular imaging of α4β2 nAChR *in vivo* has recently been reviewed (Horti et al., 2010; Sabri et al., 2008). Therefore, the current review is focussed on neuroimaging of α7 nAChRs.

2. Role of α7 nicotinic receptors in normal brain function

α7 nAChRs, discovered in 1990 (Couturier et al., 1990), belong to the superfamily of multisubunit ligand-gated ion channels and mediate the effects of the endogenous neurotransmitter acetylcholine. Homomeric α7 nAChR is functionally distinct from the heteromeric nAChRs due to lower affinity to the agonists acetylcholine and nicotine, and higher affinity to the antagonistic snake venom α-bungarotoxin (α-BGT). Agonist binding induces a change in conformation of all five subunits of the α7 nAChR and leads to opening of the cation-conducting channel across the plasma membrane, probably by cis-trans prolyl isomerisation (Lummis et al., 2005). Regarding ion selectivity, α7 nAChR is known to have the highest permeability to Ca^{2+} ions within all nAChR subtypes (Dajas-Bailador et al., 2002; Gilbert et al., 2009; Sharma & Vijayaraghavan, 2001). Therefore, the activation of α7 nAChR changes the intracellular Ca^{2+} homoestasis both directly as well as indirectly, the latter via voltage-dependent membrane-spanning Ca^{2+} channels as well as Ca^{2+} release channels and pumps in the endoplasmatic reticulum. Downstream events of this Ca^{2+} signalling result in (i) immediate effects, such as neurotransmitter release, (ii) short-term effects, such as receptor desensitisation and recovery, and (iii) long-lasting adaptive effects, such as neuroprotection or changes in the plasticity of the brain via gene expression (Leonard, 2003; Radcliffe & Dani, 1998; Shen & Yakel, 2009). Dependent on the cell-specific pattern of intracellular signalling in neurons with α7 nAChRs located post-, pre- and extrasynaptically (Berg & Conroy, 2002; Frazier et al., 1998; Schilström et al., 2000), these complex functional properties explain the involvement of the α7 nAChR in physiological processes of neurotransmission as well as its role in both acute and chronic neuropathologies (Fig. 1).

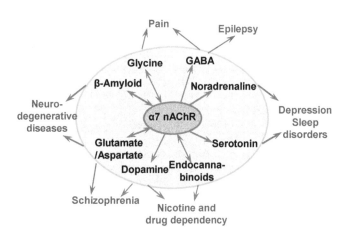

Fig. 1. Involvement of α7 nAChRs in physiological and pathophysiological processes of neurotransmission.

For example, presynaptic α7 nAChRs regulate, either directly or via modulation of glutamate release, the activity profiles of neurotransmitters such as GABA (Albuquerque et al., 1997; Liu et al., 2001), noradrenaline (Fu et al., 1999; Li et al., 1998), or dopamine (Kulak et al., 1997; Northrop et al., 2010) and thereby mediate neuronal adaptation related to development, learning, memory, attention, pain perception, and reward. Furthermore, α7 nAChRs mediate postsynaptic responses in serotonergic neurons involved in maintaining the waking state (Galindo-Charles et al., 2008). An assumed contribution of α7 nAChRs to the formation of endocannabinoids (Stella & Piomelli, 2001) and a proposed regulation of α7 nAChR activity by anandamide (van der Stelt & Di Marzo, 2005) is consistent with a functional interaction of neuromodulating systems involved in drug dependency (McPartland et al., 2008).

Species	Brain region	Radioligand, concentration	Receptor binding*	Referenz
Human	Nucleus reticularis	[^{125}I]α-BGT, 1 nM	5-12 nM	(Spurden et al., 1997)
	Nucleus geniculatis lat.	[^{125}I]α-BGT, 1 nM	2 nM	(Spurden et al., 1997)
	Dorsolateral prefrontal cortex	[^{125}I]α-BGT, 5 nM	9-12 nM	(Mathew et al., 2007)
	Cingulate cortex	[^{125}I]α-BGT, 2.6 nM	~ 16 nM	(Marutle et al., 2001)
	Temporal cortex	[^{125}I]α-BGT, 2.6 nM	~ 8 nM	(Marutle et al., 2001)
	Hippocampus	[^{125}I]α-BGT, 1.2 nM	2-8 nM	(Hellström-Lindahl & Court, 2000)
	Cerebellum	[^{125}I]α-BGT, 1 nM	1-3 nM	(Lee et al., 2002)
Monkey	Cortex	[^{125}I]iodo-MLA	6 nM (B_{max})	(Kulak et al., 2006)
	Striatum	[^{125}I]iodo-MLA	3-4 nM (B_{max})	(Kulak et al., 2006)
		[^{125}I]α-BGT, 3 nM	7.5 nM	(Quik et al., 2005)
Rat	Cortex	[^{3}H]MLA, 5 nM	6-16 nM	(Mugnaini et al., 2002)
		[^{3}H]MLA, 20 nM	~30 fmol/mg protein	(Davies et al., 1999)
		[^{125}I]α-BGT, 10 nM	~40 fmol/mg protein	(Davies et al., 1999)
		[^{125}I]α-BGT	~ 1.1 nM (B_{max})	(Christensen et al., 2010)
	Thalamus	[^{3}H]MLA, 5 nM	0.9 - 21 nM	(Mugnaini et al., 2002)
	Hippocampus	[^{3}H]MLA, 5 nM	6-182 nM	(Mugnaini et al., 2002)
		[^{3}H]MLA, 20 nM	~ 70 fmol/mg protein	(Davies et al., 1999)
		[^{125}I]α-BGT, 10 nM	~ 70 fmol/mg protein	(Davies et al., 1999)
		[^{125}I]α-BGT	~1.2 nM (B_{max})	(Christensen et al., 2010)
	Hypothalamus	[^{3}H]MLA, 5 nM	14-34 nM	(Mugnaini et al., 2002)
		[^{3}H]MLA, 20 nM	~ 55 fmol/mg protein	(Davies et al., 1999)
		[^{125}I]α-BGT, 10 nM	~ 50 fmol/mg protein	(Davies et al., 1999)
Mouse	Cortex	[^{3}H]MLA, 2 nM	1-5 fmol/mg protein	(Whiteaker et al., 1999)
		[^{125}I]α-BGT, 1.2 nM	~ 8 nM	(Svedberg et al., 2002)
		[^{125}I]α-BGT, 2 nM	0-3 fmol/mg protein	(Whiteaker et al., 1999)
	Thalamus	[^{3}H]MLA, 2 nM	1-20 fmol/mg protein	(Whiteaker et al., 1999)
		[^{125}I]α-BGT, 2 nM	0-12 fmol/mg protein	(Whiteaker et al., 1999)
		[^{125}I]α-BGT, 1.2 nM	~ 3 nM	(Svedberg et al., 2002)
	Hippocampus	[^{3}H]MLA, 2 nM	0-9 fmol/mg protein	(Whiteaker et al., 1999)
		[^{125}I]α-BGT, 2 nM	0-4 fmol/mg protein	(Whiteaker et al., 1999)
		[^{125}I]α-BGT, 1.2 nM	~ 12 nM	(Svedberg et al., 2002)
	Hypothalamus	[^{3}H]MLA, 2 nM	1-12 fmol/mg protein	(Whiteaker et al., 1999)
		[^{125}I]α-BGT, 2 nM	1-6 fmol/mg protein	(Whiteaker et al., 1999)

Table 1. Quantitative *in vitro* autoradiographic studies on α7 nAChR binding of various radioligands in the brains of different species, *nM = fmol/mg wet weight

Qualitatively, the expression pattern of α7 nAChR is similar in rodent and primate brain (Han et al., 2000), although a comprehensive and parallel quantitative analysis of α7 nAChR protein expression in the brain of different species, expected to facilitate the translation of experimental data on the imaging of α7 nAChR from *in vitro* and *in vivo* animal models into clinical application, is still warranted. In general, regions with high- to moderate-density of α7 nAChR gene expression and [125I]α-BGT binding are related to learning and memory such as thalamic and hippocampal structures, the horizontal limb of the diagonal band of Broca, and the nucleus basalis of Meynert (Alkondon et al., 2007; Breese et al., 1997; Fabian-Fine et al., 2001; Hellström-Lindahl et al., 1999; Schulz et al., 1991; Spurden et al., 1997). However, species differences exist regarding the total number of binding sites of α7 nAChR specific radioligands (Han et al., 2003) with for example a lower amount of [125I]α-BGT binding in the monkey hippocampus or the human thalamus and cortex compared with the same regions of rat brain (Breese et al., 1997) (Tab. 1).

3. Alterations of α7 nAChR in diseased brain

The World Health Organization has classified dependence on the use of drugs including tobacco as a disease in 1965. During the following decades convincing evidence was obtained that nicotine is the key factor in tobacco addiction and that nicotinic acetylcholine receptors are of importance (Stolerman, 1990). It has been suggested that α7 nAChRs in the ventral tegmental area mediate nicotine´s stimulatory effect on mesolimbocortical dopaminergic function and consequently its reinforcing and dependence-producing properties (Nomikos et al., 2000). As shown in rats, exposure to tobacco smoke not only induced nicotine dependence but increased the α7 nAChR density in the CA2/3 area (+ 25%) and the stratum oriens (+ 18%) of the hippocampus (Small et al., 2010).

With respect to clinical considerations, a close association between nicotine addiction and schizophrenia has been found (Lohr & Flynn, 1992). Consistent with the hypothesis, that a gene-mediated dysfunction of α7 nAChR (Dome et al., 2010; Freedman et al., 1997; Stephens et al., 2009) underlies impairments seen in schizophrenia (Nomikos et al., 2000), the density of hippocampal [125I]α-BGT binding sites was decreased in schizophrenic patients (Freedman et al., 1995) but was at control levels in schizophrenic smokers (Mexal et al., 2010).

Evidence for an involvement of α7 nAChR in Alzheimer's disease (AD) was obtained at about 30 years ago from data showing a significantly reduced number of [125I]α-BGT binding sites in the mid-temporal gyrus from demented patients (Davies & Feisullin, 1981). During the last decade, comparable results were obtained by analysing other neurodegenerative diseases. Lewy body dementia (DLB) and Parkinson´s disease have also been associated with alterations in the transcription or translation of the α7 subunit (Burghaus et al., 2003; Court et al., 2000; Nordberg, 2001; Wevers & Schröder, 1999), indicating a hypocholinergic tone due to for example reduced levels of α7 mRNA and protein in the hippocampus and reticular nucleus in AD and DLB (Court et al., 1999; Guan et al., 2000; Hellström-Lindahl et al., 1999). Functional interactions of β-amyloid with α7 nAChR, revealed *in vitro* (Wang et al., 2000), and the colocalization of both in AD support the hypothesis that neuronal degeneration in AD might also be triggered by β-amyloid-initiated and α7 nAChR-mediated inflammatory processes (Bencherif & Lippiello, 2010).

Interestingly, also in traumatic brain injury (TBI), regarded as risk factor for AD (Fleminger et al., 2003), significantly lowered α7 nAChR densities were found in rats and pigs (Hoffmeister et al., 2010). The resulting cholinergic hypofunction may attenuate the anti-inflammatory effect of acetylcholine (Rosas-Ballina & Tracey, 2009) and thus contribute to the process of neurodegeneration (Conejero-Goldberg et al., 2008).

Other diseases with potential involvement of α7 nAChR include epilepsy and attention deficit hyperactivity disorder (ADHD). While some forms of epilepsy have recently been associated with alterations of α4 subtype expression (Raggenbass & Bertrand, 2002), there is experimental evidence that α7 nAChR may play a role in epileptogenesis (Dobelis et al., 2003). Based on similarities between schizophrenia and ADHD with regard to a number of disturbances in attention it has been hypothesized that the α7 subunit gene may be of significance in ADHD although experimental data are still missing (Kent et al., 2001). Previous attempts to treat ADHD patients with nicotine (Levin et al., 1996; Potter & Newhouse, 2004) are currently repeated in a Phase II study with the selective α7 nAChR ligand TC-5619 by Targacept Inc.

4. α7 nAChR as target for drug development

Because the activation of α7 nAChR persistently affects synaptic transmission, multiple neurotransmitter and neuropeptide systems, and eventually brain plasticity (Leonard, 2003; Radcliffe & Dani, 1998; Shen & Yakel, 2009), α7 nAChR has been assessed as a potential target for the rational design of drugs for neuroprotective and neuropsychiatric indications. The large number of studies on receptor structure and pharmacology makes α7 nAChR an extensively investigated receptor protein and the continued development of orthosteric ligands and allosteric modulators by the pharmaceutical industry testifies the importance of efforts to assess α7 nAChR expression and functionality in the living human brain (Bunnelle et al., 2004; Mazurov et al., 2006).

Evidence of a correlation between α7 nAChR properties and brain performance has been provided by studies on the attentional and cognitive enhancement obtained by α7 nAChR agonists (Feuerbach et al., 2009; Levin et al., 1999; Roncarati et al., 2009) and positive allosteric modulators (Faghih et al., 2008; Timmermann et al., 2007) as well as on α7 nAChR related pharmacotherapeutic approaches for schizophrenia (Freedman et al., 2008; Olincy et al., 2006; Tregellas et al., 2011), and dementia (Bacher et al., 2010; Kitagawa et al., 2003; Thomsen et al., 2010). Furthermore, electrophysiological (Hurst et al., 2005; Ng et al., 2007) and behavioural data (Bitner et al., 2010; Pacini et al., 2010; Tietje et al., 2008) highlight the potential of α7 nAChR as therapeutic target for neurodegenerative diseases. The close connection between α7 nAChR signalling, inflammation, and neurodegeneration makes α7 nAChR auspicious also for medicinal control of inflammation as an epiphenomenon of many brain disorders (Conejero-Goldberg et al., 2008; de Jonge & Ulloa, 2007; Rosas-Ballina & Tracey, 2009).

5. Noninvasive imaging of α7 receptors in normal and diseased brain

Far beyond what can be analysed postmortem, the non-invasive and real-time investigation of α7 nAChR by means of molecular imaging techniques provides the assessment of temporal and spatial changes in receptor distribution and density during disease progression and drug treatments.

5.1 Technical requirements

The most advanced system for non-invasive diagnostic and therapeutic neuroreceptor imaging is positron emission tomography (PET) (Antoni & Langström, 2008; Hagooly et al., 2008; Heiss & Herholz, 2006). In PET, the quantitative detection of the distribution of radiolabeled molecules *in vivo* with high resolution and sensitivity leads to functional images of brain biochemistry and physiology (Spanoudaki & Ziegler, 2008). PET has now become an advanced nuclear medicine imaging technique integrated into routine clinical use (Galban et al., 2010) and a highly sophisticated tool for experimental animal research (Lancelot & Zimmer, 2010; Xi et al., 2011).

Receptor ligands used for PET are radiolabelled with short-lived positron-emitting isotopes such as ^{15}O, ^{13}N, ^{11}C, and ^{18}F with half-lives of 2, 10, 20.4, and 109.6 min, respectively. The spatial resolution of recently developed clinical PET systems with about 2-3 mm allows tracing of radioligand distribution even within small cerebral nuclei in human brain (Heiss et al., 2004; Lecomte, 2009; Wienhard et al., 2002), and a detailed regional analysis also in rodents (Lancelot & Zimmer, 2010; Lecomte, 2009; Xi et al., 2011) can be achieved with dedicated small-animal PET scanners. To overcome the problem of the anatomic classification of areas with increased or diminished radioligand accumulation, co-registration of brain anatomy with MRI or CT is needed. Software-based approaches used for computerized anatomical alignment have been very successful in brain imaging because of the relatively fixed and uniform structure of the head, and both manual and automated systems have been developed in the last years (Slomka & Baum, 2009). Through the use of multimodal approaches delineation of small-sized but receptor-rich brain areas is considerably improved (Heiss, 2009). During the last decade hybrid PET-CT scanners have been developed, where two gantries for PET and CT are placed back-to-back (Mawlawi & Townsend, 2009). Technically even more challenging is the development of hybrid PET-MRI scanners because of the sensitivity of the photomultiplier tubes of the standard PET detectors to even low magnetic fields. This problem has been solved only recently (Pichler et al., 2008; Pichler et al., 2006) and was first successfully accomplished for small-animal designs (Judenhofer et al., 2008). Very recently, fully integrated PET-MRI systems which allow simultaneous data acquisition have been developed as clinical research instruments, and four prototypes of integrated hybrid PET-MRI scanners were installed at two PET centres in Europe (Germany) and the United States so far. However, several technological and methodical issues have to be addressed before PET-MRI can establish itself as a routine clinical tool (von Schulthess & Schlemmer, 2009).

5.2 Radiotracer development

PET technology, using radionuclides with high specific radioactivity and the opportunity to specifically label a chemical compound by substituting a stable atom with its radioactive counterpart, combined with quantitative measurements of radioactivity, is the preferred modality for molecular imaging (Antoni & Langström, 2008). Despite of some of the limitations in instrumentation discussed above, the bottleneck for broad clinical applications in neuroimaging is the limited availability of suitable radioligands. Among positron-emitting isotopes only ^{11}C and ^{18}F are applicable for imaging of neurotransmitter-related components in the brain. Their short half-live (^{11}C: $t_{1/2}$ = 20.4 min, ^{18}F: $t_{1/2}$ = 109.6 min) allows repeated investigations in the same patient or the same animal with short time intervals. Accordingly, the patient or the animal can be considered as its own reference following a pharmacological intervention. For use in a satellite concept (i.e. with no on-site cyclotron available at the PET center), there is a special demand for PET radioisotopes with longer half-life such as [18]F.

Even though the basic mechanisms of radioligand-target interactions *in vitro* and *in vivo* are identical, *in vivo* imaging requires some additional factors that have to be taken into account. In addition to high-affinity binding and supreme selectivity towards the biological target, key requirements for all types of radioligands, suitable physicochemical properties gain special importance for brain imaging with PET. For example not only the transfer of the radioligand across the blood-brain barrier (BBB) is determined by its lipophilicity (Davson & Segal, 1996; Liu et al., 2010) but also the non-specific binding (Waterhouse, 2003). High accumulation and prolonged retention in the target region with target-to-background ratios of desirably more than 5 are closely related to both the affinity of the radioligand and the density of its potential binding sites, which are small compared to the concentration of non-target proteins. Because saturation of binding sites may be obtained at comparably low radioligand concentrations, the concentration of the radioligand applied has to be about 1000-fold lower than the pharmacological threshold. In other words, high specific activity in the range of 50-500 GBq/μmol has to be achieved, feasible nowadays with both [11]C- and [18]F- labeled radioligands (Antoni & Langström, 2008).

In summary, high target affinity, specificity, sensitivity, metabolic stability and appropriate pharmacokinetics are among the most important features for a good *in vivo* neuroreceptor-imaging agent. Despite the fact that over the past decade a great variety of α7 nAChR selective agents have been developed, so far there are only a few radioligands which fulfil at least some of these criteria and will be discussed below.

5.3 Imaging of α7 nAChR in animal and human brain

Although a radiopharmaceutical for PET imaging of α7 nAChR that fulfills all the above-mentioned pre-conditions is still missing, there is general agreement to develop ligands, which bind to the orthosteric site of the α7 nAChR. The steric and electronic requirements of this site are met by structurally diverse classes of compounds as reviewed recently (Toyohara et al., 2010a), and potential ligands originate from for example benzylidene anabasein compounds such as GTS-21 (Meyer et al., 1998), or the quinuclidine framework such as AR-R-17779, both shown in Fig. 2 (Bodnar et al., 2005; Mazurov et al., 2005; Mullen et al., 2000; Tatsumi et al., 2005). A recently developed highly selective fluorescent α7 nicotinic receptor ligand is restricted to *in vitro* studies because of its chemical structure (Hone et al., 2010).

Despite this basic knowledge and promising experimental data obtained *in vitro*, the imaging of α7 nAChR *in vivo* is still in its infancy. This is not only due to the inadequate *in vivo* performance caused by an insufficient target specificity of radioligands such as the non-negligible 5HT$_3$R binding of otherwise promising quinuclidine-based tracers (Pomper et al., 2005) (Table 2).

Compared to the heteromeric α4β2 nAChRs, imaging of α7 nAChR is challenged by the much lower expression of this target, which is illustrated by the up to 100-fold lower density of binding sites of α7-specific [^{125}I]α-BGT in comparison to α4β2-specific [^{3}H]nicotine in different nuclei of human thalamus (Spurden et al., 1997). Furthermore, the outcome of preclinical studies in primates can hardly be predicted from biodistribution studies in rodents. While in the monkey brain high target-to-nontarget ratios were obtained for the diazabicyclooctane derivatives [¹¹C]A-582941 and [¹¹C]A-844606, both failed with regard to regional distribution and selectivity in the mouse brain (Toyohara et al., 2010b) (Tab. 2).

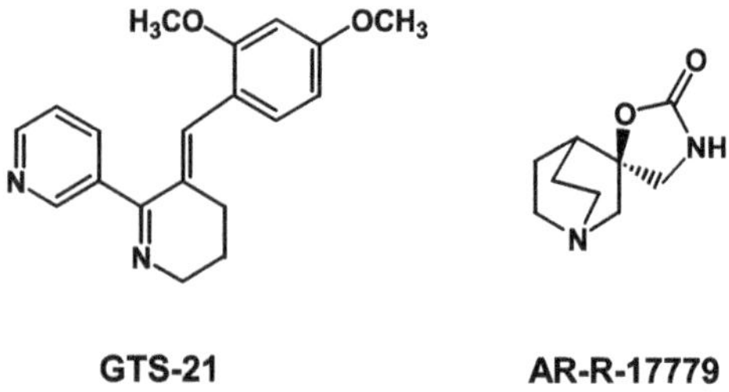

GTS-21   **AR-R-17779**

Fig. 2. Lead structures for development of radioligands for neuroimaging of α7 nAChR

Recently, the 1,4-diazabicyclo-[3.2.2]nonane skeleton (Bunnelle et al., 2004) has been identified as new structure to improve the receptor-ligand interaction, and both ¹⁸F-substituted compounds such as [¹⁸F]NS10743 (Peters et al., 2007) and those for labelling with ¹¹C such as [¹¹C]CHIBA-1001 (Hashimoto et al., 2008; Toyohara et al., 2009) and [¹¹C]NS12857 (Lehel et al., 2009) have been designed (Table 2). As illustrated by the data in Tab. 2, the general suitability of these derivatives for imaging of α7 nAChR is supported by preclinical PET studies in pigs (Deuther-Conrad et al., 2011; Lehel et al., 2009) and non-human primates (Hashimoto et al., 2008) as well as a first clinical study (Toyohara et al., 2009). However, substantial enhancement in the affinity of the α7 nAChR PET ligands is required to improve image analysis, modelling, and eventually quantification of α7 nAChR in brain diseases. Considering the low density of α7 nAChR in brain, the target affinity of the currently most promising tracers [¹¹C]CHIBA-1001 (K_i ~ 35 nM; (Hashimoto et al., 2008; Toyohara et al., 2009) and [¹⁸F]NS10743 (K_i ~ 10 nM; (Deuther-Conrad et al., 2009) has proved insufficient, because dissociation constants of ≥ 10 nM result in baseline binding potential values considerably lower than the threshold value of 2 (Koeppe, 2001). NS14490, a novel diazabicyclononane derivative which has been developed by NeuroSearch and radiolabelled in collaboration with the authors, possesses a K_i value of ~ 3 nM *in vitro* (Deuther-Conrad and colleagues, unpublished), and the ligand distribution pattern of [¹⁸F]NS14490 has been assessed in a first proof-of-principle experiment (Fig. 3).

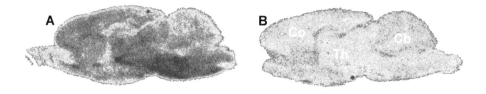

Fig. 3. *In vitro* autoradiography on the distribution of [¹⁸F]NS14490 in rat brain (sagittal slices, 12 μm). A = [¹⁸F]NS14490, total binding; B = Co-incubation of [¹⁸F]NS14490 with 20 μM methyllycaconitine; Abbreviations: Co=cortex; Cb=cerebellum; Th=thalamus.

PET radioligand	Species; Study type	Main findings	Reference
[^{125}I]4	CD1 mice Biodistribution	Very limited uptake of radioactivity in the brain; No evidence of receptor blockade	(Pomper et al., 2005)
[^{11}C]1	SPRD rats Biodistribution	No regionally selective or specific binding	(Dolle et al., 2001)
[^{11}C]NS12857	*Sus scrofa domestica* Dynamic PET scan	High uptake in the pig brain; Distribution as reported in primates; Lack of *in vivo* displacement	(Lehel et al., 2009)
[^{18}F]NS10743	*Sus scrofa domestica* Dynamic PET scan	High uptake in the pig brain; Blocking significantly reduced binding potential in regions with high radioactivity uptake	(Deuther-Conrad et al., 2011)
[2/4-methoxy-^{11}C]GTS-21	*Papio anubis* Dynamic PET scan	Very high initial uptake followed by rapid clearance; Radiometa-bolites penetrate the BBB; High nonspecific binding consistent with the low affinity for α7 nAChR	(Kim et al., 2007)
[^{11}C]MeQAA	*Macaca mulatta* Dynamic PET scan	R-enantiomer with high uptake of radioactivity in the brain and α7 nAChR-related distribution	(Ogawa et al., 2010)
[^{76}Br]SSR180711	*Macaca mulatta* Dynamic PET scan	Substantial and heterogenous brain accumulation; Uptake reduced to background level of the cerebellum by pretreatment with the α7 nAChR agonist SSR180711	(Hashimoto et al., 2008)
[^{11}C]A-582941 [^{11}C]A-844606	*Macaca mulatta* Dynamic PET scan	Regional distribution consistent with α7 nAChR expression	(Toyohara et al., 2010b)
[^{11}C]CHIBA-1001	Clinical PET study (one healthy male subject)	Selective uptake in the regions of the hippocampus, cortex and basal ganglia; gradual washouts; cerebellum with lowest binding	(Toyohara et al., 2009)

Table 2. Findings on *in vivo* biodistribution and PET imaging studies on the binding of α7 nAChR specific radioligands in brain of different species.

6. Noninvasive imaging of α7 nAChR in other diseases – Reality and vision

For another derivative, NS14492, an IC_{50} value of 4.5 nM was reported. It was radiolabelled with ^{11}C and investigated in pigs, where the radioligand showed the capability of measuring *in vivo* occupancy at α7 nAChR (Ettrup et al., 2010).

With regard to molecular imaging, the development of quantitative approaches to visualise α7 nAChR outside the brain is another big challenge because comparably low receptor densities have to be expected also in peripheral organs. Experimental radiotracer studies discussed above provided evidence of specific α7 receptor binding not only in the adrenals with reported receptor densities of less than 10 fmol/mg in human tissue (Mousavi et al., 2001) but also in heart, muscle, gut, kidney, thymus, pancreas and liver (Deuther-Conrad et al., 2009).

In general, imaging the concentration, distribution and occupancy of neuroreceptors involved in respiratory and cardiovascular disorders is a very attractive research area as it can provide new insights in the aetiology of these diseases as well as means to diagnose them (Hagooly et al., 2008). Regarding α7 nAChR, the presence of these receptors in microvascular endothelial cells has been shown and their involvement in the regulation of microvascular permeability and angiogenesis has been suggested (Egleton et al., 2009; Li & Wang, 2006; Moccia et al., 2004).

Furthermore, nicotinic α7 receptors are part of a neural circuit where acetylcholine transmitted via the vagus nerve is thought to control cytokine release as part of the cholinergic anti-inflammatory pathway (Tracey, 2002). This pathway may protect organs such as heart or kidney from ischemic injury (Li et al., 2010; Sadis et al., 2007; Yeboah et al., 2008) and could be of importance in patients with autoimmune diseases known to be characterized by suppressed vagus nerve activity (Bruchfeld et al., 2010). Accordingly, neuroimmunomodulation mediated by α7 nAChR agonists is regarded as a future therapeutic approach (Bencherif et al., 2011; Kumar & Sharma, 2010).

Nicotinic α7 receptors are also regarded as a powerful regulator of responses that stimulate cancer cells (Egleton et al., 2008; Schuller, 2009). In particular, evidence of the involvement of nicotinic α7 receptors in the control of basal cell proliferation and differentiation pathways in lung and the participation of these receptors in airway remodelling during brochopulmonary diseases led to the assumption that α7 nAChRs are of relevance for lung development, injury, repair, and carcinogenesis (Maouche et al., 2009). Because the α7 nAChR is the most predominantly expressed nAChR subtype in bronchial epithelial cells (Paleari et al., 2009) and mRNA for α7 nAChR has been detected not only in normal lung cells but in most human lung cancer cell lines (Egleton et al., 2008; Plummer et al., 2005), it has been hypothesized that a desensitization of α7 nAChR in heavy smokers with a prolonged exposure to nicotine could lead to squamous metaplasia (Tournier & Birembaut, 2011). While in an early investigation of small cell carcinomas of the lung no specific [^{125}I]-α-bungarotoxin binding could be demonstrated, probably due to a sub-threshold density of the α7 receptor protein related to this particular type of cancer (Cunningham et al., 1985), not only all of 50 investigated non-small cell lung cancer (NSCLC) cell lines expressed the α7 subtype (Paleari et al., 2009) but also all out of 52 investigated NSCLC patients expressed α7 receptor mRNA and protein and the values were higher in smoking patients with squamous carcinomas than those with adenocarcinomas (Paleari et al., 2008).

Besides lung cancer, α7 nAChR-mediated signalling has been implicated in the growth and metastasis of colon cancer (Wei et al., 2009; Wei et al., 2011; Ye et al., 2004), probably due to the activity of the endogenous allosteric α7 nAChR modulator SLURP-1 and the upregulation of the downstream signalling molecule NF-κB (Chernyavsky et al., 2010; Pettersson et al., 2008; Ye et al., 2004). Also the development of keratinocyte carcinoma, the most prevalent skin cancer and the most common cancer in United States (Albert & Weinstock, 2003), may depend on α7 nAChR expression and regulation. Interestingly, antagonisation of nAChR activity by SLURP-1 and -2 prevented the tobacco nitrosamine-induced malignant transformation of oral keratinocytes (Arredondo et al., 2007), cells known to express α7 nAChR (Chernyavsky et al., 2010). Further cancers with known α7 nAChR expression include breast, pancreas, and prostate carcinomas (Al-Wadei et al., 2009; Dasgupta et al., 2009; Hirata et al., 2010; Hruska et al., 2009).

Based on this evidence, α7 nAChR is considered a primary target in ongoing research on pathogenesis of a variety of cancers. Furthermore, the quantitative imaging of disease-related changes in the expression of peripheral α7 nAChR by PET is highly desirable for the validation of novel approaches in diagnostics and development of cancer-specific therapy.

7. Conclusion

Generally, the development of imaging approaches to non-invasively quantify α7 nAChR receptors in and outside the brain is expected to help in the generation and testing of novel hypotheses supporting the understanding of pathogenetic processes and promoting novel diagnostic and therapeutic concepts. The clinical significance of a malfunction of α7 nAChR, involved in particular cell-type and pathology specific modulating and signalling cascades, can be assessed on molecular level with an imaging-supported spatiotemporal quantification of α7 nAChR protein. In this context, the imaging technique must be sensitive enough not only to identify but also to assess the dynamics and quantity of even subtle changes in the amount of functional α7 nAChR, which is despite its physiological importance expressed at comparably low levels in the brain and periphery. PET techniques offer the highest achievable resolution of functional processes in the body in four dimensions by imaging of α7 nAChR with further optimised PET radiotracers, which might be based for instance on the currently most promising diazabicyclononane derivatives.

8. References

Al-Wadei, H. A., Al-Wadei, M. H. & Schuller, H. M. (2009). Prevention of pancreatic cancer by the beta-blocker propranolol. *Anti-Cancer Drugs*, Vol.20, No.6, (July 2009), pp 477-482, ISSN 0959-4973

Albert, M. R. & Weinstock, M. A. (2003). Keratinocyte carcinoma. *CA: A Cancer Journal for Clinicians*, Vol.53, No.5, (September 2003), pp 292-302, ISSN 0007-9235

Albuquerque, E. X., Pereira, E. F., Alkondon, M. & Rogers, S. W. (2009). Mammalian nicotinic acetylcholine receptors: from structure to function. *Physiological Reviews*, Vol.89, No.1, (Jan 2009), pp 73-120, ISSN 0031-9333

Albuquerque, E. X., Alkondon, M., Pereira, E. F., Castro, N. G., Schrattenholz, A., Barbosa, C. T., Bonfante-Cabarcas, R., Aracava, Y., Eisenberg, H. M. & Maelicke, A. (1997). Properties of neuronal nicotinic acetylcholine receptors: pharmacological characterization and modulation of synaptic function. *Journal of Pharmacology and Experimental Therapeutics*, Vol.280, No.3, (March 1997), pp 1117-1136, ISSN 0022-3565

Alkondon, M., Pereira, E. F. & Albuquerque, E. X. (2007). Age-dependent changes in the functional expression of two nicotinic receptor subtypes in CA1 stratum radiatum interneurons in the rat hippocampus. *Biochemical Pharmacology*, Vol.74, No.8, (October 2007), pp 1134-1144, ISSN 0006-2952

Allen, D. D. & Lockman, P. R. (2003). The blood-brain barrier choline transporter as a brain drug delivery vector. *Life Sciences*, Vol.73, No.13, (August 2003), pp 1609-1615, ISSN 0024-3205

Antoni, G. & Langström, B. (2008). Radiopharmaceuticals: molecular imaging using positron emission tomography. *Handb Exp Pharmacol*, No.185 Pt 1, 2008), pp 177-201, ISSN 0171-2004

Arredondo, J., Chernyavsky, A. I. & Grando, S. A. (2007). SLURP-1 and -2 in normal, immortalized and malignant oral keratinocytes. *Life Sciences*, Vol.80, No.24-25, (May 2007), pp 2243-2247, ISSN 0024-3205

Bacher, I., Rabin, R., Woznica, A., Sacco, K. A. & George, T. P. (2010). Nicotinic receptor mechanisms in neuropsychiatric disorders: Therapeutic Implications. *Primary Psychiatry*, Vol.17, No.1, (January 2010), pp 35-41, ISSN 1082-6319

Bencherif, M. & Lippiello, P. M. (2010). Alpha7 neuronal nicotinic receptors: the missing link to understanding Alzheimer's etiopathology? *Medical Hypotheses*, Vol.74, No.2, (February 2010), pp 281-285, ISSN 0306-9877

Bencherif, M., Lippiello, P. M., Lucas, R. & Marrero, M. B. (2011). Alpha7 nicotinic receptors as novel therapeutic targets for inflammation-based diseases. *Cellular and Molecular Life Sciences*, Vol.68, No.6, (March 2011), pp 931-949, ISSN 1420-682X

Berg, D. K. & Conroy, W. G. (2002). Nicotinic α7 receptors: synaptic options and downstream signaling in neurons. *Journal of Neurobiology*, Vol.53, No.4, (December 2002), pp 512-523, ISSN 0022-3034

Bitner, R. S., Bunnelle, W. H., Decker, M. W., Drescher, K. U., Kohlhaas, K. L., Markosyan, S., Marsh, K. C., Nikkel, A. L., Browman, K., Radek, R., Anderson, D. J., Buccafusco, J. & Gopalakrishnan, M. (2010). In vivo pharmacological characterization of a novel selective α7 neuronal nicotinic acetylcholine receptor agonist ABT-107: preclinical considerations in Alzheimer's disease. *Journal of Pharmacology and Experimental Therapeutics*, Vol.334, No.3, (September 2010), pp 875-886, ISSN 0022-3565

Bodnar, A. L., Cortes-Burgos, L. A., Cook, K. K., Dinh, D. M., Groppi, V. E., Hajos, M., Higdon, N. R., Hoffmann, W. E., Hurst, R. S., Myers, J. K., Rogers, B. N., Wall, T. M., Wolfe, M. L. & Wong, E. (2005). Discovery and structure-activity relationship of quinuclidine benzamides as agonists of α7 nicotinic acetylcholine receptors. *Journal of Medicinal Chemistry*, Vol.48, No.4, (February 2005), pp 905-908, ISSN 0022-2623

Breese, C. R., Adams, C., Logel, J., Drebing, C., Rollins, Y., Barnhart, M., Sullivan, B., Demasters, B. K., Freedman, R. & Leonard, S. (1997). Comparison of the regional expression of nicotinic acetylcholine receptor alpha7 mRNA and [125I]-α-bungarotoxin binding in human postmortem brain. *Journal of Comparative Neurology*, Vol.387, No.3, (October 1997), pp 385-398, ISSN 0021-9967

Bruchfeld, A., Goldstein, R. S., Chavan, S., Patel, N. B., Rosas-Ballina, M., Kohn, N., Qureshi, A. R. & Tracey, K. J. (2010). Whole blood cytokine attenuation by cholinergic agonists ex vivo and relationship to vagus nerve activity in rheumatoid arthritis. *Journal of Internal Medicine*, Vol.268, No.1, (July 2010), pp 94-101, ISSN 0955-7873

Bunnelle, W. H., Dart, M. J. & Schrimpf, M. R. (2004). Design of ligands for the nicotinic acetylcholine receptors: the quest for selectivity. *Curr Top Med Chem*, Vol.4, No.3, (February 2004), pp 299-334, ISSN 1568-0266

Burghaus, L., Schütz, U., Krempel, U., Lindstrom, J. & Schröder, H. (2003). Loss of nicotinic acetylcholine receptor subunits α4 and α7 in the cerebral cortex of Parkinson patients. *Parkinsonism Relat Disord*, Vol.9, No.5, (June 2003), pp 243-246, ISSN 1353-8020

Changeux, J. P. (2010). Nicotine addiction and nicotinic receptors: lessons from genetically modified mice. *Nature Reviews Neuroscience*, Vol.11, No.6, (June 2010), pp 389-401, ISSN 1471-003X

Chernyavsky, A. I., Arredondo, J., Galitovskiy, V., Qian, J. & Grando, S. A. (2010). Upregulation of nuclear factor-κB expression by SLURP-1 is mediated by α7-nicotinic acetylcholine receptor and involves both ionic events and activation of protein kinases. *Am J Physiol Cell Physiol*, Vol.299, No.5, (November 2010), pp C903-911, ISSN 0363-6143

Christensen, D. Z., Mikkelsen, J. D., Hansen, H. H. & Thomsen, M. S. (2010). Repeated administration of α7 nicotinic acetylcholine receptor (nAChR) agonists, but not positive allosteric modulators, increases α7 nAChR levels in the brain. *Journal of Neurochemistry*, Vol.114, No.4, (August 2010), pp 1205-1216, ISSN 0022-3042

Conejero-Goldberg, C., Davies, P. & Ulloa, L. (2008). Alpha7 nicotinic acetylcholine receptor: A link between inflammation and neurodegeneration. *Neuroscience and Biobehavioral Reviews*, Vol.32, No.4, (April 2008), pp 693-706, ISSN 0149-7634

Court, J., Spurden, D., Lloyd, S., McKeith, I., Ballard, C., Cairns, N., Kerwin, R., Perry, R. & Perry, E. (1999). Neuronal nicotinic receptors in dementia with Lewy bodies and schizophrenia: α-bungarotoxin and nicotine binding in the thalamus. *Journal of Neurochemistry*, Vol.73, No.4, (October 1999), pp 1590-1597, ISSN 0022-3042

Court, J. A., Martin-Ruiz, C., Graham, A. & Perry, E. (2000). Nicotinic receptors in human brain: topography and pathology. *Journal of Chemical Neuroanatomy*, Vol.20, No.3-4, (December 2000), pp 281-298, ISSN 0891-0618

Couturier, S., Bertrand, D., Matter, J. M., Hernandez, M. C., Bertrand, S., Millar, N., Valera, S., Barkas, T. & Ballivet, M. (1990). A neuronal nicotinic acetylcholine receptor subunit (α7) is developmentally regulated and forms a homo-oligomeric channel blocked by alpha-BTX. *Neuron*, Vol.5, No.6, (December 1990), pp 847-856, ISSN 0896-6273

Cunningham, J. M., Lennon, V. A., Lambert, E. H. & Scheithauer, B. (1985). Acetylcholine receptors in small cell carcinomas. *Journal of Neurochemistry*, Vol.45, No.1, (July 1985), pp 159-167, ISSN 0022-3042

Dajas-Bailador, F. A., Mogg, A. J. & Wonnacott, S. (2002). Intracellular Ca^{2+} signals evoked by stimulation of nicotinic acetylcholine receptors in SH-SY5Y cells: contribution of voltage-operated Ca^{2+} channels and Ca^{2+} stores. *Journal of Neurochemistry*, Vol.81, No.3, (May 2002), pp 606-614, ISSN 0022-3042

Dasgupta, P., Rizwani, W., Pillai, S., Kinkade, R., Kovacs, M., Rastogi, S., Banerjee, S., Carless, M., Kim, E., Coppola, D., Haura, E. & Chellappan, S. (2009). Nicotine induces cell proliferation, invasion and epithelial-mesenchymal transition in a variety of human cancer cell lines. *International Journal of Cancer*, Vol.124, No.1, (January 2009), pp 36-45, ISSN 0020-7136

Davies, A. R., Hardick, D. J., Blagbrough, I. S., Potter, B. V., Wolstenholme, A. J. & Wonnacott, S. (1999). Characterisation of the binding of [³H]methyllycaconitine: a new radioligand for labelling α7-type neuronal nicotinic acetylcholine receptors. *Neuropharmacology*, Vol.38, No.5, (May 1999), pp 679-690, ISSN 0028-3908

Davies, P. & Feisullin, S. (1981). Postmortem stability of α-bungarotoxin binding sites in mouse and human brain. *Brain Research*, Vol.216, No.2, (July 1981), pp 449-454, ISSN 0006-8993

Davson, H. & Segal, M. B. (1996). *Physiology of the CSF and blood-brain barriers*, CRC Press, ISBN 0849344727, Boca Raton, USA

de Jonge, W. J. & Ulloa, L. (2007). The α7 nicotinic acetylcholine receptor as a pharmacological target for inflammation. *British Journal of Pharmacology*, Vol.151, No.7, (August 2007), pp 915-929, ISSN 0007-1188

De Simone, R., Ajmone-Cat, M. A., Carnevale, D. & Minghetti, L. (2005). Activation of alpha7 nicotinic acetylcholine receptor by nicotine selectively up-regulates cyclooxygenase-2 and prostaglandin E2 in rat microglial cultures. *Journal of Neuroinflammation*, Vol.2, No.4, (January 2005), pp 1-10, ISSN 1742-2094

Deuther-Conrad, W., Fischer, S., Hiller, A., Nielsen, E. O., Timmermann, D. B., Steinbach, J., Sabri, O., Peters, D. & Brust, P. (2009). Molecular imaging of α7 nicotinic acetylcholine receptors: design and evaluation of the potent radioligand [¹⁸F]NS10743. *Eur J Nucl Med Mol Imaging*, Vol.36, No.5, (May 2009), pp 791-800, ISSN 1619-7070

Deuther-Conrad, W., Fischer, S., Hiller, A., Becker, G., Cumming, P., Xiong, G., Funke, U., Sabri, O., Peters, D. & Brust, P. (2011). Assessment of α7 nicotinic acetylcholine receptor availability in porcine brain with [¹⁸F]NS10743. . *Eur J Nucl Med Mol Imaging*, (March 2011), p in press, ISSN 1619-7070

Dobelis, P., Hutton, S., Lu, Y. & Collins, A. C. (2003). GABAergic systems modulate nicotinic receptor-mediated seizures in mice. *Journal of Pharmacology and Experimental Therapeutics*, Vol.306, No.3, (September 2003), pp 1159-1166, ISSN 0022-3565

Dolle, F., Valette, H., Hinnen, F., Vaufrey, F., Demphel, S., Coulon, C., Ottaviani, M., Bottlaender, M. & Crouzel, C. (2001). Synthesis and preliminary evaluation of a carbon-11-labelled agonist of the α7 nicotinic acetylcholine receptor. *Journal of Labelled Compounds & Radiopharmaceuticals*, Vol.44, No.11, (October 2001), pp 785-795, ISSN 0362-4803

Dome, P., Lazary, J., Kalapos, M. P. & Rihmer, Z. (2010). Smoking, nicotine and neuropsychiatric disorders. *Neuroscience and Biobehavioral Reviews*, Vol.34, No.3, (March 2010), pp 295-342, ISSN 0149-7634

Egleton, R. D., Brown, K. C. & Dasgupta, P. (2008). Nicotinic acetylcholine receptors in cancer: multiple roles in proliferation and inhibition of apoptosis. *Trends in Pharmacological Sciences*, Vol.29, No.3, (March 2008), pp 151-158, ISSN 0165-6147

Egleton, R. D., Brown, K. C. & Dasgupta, P. (2009). Angiogenic activity of nicotinic acetylcholine receptors: implications in tobacco-related vascular diseases. *Pharmacology and Therapeutics*, Vol.121, No.2, (February 2009), pp 205-223, ISSN 0163-7258

Ettrup, A., Mikkelsen, J. D., Palner, M., Lehel, S., Madsen, J., Timmermann, D. B., Peters, D. & Knudsen, G. M. (2010) [¹¹C]NS14492 as a novel PET ligand for imaging cerebral α7 nicotinic receptors: in vivo evaluation and drug occupancy measurements (abstract). *Society of Neuroscience* San Diego:November 13-17, 2010, F39.

Fabian-Fine, R., Skehel, P., Errington, M. L., Davies, H. A., Sher, E., Stewart, M. G. & Fine, A. (2001). Ultrastructural distribution of the α7 nicotinic acetylcholine receptor subunit in rat hippocampus. *Journal of Neuroscience*, Vol.21, No.20, (October 2001), pp 7993-8003, ISSN 0270-6474

Faghih, R., Gopalakrishnan, M. & Briggs, C. A. (2008). Allosteric modulators of the α7 nicotinic acetylcholine receptor. *Journal of Medicinal Chemistry*, Vol.51, No.4, (February 2008), pp 701-712, ISSN 0022-2623

Feuerbach, D., Lingenhoehl, K., Olpe, H. R., Vassout, A., Gentsch, C., Chaperon, F., Nozulak, J., Enz, A., Bilbe, G., McAllister, K. & Hoyer, D. (2009). The selective nicotinic acetylcholine receptor α7 agonist JN403 is active in animal models of cognition, sensory gating, epilepsy and pain. *Neuropharmacology*, Vol.56, No.1, (January 2009), pp 254-263, ISSN 0028-3908

Fleminger, S., Oliver, D. L., Lovestone, S., Rabe-Hesketh, S. & Giora, A. (2003). Head injury as a risk factor for Alzheimer's disease: the evidence 10 years on; a partial replication. *Journal of Neurology, Neurosurgery and Psychiatry*, Vol.74, No.7, (July 2003), pp 857-862, ISSN 0022-3050

Frazier, C. J., Rollins, Y. D., Breese, C. R., Leonard, S., Freedman, R. & Dunwiddie, T. V. (1998). Acetylcholine activates an α-bungarotoxin-sensitive nicotinic current in rat hippocampal interneurons, but not pyramidal cells. *Journal of Neuroscience*, Vol.18, No.4, (February 1998), pp 1187-1195, ISSN 0270-6474

Freedman, R., Hall, M., Adler, L. E. & Leonard, S. (1995). Evidence in postmortem brain tissue for decreased numbers of hippocampal nicotinic receptors in schizophrenia. *Biological Psychiatry*, Vol.38, No.1, (July 1995), pp 22-33, ISSN 0006-3223

Freedman, R., Olincy, A., Buchanan, R. W., Harris, J. G., Gold, J. M., Johnson, L., Allensworth, D., Guzman-Bonilla, A., Clement, B., Ball, M. P., Kutnick, J., Pender, V., Martin, L. F., Stevens, K. E., Wagner, B. D., Zerbe, G. O., Soti, F. & Kem, W. R. (2008). Initial phase 2 trial of a nicotinic agonist in schizophrenia. *American Journal of Psychiatry*, Vol.165, No.8, (August 2008), pp 1040-1047, ISSN 0002-953X

Freedman, R., Coon, H., Myles-Worsley, M., Orr-Urtreger, A., Olincy, A., Davis, A., Polymeropoulos, M., Holik, J., Hopkins, J., Hoff, M., Rosenthal, J., Waldo, M. C., Reimherr, F., Wender, P., Yaw, J., Young, D. A., Breese, C. R., Adams, C., Patterson, D., Adler, L. E., Kruglyak, L., Leonard, S. & Byerley, W. (1997). Linkage of a neurophysiological deficit in schizophrenia to a chromosome 15 locus. *Proceedings of the National Academy of Sciences of the United States of America*, Vol.94, No.2, (January 1997), pp 587-592, ISSN 0027-8424

Fu, Y., Matta, S. G. & Sharp, B. M. (1999). Local α-bungarotoxin-sensitive nicotinic receptors modulate hippocampal norepinephrine release by systemic nicotine. *Journal of Pharmacology and Experimental Therapeutics*, Vol.289, No.1, (April 1999), pp 133-139, ISSN 0022-3565

Galban, C. J., Galban, S., Van Dort, M. E., Luker, G. D., Bhojani, M. S., Rehemtulla, A. & Ross, B. D. (2010). Applications of molecular imaging. *Prog Mol Biol Transl Sci*, Vol.95, (September 2010), pp 237-298, ISSN 1877-1173

Galindo-Charles, L., Hernandez-Lopez, S., Galarraga, E., Tapia, D., Bargas, J., Garduno, J., Frias-Dominguez, C., Drucker-Colin, R. & Mihailescu, S. (2008). Serotoninergic dorsal raphe neurons possess functional postsynaptic nicotinic acetylcholine receptors. *Synapse*, Vol.62, No.8, (August 2008), pp 601-615, ISSN 0887-4476

Gilbert, D., Lecchi, M., Arnaudeau, S., Bertrand, D. & Demaurex, N. (2009). Local and global calcium signals associated with the opening of neuronal α7 nicotinic acetylcholine receptors. *Cell Calcium*, Vol.45, No.2, (February 2009), pp 198-207, ISSN 0143-4160

Graef, S., Schönknecht, P., Sabri, O. & Hegerl, U. (2011). Cholinergic receptor subtypes and their role in cognition, emotion, and vigilance control: An overview of preclinical and clinical findings. *Psychopharmacology*, Vol.DOI: 10.1007/s00213-010-2153-8, (January 2011)ISSN 0033-3158

Guan, Z. Z., Zhang, X., Ravid, R. & Nordberg, A. (2000). Decreased protein levels of nicotinic receptor subunits in the hippocampus and temporal cortex of patients with Alzheimer's disease. *Journal of Neurochemistry*, Vol.74, No.1, (January 2000), pp 237-243, ISSN 0022-3042

Hagooly, A., Rossin, R. & Welch, M. J. (2008). Small molecule receptors as imaging targets. *Handb Exp Pharmacol*, No.185 Pt 2, 2008), pp 93-129, ISSN 0171-2004

Han, Z. Y., Le Novere, N., Zoli, M., Hill, J. A., Jr., Champtiaux, N. & Changeux, J. P. (2000). Localization of nAChR subunit mRNAs in the brain of Macaca mulatta. *European Journal of Neuroscience*, Vol.12, No.10, (October 2000), pp 3664-3674, ISSN 0953-816x

Han, Z. Y., Zoli, M., Cardona, A., Bourgeois, J. P., Changeux, J. P. & Le Novere, N. (2003). Localization of [3H]nicotine, [3H]cytisine, [3H]epibatidine, and [125I]alpha-bungarotoxin binding sites in the brain of Macaca mulatta. *Journal of Comparative Neurology*, Vol.461, No.1, (June 2003), pp 49-60, ISSN 0021-9967

Hashimoto, K., Nishiyama, S., Ohba, H., Matsuo, M., Kobashi, T., Takahagi, M., Iyo, M., Kitashoji, T. & Tsukada, H. (2008). [11C]CHIBA-1001 as a novel PET ligand for α7 nicotinic receptors in the brain: a PET study in conscious monkeys. *PLoS ONE*, Vol.3, No.9, 2008), p e3231, ISSN 1932-6203

Hawkins, B. T., Egleton, R. D. & Davis, T. P. (2005). Modulation of cerebral microvascular permeability by endothelial nicotinic acetylcholine receptors. *American Journal of Physiology - Heart and Circulatory Physiology*, Vol.289, No.1, (July 2005), pp H212-219, ISSN 0363-6135

Heiss, W. D. (2009). The potential of PET/MR for brain imaging. *European Journal of Nuclear Medicine and Molecular Imaging*, Vol.36 Suppl 1, (March 2009), pp S105-112, ISSN 1619-7070

Heiss, W. D. & Herholz, K. (2006). Brain receptor imaging. *Journal of Nuclear Medicine*, Vol.47, No.2, (February 2006), pp 302-312, ISSN 0161-5505

Heiss, W. D., Habedank, B., Klein, J. C., Herholz, K., Wienhard, K., Lenox, M. & Nutt, R. (2004). Metabolic rates in small brain nuclei determined by high-resolution PET. *Journal of Nuclear Medicine*, Vol.45, No.11, (November 2004), pp 1811-1815, ISSN 0161-5505

Hellström-Lindahl, E. & Court, J. A. (2000). Nicotinic acetylcholine receptors during prenatal development and brain pathology in human aging. *Behavioural Brain Research*, Vol.113, No.1-2, (August 2000), pp 159-168, ISSN 0166-4328

Hellström-Lindahl, E., Mousavi, M., Zhang, X., Ravid, R. & Nordberg, A. (1999). Regional distribution of nicotinic receptor subunit mRNAs in human brain: comparison between Alzheimer and normal brain. *Brain Research. Molecular Brain Research*, Vol.66, No.1-2, (March 1999), pp 94-103, ISSN 0169-328x

Hirata, N., Sekino, Y. & Kanda, Y. (2010). Nicotine increases cancer stem cell population in MCF-7 cells. *Biochemical and Biophysical Research Communications*, Vol.403, No.1, (December 2010), pp 138-143, ISSN 0006-291X

Hoffmeister, P. G., Donat, C. K., Schuhmann, M. U., Voigt, C., Walter, B., Nieber, K., Meixensberger, J., Bauer, R. & Brust, P. (2010). Traumatic Brain Injury Elicits Similar Alterations in alpha7 Nicotinic Receptor Density in Two Different Experimental Models. *NeuroMolecular Medicine*, Vol.DOI: 10.1007/s12017-010-8136-4, (September 2010)ISSN 1535-1084

Hone, A. J., Whiteaker, P., Mohn, J. L., Jacob, M. H. & McIntosh, J. M. (2010). Alexa Fluor 546-ArIB[V11L;V16A] is a potent ligand for selectively labeling alpha 7 nicotinic acetylcholine receptors. *Journal of Neurochemistry*, Vol.114, No.4, (August 2010), pp 994-1006, ISSN 0022-3042

Horti, A. G., Gao, Y., Kuwabara, H. & Dannals, R. F. (2010). Development of radioligands with optimized imaging properties for quantification of nicotinic acetylcholine receptors by positron emission tomography. *Life Sciences*, Vol.86, No.15-16, (April 2010), pp 575-584, ISSN 0024-3205

Hruska, M., Keefe, J., Wert, D., Tekinay, A. B., Hulce, J. J., Ibanez-Tallon, I. & Nishi, R. (2009). Prostate stem cell antigen is an endogenous lynx1-like prototoxin that antagonizes α7-containing nicotinic receptors and prevents programmed cell death of parasympathetic neurons. *Journal of Neuroscience*, Vol.29, No.47, (November 2009), pp 14847-14854, ISSN 0270-6474

Hurst, R. S., Hajos, M., Raggenbass, M., Wall, T. M., Higdon, N. R., Lawson, J. A., Rutherford-Root, K. L., Berkenpas, M. B., Hoffmann, W. E., Piotrowski, D. W., Groppi, V. E., Allaman, G., Ogier, R., Bertrand, S., Bertrand, D. & Arneric, S. P. (2005). A novel positive allosteric modulator of the α7 neuronal nicotinic acetylcholine receptor: in vitro and in vivo characterization. *Journal of Neuroscience*, Vol.25, No.17, (April 2005), pp 4396-4405, ISSN 0270-6474

Judenhofer, M. S., Wehrl, H. F., Newport, D. F., Catana, C., Siegel, S. B., Becker, M., Thielscher, A., Kneilling, M., Lichy, M. P., Eichner, M., Klingel, K., Reischl, G., Widmaier, S., Rocken, M., Nutt, R. E., Machulla, H. J., Uludag, K., Cherry, S. R., Claussen, C. D. & Pichler, B. J. (2008). Simultaneous PET-MRI: a new approach for functional and morphological imaging. *Nature Medicine*, Vol.14, No.4, (April 2008), pp 459-465, ISSN 1078-8956

Kent, L., Green, E., Holmes, J., Thapar, A., Gill, M., Hawi, Z., Fitzgerald, M., Asherson, P., Curran, S., Mills, J., Payton, A. & Craddock, N. (2001). No association between CHRNA7 microsatellite markers and attention-deficit hyperactivity disorder. *American Journal of Medical Genetics*, Vol.105, No.8, (December 2001), pp 686-689, ISSN 0148-7299

Kim, S. W., Ding, Y. S., Alexoff, D., Patel, V., Logan, J., Lin, K. S., Shea, C., Muench, L., Xu, Y., Carter, P., King, P., Constanzo, J. R., Ciaccio, J. A. & Fowler, J. S. (2007). Synthesis and positron emission tomography studies of C-11-labeled isotopomers and metabolites of GTS-21, a partial alpha7 nicotinic cholinergic agonist drug. *Nuclear Medicine and Biology*, Vol.34, No.5, (July 2007), pp 541-551, ISSN 0969-8051

Kitagawa, H., Takenouchi, T., Azuma, R., Wesnes, K. A., Kramer, W. G., Clody, D. E. & Burnett, A. L. (2003). Safety, pharmacokinetics, and effects on cognitive function of multiple doses of GTS-21 in healthy, male volunteers. *Neuropsychopharmacology*, Vol.28, No.3, (March 2003), pp 542-551, ISSN 0893-133X

Koeppe, R. A. (2001). A panel discussion on the future of pharmacology and experimental tomography, In: *Physiological imaging of the brain with PET*, A. Gjedde, S. B. Hansen, G. M. Knudsen & O. B. Paulson, (Eds.), 402, Academic Press, ISBN 0-12-285751-8, New York, USA

Kulak, J. M., Carroll, F. I. & Schneider, J. S. (2006). [^{125}I]Iodomethyllycaconitine binds to α7 nicotinic acetylcholine receptors in monkey brain. *European Journal of Neuroscience*, Vol.23, No.10, (May 2006), pp 2604-2610, ISSN 0953-816X

Kulak, J. M., Nguyen, T. A., Olivera, B. M. & McIntosh, J. M. (1997). Alpha-conotoxin MII blocks nicotine-stimulated dopamine release in rat striatal synaptosomes. *Journal of Neuroscience*, Vol.17, No.14, (July 1997), pp 5263-5270, ISSN 0270-6474

Kumar, V. & Sharma, A. (2010). Is neuroimmunomodulation a future therapeutic approach for sepsis? *International Immunopharmacology*, Vol.10, No.1, (January 2010), pp 9-17, ISSN 1567-5769

Lancelot, S. & Zimmer, L. (2010). Small-animal positron emission tomography as a tool for neuropharmacology. *Trends in Pharmacological Sciences*, Vol.31, No.9, (September 2010), pp 411-417, ISSN 0165-6147

Langley, J. N. (1906). Croonian Lecture, 1906: On Nerve Endings and on Special Excitable Substances in Cells. *Proceedings of the Royal Society of London. Series B: Biological Sciences*, Vol.78, No.524, (September 1906), pp 170-194 Online ISSN 1471-2954

Lecomte, R. (2009). Novel detector technology for clinical PET. *European Journal of Nuclear Medicine and Molecular Imaging*, Vol.36 Suppl 1, (March 2009), pp S69-85, ISSN 1619-7070

Lee, M., Martin-Ruiz, C., Graham, A., Court, J., Jaros, E., Perry, R., Iversen, P., Bauman, M. & Perry, E. (2002). Nicotinic receptor abnormalities in the cerebellar cortex in autism. *Brain*, Vol.125, No.Pt 7, (July 2002), pp 1483-1495, ISSN 0006-8950

Lehel, S., Madsen, J., Ettrup, A., Mikkelsen, J. D., Timmermann, D. B., Peters, D. & Knudsen, G. M. (2009). [^{11}C]NS-12857: A novel PET ligand for α7-nicotinergic receptors. *Journal of Labelled Compounds & Radiopharmaceuticals*, Vol.52, (2009), pp S379-S379, ISSN 0362-4803

Leonard, S. (2003). Consequences of low levels of nicotinic acetylcholine receptors in schizophrenia for drug development. *Drug Development Research*, Vol.60, No.2, (October 2003), pp 127-136, ISSN (electronic) 1098-2299

Levin, E. D., Bettegowda, C., Blosser, J. & Gordon, J. (1999). AR-R17779, and α7 nicotinic agonist, improves learning and memory in rats. *Behavioural Pharmacology*, Vol.10, No.6-7, (November 1999), pp 675-680, ISSN 0955-8810

Levin, E. D., Conners, C. K., Sparrow, E., Hinton, S. C., Erhardt, D., Meck, W. H., Rose, J. E. & March, J. (1996). Nicotine effects on adults with attention-deficit/hyperactivity disorder. *Psychopharmacology*, Vol.123, No.1, (January 1996), pp 55-63, ISSN 0033-3158

Li, D. L., Liu, B. H., Sun, L., Zhao, M., He, X., Yu, X. J. & Zang, W. J. (2010). Alterations of muscarinic acetylcholine receptors-2, 4 and α7-nicotinic acetylcholine receptor expression after ischaemia / reperfusion in the rat isolated heart. *Clinical and Experimental Pharmacology and Physiology*, Vol.37, No.12, (December 2010), pp 1114-1119, ISSN 0143-9294

Li, X., Rainnie, D. G., McCarley, R. W. & Greene, R. W. (1998). Presynaptic nicotinic receptors facilitate monoaminergic transmission. *Journal of Neuroscience*, Vol.18, No.5, (March 1998), pp 1904-1912, ISSN 0270-6474

Li, X. W. & Wang, H. (2006). Non-neuronal nicotinic α7 receptor, a new endothelial target for revascularization. *Life Sciences*, Vol.78, No.16, (March 2006), pp 1863-1870, ISSN 0024-3205

Liu, X., Testa, B. & Fahr, A. (2010). Lipophilicity and its relationship with passive drug permeation. *Pharmaceutical Research*, Vol.DOI: 10.1007/s11095-010-0303-7, (October 2010)ISSN 0724-8741

Liu, Y., Ford, B., Mann, M. A. & Fischbach, G. D. (2001). Neuregulins increase α7 nicotinic acetylcholine receptors and enhance excitatory synaptic transmission in GABAergic interneurons of the hippocampus. *Journal of Neuroscience*, Vol.21, No.15, (August 2001), pp 5660-5669, ISSN 0270-6474

Lohr, J. B. & Flynn, K. (1992). Smoking and schizophrenia. *Schizophrenia Research*, Vol.8, No.2, (December 1992), pp 93-102, ISSN 0920-9964

Lummis, S. C., Beene, D. L., Lee, L. W., Lester, H. A., Broadhurst, R. W. & Dougherty, D. A. (2005). Cis-trans isomerization at a proline opens the pore of a neurotransmitter-gated ion channel. *Nature*, Vol.438, No.7065, (November 2005), pp 248-252, ISSN 1476-4687

Maouche, K., Polette, M., Jolly, T., Medjber, K., Cloez-Tayarani, I., Changeux, J. P., Burlet, H., Terryn, C., Coraux, C., Zahm, J. M., Birembaut, P. & Tournier, J. M. (2009). α7 nicotinic acetylcholine receptor regulates airway epithelium differentiation by controlling basal cell proliferation. *American Journal of Pathology*, Vol.175, No.5, (November 2009), pp 1868-1882, ISSN 1525-2191

Marutle, A., Zhang, X., Court, J., Piggott, M., Johnson, M., Perry, R., Perry, E. & Nordberg, A. (2001). Laminar distribution of nicotinic receptor subtypes in cortical regions in schizophrenia. *Journal of Chemical Neuroanatomy*, Vol.22, No.1-2, (July 2001), pp 115-126, ISSN 0891-0618

Mathew, S. V., Law, A. J., Lipska, B. K., Davila-Garcia, M. I., Zamora, E. D., Mitkus, S. N., Vakkalanka, R., Straub, R. E., Weinberger, D. R., Kleinman, J. E. & Hyde, T. M. (2007). Alpha7 nicotinic acetylcholine receptor mRNA expression and binding in postmortem human brain are associated with genetic variation in neuregulin 1. *Human Molecular Genetics*, Vol.16, No.23, (December 2007), pp 2921-2932, ISSN 0964-6906

Mawlawi, O. & Townsend, D. W. (2009). Multimodality imaging: an update on PET/CT technology. *European Journal of Nuclear Medicine and Molecular Imaging*, Vol.36 Suppl 1, (March 2009), pp S15-29, ISSN 1619-7070

Mazurov, A., Hauser, T. & Miller, C. H. (2006). Selective α7 nicotinic acetylcholine receptor ligands. *Current Medicinal Chemistry*, Vol.13, No.13, (October 2006), pp 1567-1584, ISSN 0929-8673

Mazurov, A., Klucik, J., Miao, L., Phillips, T. Y., Seamans, A., Schmitt, J. D., Hauser, T. A., Johnson, R. T., Jr. & Miller, C. (2005). 2-(Arylmethyl)-3-substituted quinuclidines as selective α7 nicotinic receptor ligands. *Bioorganic and Medicinal Chemistry Letters*, Vol.15, No.8, (April 2005), pp 2073-2077, ISSN 0960-894X

McPartland, J. M., Blanchon, D. J. & Musty, R. E. (2008). Cannabimimetic effects modulated by cholinergic compounds. *Addiction Biology*, Vol.13, No.3-4, (September 2008), pp 411-415, ISSN 1355-6215

Mexal, S., Berger, R., Logel, J., Ross, R. G., Freedman, R. & Leonard, S. (2010). Differential regulation of α7 nicotinic receptor gene (*CHRNA7*) expression in schizophrenic smokers. *Journal of Molecular Neuroscience*, Vol.40, No.1-2, (January 2010), pp 185-195, ISSN 0895-8696

Meyer, E. M., Kuryatov, A., Gerzanich, V., Lindstrom, J. & Papke, R. L. (1998). Analysis of 3-(4-hydroxy, 2-methoxybenzylidene)anabaseine selectivity and activity at human and rat α7 nicotinic receptors. *Journal of Pharmacology and Experimental Therapeutics*, Vol.287, No.3, (December 1998), pp 918-925, ISSN 0022-3565

Moccia, F., Frost, C., Berra-Romani, R., Tanzi, F. & Adams, D. J. (2004). Expression and function of neuronal nicotinic ACh receptors in rat microvascular endothelial cells. *Am J Physiol Heart Circ Physiol*, Vol.286, No.2, (February 2004), pp H486-491, ISSN 0363-6135

Mousavi, M., Hellström-Lindahl, E., Guan, Z. Z., Bednar, I. & Nordberg, A. (2001). Expression of nicotinic acetylcholine receptors in human and rat adrenal medulla. *Life Sciences*, Vol.70, No.5, (December 2001), pp 577-590, ISSN 0024-3205

Mugnaini, M., Tessari, M., Tarter, G., Merlo Pich, E., Chiamulera, C. & Bunnemann, B. (2002). Upregulation of [^{3}H]methyllycaconitine binding sites following continuous infusion of nicotine, without changes of α7 or α6 subunit mRNA: an autoradiography and in situ hybridization study in rat brain. *European Journal of Neuroscience*, Vol.16, No.9, (November 2002), pp 1633-1646, ISSN 0953-816X

Mullen, G., Napier, J., Balestra, M., DeCory, T., Hale, G., Macor, J., Mack, R., Loch, J., 3rd, Wu, E., Kover, A., Verhoest, P., Sampognaro, A., Phillips, E., Zhu, Y., Murray, R., Griffith, R., Blosser, J., Gurley, D., Machulskis, A., Zongrone, J., Rosen, A. & Gordon, J. (2000). (-)-Spiro[1-azabicyclo[2.2.2]octane-3,5'-oxazolidin-2'-one], a conformationally restricted analogue of acetylcholine, is a highly selective full agonist at the α7 nicotinic acetylcholine receptor. *Journal of Medicinal Chemistry*, Vol.43, No.22, (November 2000), pp 4045-4050, ISSN 0022-2623

Ng, H. J., Whittemore, E. R., Tran, M. B., Hogenkamp, D. J., Broide, R. S., Johnstone, T. B., Zheng, L., Stevens, K. E. & Gee, K. W. (2007). Nootropic α7 nicotinic receptor allosteric modulator derived from GABA$_A$ receptor modulators. *Proceedings of the National Academy of Sciences of the United States of America*, Vol.104, No.19, (May 2007), pp 8059-8064, ISSN 0027-8424

Nomikos, G. G., Schilström, B., Hildebrand, B. E., Panagis, G., Grenhoff, J. & Svensson, T. H. (2000). Role of α7 nicotinic receptors in nicotine dependence and implications for psychiatric illness. *Behavioural Brain Research*, Vol.113, No.1-2, (August 2000), pp 97-103, ISSN 0166-4328

Nordberg, A. (2001). Nicotinic receptor abnormalities of Alzheimer's disease: therapeutic implications. *Biological Psychiatry*, Vol.49, No.3, (February 2001), pp 200-210, ISSN 0006-3223

Northrop, N. A., Smith, L. P., Yamamoto, B. K. & Eyerman, D. J. (2010). Regulation of glutamate release by α7 nicotinic receptors: differential role in methamphetamine-induced damage to dopaminergic and serotonergic terminals. *Journal of*

Pharmacology and Experimental Therapeutics, Vol.DOI:10.1124/jpet.110.177287, (December 2010)ISSN 0022-3565

Ogawa, M., Nishiyama, S., Tsukada, H., Hatano, K., Fuchigami, T., Yamaguchi, H., Matsushima, Y., Ito, K. & Magata, Y. (2010). Synthesis and evaluation of new imaging agent for central nicotinic acetylcholine receptor α7 subtype. *Nuclear Medicine and Biology*, Vol.37, No.3, (April 2010), pp 347-355, ISSN 0969-8051

Oldendorf, W., Braun, L. & Cornford, E. (1979). pH dependence of blood-brain barrier permeability to lactate and nicotine. *Stroke*, Vol.10, No.5, (September 1979), pp 577-581, ISSN 0039-2499

Olincy, A., Harris, J. G., Johnson, L. L., Pender, V., Kongs, S., Allensworth, D., Ellis, J., Zerbe, G. O., Leonard, S., Stevens, K. E., Stevens, J. O., Martin, L., Adler, L. E., Soti, F., Kem, W. R. & Freedman, R. (2006). Proof-of-concept trial of an α7 nicotinic agonist in schizophrenia. *Archives of General Psychiatry*, Vol.63, No.6, (Jun 2006), pp 630-638, ISSN 0003-990X

Pacini, A., Mannelli, L. D., Bonaccini, L., Ronzoni, S., Bartolini, A. & Ghelardini, C. (2010). Protective effect of alpha7 nAChR: Behavioural and morphological features on neuropathy. *Pain*, Vol.150, No.3, (September 2010), pp 542-549, ISSN 0304-3959

Paleari, L., Cesario, A., Fini, M. & Russo, P. (2009). α7-Nicotinic receptor antagonists at the beginning of a clinical era for NSCLC and Mesothelioma? *Drug Discov Today*, Vol.14, No.17-18, (September 2009), pp 822-836, ISSN 1359-6446

Paleari, L., Catassi, A., Ciarlo, M., Cavalieri, Z., Bruzzo, C., Servent, D., Cesario, A., Chessa, L., Cilli, M., Piccardi, F., Granone, P. & Russo, P. (2008). Role of α7-nicotinic acetylcholine receptor in human non-small cell lung cancer proliferation. *Cell Proliferation*, Vol.41, No.6, (December 2008), pp 936-959, ISSN 0960-7722

Peters, D., Olsen, G. M., Nielsen, E. O., Timmermann, D. B., Loechel, S. C., Mikkelsen, J. D., Hansen, H. B., Redrobe, J. P., Christensen, J. K. & Dyhring, T. (2007). Novel 1,4-diaza-bicyclo[3.2.2]nonyl oxadiazolyl derviatives and their medical use, WO/2007/138037

Pettersson, A., Nordlander, S., Nylund, G., Khorram-Manesh, A., Nordgren, S. & Delbro, D. S. (2008). Expression of the endogenous, nicotinic acetylcholine receptor ligand, SLURP-1, in human colon cancer. *Autonomic and Autacoid Pharmacology*, Vol.28, No.4, (October 2008), pp 109-116, ISSN1474-8665

Pichler, B. J., Judenhofer, M. S. & Pfannenberg, C. (2008). Multimodal imaging approaches: PET/CT and PET/MRI. *Handb Exp Pharmacol*, No.185 Pt 1, 2008), pp 109-132, ISSN 0171-2004

Pichler, B. J., Judenhofer, M. S., Catana, C., Walton, J. H., Kneilling, M., Nutt, R. E., Siegel, S. B., Claussen, C. D. & Cherry, S. R. (2006). Performance test of an LSO-APD detector in a 7-T MRI scanner for simultaneous PET/MRI. *Journal of Nuclear Medicine*, Vol.47, No.4, (April 2006), pp 639-647, ISSN 0161-5505

Pictet, A. (1903). Synthese de la nicotine. *Comptes Rendus de l Academie des Sciences*, Vol.137, (November 1903), pp 860-862, ISSN 0764-4469

Pinner, A. (1893). Ueber Nicotin. Die Constitution des Alkaloids. V. Mittheilung. *Berichte der deutschen chemischen Gesellschaft*, Vol.26, No.1, (January 1893), pp 292-305, ISSN 1099-0682

Pinner, A. & Wolffenstein, R. (1891). Ueber Nicotin. *Berichte der deutschen chemischen Gesellschaft*, Vol.24, No.1, (January 1891), pp 61-67, ISSN 1099-0682

Plummer, H. K., 3rd, Dhar, M. & Schuller, H. M. (2005). Expression of the α7 nicotinic acetylcholine receptor in human lung cells. *Respiration Research*, Vol.6, (April 2005), p 29, ISSN 1465-993X

Pomper, M. G., Phillips, E., Fan, H., McCarthy, D. J., Keith, R. A., Gordon, J. C., Scheffel, U., Dannals, R. F. & Musachio, J. L. (2005). Synthesis and biodistribution of radiolabeled α7 nicotinic acetylcholine receptor ligands. *Journal of Nuclear Medicine*, Vol.46, No.2, (February 2005), pp 326-334, ISSN 0161-5505

Posselt, W. & Reimann, L. (1828). Chemische Untersuchungen des Tabaks und Darstellung des eigenthümlichen wirksamen Princips dieser Pflanze. *Geiger´s Magazin für Pharmacie und die dahin einschlagenden Wissenschaften*, Vol.24, 1828), pp 138-161,

Potter, A. S. & Newhouse, P. A. (2004). Effects of acute nicotine administration on behavioral inhibition in adolescents with attention-deficit/hyperactivity disorder. *Psychopharmacology*, Vol.176, No.2, (November 2004), pp 182-194, ISSN 0033-3158

Prakash, N. & Frostig, R. D. (2005). What has intrinsic signal optical imaging taught us about NGF-induced rapid plasticity in adult cortex and its relationship to the cholinergic system? *Molecular Imaging and Biology*, Vol.7, No.1, (January 2005), pp 14-21, ISSN 1536-1632

Quik, M., Vailati, S., Bordia, T., Kulak, J. M., Fan, H., McIntosh, J. M., Clementi, F. & Gotti, C. (2005). Subunit composition of nicotinic receptors in monkey striatum: effect of treatments with 1-methyl-4-phenyl-1,2,3,6-tetrahydropyridine or L-DOPA. *Molecular Pharmacology*, Vol.67, No.1, (January 2005), pp 32-41, ISSN 0026-895X

Radcliffe, K. A. & Dani, J. A. (1998). Nicotinic stimulation produces multiple forms of increased glutamatergic synaptic transmission. *Journal of Neuroscience*, Vol.18, No.18, (September 1998), pp 7075-7083, ISSN 0270-6474

Raggenbass, M. & Bertrand, D. (2002). Nicotinic receptors in circuit excitability and epilepsy. *Journal of Neurobiology*, Vol.53, No.4, (December 2002), pp 580-589, ISSN 0022-3034

Roncarati, R., Scali, C., Comery, T. A., Grauer, S. M., Aschmi, S., Bothmann, H., Jow, B., Kowal, D., Gianfriddo, M., Kelley, C., Zanelli, U., Ghiron, C., Haydar, S., Dunlop, J. & Terstappen, G. C. (2009). Procognitive and neuroprotective activity of a novel α7 nicotinic acetylcholine receptor agonist for treatment of neurodegenerative and cognitive disorders. *Journal of Pharmacology and Experimental Therapeutics*, Vol.329, No.2, (May 2009), pp 459-468, ISSN 0022-3565

Rosas-Ballina, M. & Tracey, K. J. (2009). The neurology of the immune system: neural reflexes regulate immunity. *Neuron*, Vol.64, No.1, (October 2009), pp 28-32, ISSN 0896-6273

Rose, J. E., Mukhin, A. G., Lokitz, S. J., Turkington, T. G., Herskovic, J., Behm, F. M., Garg, S. & Garg, P. K. (2010). Kinetics of brain nicotine accumulation in dependent and nondependent smokers assessed with PET and cigarettes containing ^{11}C-nicotine. *Proceedings of the National Academy of Sciences of the United States of America*, Vol.107, No.11, (Mar 16 2010), pp 5190-5195, ISSN 0027-8424

Ross, R. G., Stevens, K. E., Proctor, W. R., Leonard, S., Kisley, M. A., Hunter, S. K., Freedman, R. & Adams, C. E. (2010). Research review: Cholinergic mechanisms, early brain development, and risk for schizophrenia. *Journal of Child Psychology and Psychiatry and Allied Disciplines*, Vol.51, No.5, (May 2010), pp 535-549, ISSN 0021-9630

Sabri, O., Kendziorra, K., Wolf, H., Gertz, H. J. & Brust, P. (2008). Acetylcholine receptors in dementia and mild cognitive impairment. *Eur J Nucl Med Mol Imaging*, Vol.35 Suppl 1, (March 2008), pp S30-45, ISSN 1619-7070

Sadis, C., Teske, G., Stokman, G., Kubjak, C., Claessen, N., Moore, F., Loi, P., Diallo, B., Barvais, L., Goldman, M., Florquin, S. & Le Moine, A. (2007). Nicotine protects kidney from renal ischemia/reperfusion injury through the cholinergic anti-inflammatory pathway. *PLoS ONE*, Vol.2, No.5, (May 2007), pp e469 (461-468), ISSN 1932-6203

Schep, L. J., Slaughter, R. J. & Beasley, D. M. (2009). Nicotinic plant poisoning. *Clinical Toxicology (Philadelphia)*, Vol.47, No.8, (September 2009), pp 771-781, ISSN 1556-3650

Schilström, B., Fagerquist, M. V., Zhang, X., Hertel, P., Panagis, G., Nomikos, G. G. & Svensson, T. H. (2000). Putative role of presynaptic α7* nicotinic receptors in nicotine stimulated increases of extracellular levels of glutamate and aspartate in the ventral tegmental area. *Synapse*, Vol.38, No.4, (December 2000), pp 375-383, ISSN 0887-4476

Schuller, H. M. (2009). Is cancer triggered by altered signalling of nicotinic acetylcholine receptors? *Nature Reviews Cancer*, Vol.9, No.3, (March 2009), pp 195-205, ISSN 1474-175X

Schulz, D. W., Loring, R. H., Aizenman, E. & Zigmond, R. E. (1991). Autoradiographic localization of putative nicotinic receptors in the rat brain using 125I-neuronal bungarotoxin. *Journal of Neuroscience*, Vol.11, No.1, (January 1991), pp 287-297, ISSN 0270-6474

Sharma, G. & Vijayaraghavan, S. (2001). Nicotinic cholinergic signaling in hippocampal astrocytes involves calcium-induced calcium release from intracellular stores. *Proceedings of the National Academy of Sciences of the United States of America*, Vol.98, No.7, (March 2001), pp 4148-4153, ISSN 0027-8424

Sharma, G. & Vijayaraghavan, S. (2002). Nicotinic receptor signaling in nonexcitable cells. *Journal of Neurobiology*, Vol.53, No.4, (December 2002), pp 524-534, ISSN 0022-3034

Shen, J. X. & Yakel, J. L. (2009). Nicotinic acetylcholine receptor-mediated calcium signaling in the nervous system. *Acta Pharmacol Sin*, Vol.30, No.6, (June 2009), pp 673-680, ISSN 1671-4083

Siegmund, B., Leitner, E. & Pfannhauser, W. (1999). Determination of the nicotine content of various edible nightshades (Solanaceae) and their products and estimation of the associated dietary nicotine intake. *Journal of Agricultural and Food Chemistry*, Vol.47, No.8, (August 1999), pp 3113-3120, ISSN 0021-8561

Slomka, P. J. & Baum, R. P. (2009). Multimodality image registration with software: state-of-the-art. *European Journal of Nuclear Medicine and Molecular Imaging*, Vol.36 Suppl 1, (March 2009), pp S44-55, ISSN 1619-7070

Small, E., Shah, H. P., Davenport, J. J., Geier, J. E., Yavarovich, K. R., Yamada, H., Sabarinath, S. N., Derendorf, H., Pauly, J. R., Gold, M. S. & Bruijnzeel, A. W. (2010). Tobacco smoke exposure induces nicotine dependence in rats. *Psychopharmacology*, Vol.208, No.1, (January 2010), pp 143-158, ISSN 0033-3158

Spanoudaki, V. C. & Ziegler, S. I. (2008). PET & SPECT instrumentation. *Handb Exp Pharmacol*, No.185 Pt 1, 2008), pp 53-74, ISSN 0171-2004

Spurden, D. P., Court, J. A., Lloyd, S., Oakley, A., Perry, R., Pearson, C., Pullen, R. G. & Perry, E. K. (1997). Nicotinic receptor distribution in the human thalamus:

autoradiographical localization of [³H]nicotine and [¹²⁵I] alpha-bungarotoxin binding. *Journal of Chemical Neuroanatomy*, Vol.13, No.2, (July 1997), pp 105-113, ISSN 0891-0618

Stella, N. & Piomelli, D. (2001). Receptor-dependent formation of endogenous cannabinoids in cortical neurons. *European Journal of Pharmacology*, Vol.425, No.3, (August 2001), pp 189-196, ISSN 0014-2999

Stephens, S. H., Logel, J., Barton, A., Franks, A., Schultz, J., Short, M., Dickenson, J., James, B., Fingerlin, T. E., Wagner, B., Hodgkinson, C., Graw, S., Ross, R. G., Freedman, R. & Leonard, S. (2009). Association of the 5'-upstream regulatory region of the α7 nicotinic acetylcholine receptor subunit gene (CHRNA7) with schizophrenia. *Schizophrenia Research*, Vol.109, No.1-3, (April 2009), pp 102-112, ISSN 0920-9964

Stolerman, I. P. (1990). Behavioural pharmacology of nicotine: implications for multiple brain nicotinic receptors. *Ciba Foundation Symposium*, Vol.152, (June 1990), pp 3-16; discussion 16-22, ISSN 0300-5208

Suzuki, T., Hide, I., Matsubara, A., Hama, C., Harada, K., Miyano, K., Andra, M., Matsubayashi, H., Sakai, N., Kohsaka, S., Inoue, K. & Nakata, Y. (2006). Microglial α7 nicotinic acetylcholine receptors drive a phospholipase C/IP3 pathway and modulate the cell activation toward a neuroprotective role. *Journal of Neuroscience Research*, Vol.83, No.8, (June 2006), pp 1461-1470, ISSN 0360-4012

Svedberg, M. M., Svensson, A. L., Johnson, M., Lee, M., Cohen, O., Court, J., Soreq, H., Perry, E. & Nordberg, A. (2002). Upregulation of neuronal nicotinic receptor subunits α4, β2, and α7 in transgenic mice overexpressing human acetylcholinesterase. *Journal of Molecular Neuroscience*, Vol.18, No.3, (June 2002), pp 211-222, ISSN 0895-8696

Tatsumi, R., Fujio, M., Satoh, H., Katayama, J., Takanashi, S., Hashimoto, K. & Tanaka, H. (2005). Discovery of the α7 nicotinic acetylcholine receptor agonists. (R)-3'-(5-Chlorothiophen-2-yl)spiro-1-azabicyclo[2.2.2]octane-3,5'-[1',3'] oxazolidin-2'-one as a novel, potent, selective, and orally bioavailable ligand. *Journal of Medicinal Chemistry*, Vol.48, No.7, (April 2005), pp 2678-2686, ISSN 0022-2623

Thomsen, M. S., Hansen, H. H., Timmerman, D. B. & Mikkelsen, J. D. (2010). Cognitive improvement by activation of α7 nicotinic acetylcholine receptors: from animal models to human pathophysiology. *Current Pharmaceutical Design*, Vol.16, No.3, (January 2010), pp 323-343, ISSN 1381-6128

Tietje, K. R., Anderson, D. J., Bitner, R. S., Blomme, E. A., Brackemeyer, P. J., Briggs, C. A., Browman, K. E., Bury, D., Curzon, P., Drescher, K. U., Frost, J. M., Fryer, R. M., Fox, G. B., Gronlien, J. H., Hakerud, M., Gubbins, E. J., Halm, S., Harris, R., Helfrich, R. J., Kohlhaas, K. L., Law, D., Malysz, J., Marsh, K. C., Martin, R. L., Meyer, M. D., Molesky, A. L., Nikkel, A. L., Otte, S., Pan, L., Puttfarcken, P. S., Radek, R. J., Robb, H. M., Spies, E., Thorin-Hagene, K., Waring, J. F., Ween, H., Xu, H., Gopalakrishnan, M. & Bunnelle, W. H. (2008). Preclinical characterization of A-582941: a novel α7 neuronal nicotinic receptor agonist with broad spectrum cognition-enhancing properties. *CNS Neuroscience & Therapeutics*, Vol.14, No.1, (Spring 2008), pp 65-82, ISSN 1755-5930

Timmermann, D. B., Gronlien, J. H., Kohlhaas, K. L., Nielsen, E. O., Dam, E., Jorgensen, T. D., Ahring, P. K., Peters, D., Holst, D., Chrsitensen, J. K., Malysz, J., Briggs, C. A., Gopalakrishnan, M. & Olsen, G. M. (2007). An allosteric modulator of the α7 nicotinic acetylcholine receptor possessing cognition-enhancing properties in vivo. *Journal of Pharmacology and Experimental Therapeutics*, Vol.323, No.1, (October 2007), pp 294-307, ISSN 0022-3565

Tournier, J. M. & Birembaut, P. (2011). Nicotinic acetylcholine receptors and predisposition to lung cancer. *Current Opinion in Oncology*, Vol.23, No.1, (January 2011), pp 83-87, ISSN 1040-8746

Toyohara, J., Wu, J. & Hashimoto, K. (2010a). Recent development of radioligands for imaging α7 nicotinic acetylcholine receptors in the brain. *Curr Top Med Chem*, Vol.10, No.15, (October 2010a), pp 1544-1557, ISSN 1568-0266

Toyohara, J., Ishiwata, K., Sakata, M., Wu, J., Nishiyama, S., Tsukada, H. & Hashimoto, K. (2010b). In vivo evaluation of α7 nicotinic acetylcholine receptor agonists [^{11}C]A-582941 and [^{11}C]A-844606 in mice and conscious monkeys. *PLoS ONE*, Vol.5, No.2, (February 2010b), p e8961, ISSN 1932-6203

Toyohara, J., Sakata, M., Wu, J., Ishikawa, M., Oda, K., Ishii, K., Iyo, M., Hashimoto, K. & Ishiwata, K. (2009). Preclinical and the first clinical studies on [^{11}C]CHIBA-1001 for mapping α7 nicotinic receptors by positron emission tomography. *Annals of Nuclear Medicine*, Vol.23, No.3, (May 2009), pp 301-309, ISSN 0914-7187

Tracey, K. J. (2002). The inflammatory reflex. *Nature*, Vol.420, No.6917, (December 2002), pp 853-859, ISSN 0028-0836

Tregellas, J. R., Tanabe, J., Rojas, D. C., Shatti, S., Olincy, A., Johnson, L., Martin, L. F., Soti, F., Kem, W. R., Leonard, S. & Freedman, R. (2011). Effects of an alpha 7-nicotinic agonist on default network activity in schizophrenia. *Biological Psychiatry*, Vol.69, No.1, (January 2011), pp 7-11, ISSN 0006-3223

van der Stelt, M. & Di Marzo, V. (2005). Anandamide as an intracellular messenger regulating ion channel activity. *Prostaglandins and Other Lipid Mediators*, Vol.77, No.1-4, (September 2005), pp 111-122, ISSN 1098-8823

von Schulthess, G. K. & Schlemmer, H. P. (2009). A look ahead: PET/MR versus PET/CT. *European Journal of Nuclear Medicine and Molecular Imaging*, Vol.36 Suppl 1, (March 2009), pp S3-9, ISSN 1619-7070

Wang, H. Y., Lee, D. H., D'Andrea, M. R., Peterson, P. A., Shank, R. P. & Reitz, A. B. (2000). β-Amyloid(1-42) binds to α7 nicotinic acetylcholine receptor with high affinity. Implications for Alzheimer's disease pathology. *Journal of Biological Chemistry*, Vol.275, No.8, (Feb 25 2000), pp 5626-5632,

Waterhouse, R. N. (2003). Determination of lipophilicity and its use as a predictor of blood-brain barrier penetration of molecular imaging agents. *Mol Imaging Biol*, Vol.5, No.6, (November 2003), pp 376-389, ISSN 1536-1632

Wei, P. L., Chang, Y. J., Ho, Y. S., Lee, C. H., Yang, Y. Y., An, J. & Lin, S. Y. (2009). Tobacco-specific carcinogen enhances colon cancer cell migration through α7-nicotinic acetylcholine receptor. *Annals of Surgery*, Vol.249, No.6, (June 2009), pp 978-985, ISSN 0003-4932

Wei, P. L., Kuo, L. J., Huang, M. T., Ting, W. C., Ho, Y. S., Wang, W., An, J. & Chang, Y. J. (2011). Nicotine enhances colon cancer cell migration by induction of fibronectin. *Annals of Surgical Oncology*, Vol.DOI: 10.1245/s10434-010-1504-3, (January 2011)ISSN 1068-9265

Wevers, A. & Schröder, H. (1999). Nicotinic acetylcholine receptors in Alzheimer's disease. *J Alzheimers Dis*, Vol.1, No.4-5, (November 1999), pp 207-219, ISSN 1387-2877

Whiteaker, P., Davies, A. R., Marks, M. J., Blagbrough, I. S., Potter, B. V., Wolstenholme, A.
    J., Collins, A. C. & Wonnacott, S. (1999). An autoradiographic study of the
    distribution of binding sites for the novel α7-selective nicotinic radioligand [³H]-
    methyllycaconitine in the mouse brain. *European Journal of Neuroscience*, Vol.11,
    No.8, (August 1999), pp 2689-2696, ISSN 0953-816X
Wienhard, K., Schmand, M., Casey, M. E., Baker, K., Bao, J., Eriksson, L., Jones, W. F.,
    Knoess, C., Lenox, M., Lercher, M., Luk, P., Michel, C., Reed, J. H., Richerzhagen,
    N., Treffert, J., Vollmar, S., Young, J. W., Heiss, W. D. & Nutt, R. (2002). The ECAT
    HRRT: Performance and first clinical application of the new high resolution
    research tomograph. *Ieee Transactions on Nuclear Science*, Vol.49, No.1, (February
    2002), pp 104-110, ISSN 0018-9499
Xi, W., Tian, M. & Zhang, H. (2011). Molecular imaging in neuroscience research with small-
    animal PET in rodents. *Neuroscience Research*, Vol.doi:10.1016/j.neures.2010.12.017,
    (January 2011)ISSN 0168-0102
Ye, Y. N., Liu, E. S., Shin, V. Y., Wu, W. K. & Cho, C. H. (2004). The modulating role of
    nuclear factor-κB in the action of α7-nicotinic acetylcholine receptor and cross-talk
    between 5-lipoxygenase and cyclooxygenase-2 in colon cancer growth induced by
    4-(N-methyl-N-nitrosamino)-1-(3-pyridyl)-1-butanone. *Journal of Pharmacology and
    Experimental Therapeutics*, Vol.311, No.1, (October 2004), pp 123-130, ISSN 0022-3565
Yeboah, M. M., Xue, X. Y., Javdan, M., Susin, M. & Metz, C. N. (2008). Nicotinic
    acetylcholine receptor expression and regulation in the rat kidney after ischemia-
    reperfusion injury. *American Journal of Physiology-Renal Physiology*, Vol.295, No.3,
    (September 2008), pp F654-F661, ISSN 0363-6127

Permissions

The contributors of this book come from diverse backgrounds, making this book a truly international effort. This book will bring forth new frontiers with its revolutionizing research information and detailed analysis of the nascent developments around the world.

We would like to thank Peter Bright, for lending his expertise to make the book truly unique. He has played a crucial role in the development of this book. Without his invaluable contribution this book wouldn't have been possible. He has made vital efforts to compile up to date information on the varied aspects of this subject to make this book a valuable addition to the collection of many professionals and students.

This book was conceptualized with the vision of imparting up-to-date information and advanced data in this field. To ensure the same, a matchless editorial board was set up. Every individual on the board went through rigorous rounds of assessment to prove their worth. After which they invested a large part of their time researching and compiling the most relevant data for our readers. Conferences and sessions were held from time to time between the editorial board and the contributing authors to present the data in the most comprehensible form. The editorial team has worked tirelessly to provide valuable and valid information to help people across the globe.

Every chapter published in this book has been scrutinized by our experts. Their significance has been extensively debated. The topics covered herein carry significant findings which will fuel the growth of the discipline. They may even be implemented as practical applications or may be referred to as a beginning point for another development. Chapters in this book were first published by InTech; hereby published with permission under the Creative Commons Attribution License or equivalent.

The editorial board has been involved in producing this book since its inception. They have spent rigorous hours researching and exploring the diverse topics which have resulted in the successful publishing of this book. They have passed on their knowledge of decades through this book. To expedite this challenging task, the publisher supported the team at every step. A small team of assistant editors was also appointed to further simplify the editing procedure and attain best results for the readers.

Our editorial team has been hand-picked from every corner of the world. Their multi-ethnicity adds dynamic inputs to the discussions which result in innovative outcomes. These outcomes are then further discussed with the researchers and contributors who give their valuable feedback and opinion regarding the same. The feedback is then collaborated with the researches and they are edited in a comprehensive manner to aid the understanding of the subject.

Apart from the editorial board, the designing team has also invested a significant amount of their time in understanding the subject and creating the most relevant covers. They scrutinized every image to scout for the most suitable representation of the subject and create an appropriate cover for the book.

The publishing team has been involved in this book since its early stages. They were actively engaged in every process, be it collecting the data, connecting with the contributors or procuring relevant information. The team has been an ardent support to the editorial, designing and production team. Their endless efforts to recruit the best for this project, has resulted in the accomplishment of this book. They are a veteran in the field of academics and their pool of knowledge is as vast as their experience in printing. Their expertise and guidance has proved useful at every step. Their uncompromising quality standards have made this book an exceptional effort. Their encouragement from time to time has been an inspiration for everyone.

The publisher and the editorial board hope that this book will prove to be a valuable piece of knowledge for researchers, students, practitioners and scholars across the globe.

List of Contributors

Eldar Rosenfeld and Anat Kesler
Neuro-ophthalmology Unit, Department of Ophthalmology, Tel-Aviv Medical Center, Sackler School of Medicine, Tel Aviv University, Tel Aviv, Israel

Laia Rodriguez-Revenga and Montserrat Mila
Biochemistry and Molecular Genetics Department, Hospital Clinic, IDIBAPS Barcelona, Spain
CIBER de Enfermedades Raras (CIBERER), Barcelona, Spain

Esther Granell Moreno
Neuroradiology Unit, Radiology Department, Hospital Sant Pau, Barcelona, Spain

Beatriz Gómez-Ansón
Neuroradiology Unit, Radiology Department, Hospital Sant Pau, Barcelona, Spain
CIBER de Enfermedades Neurodegenerativas (CIBERNED), Barcelona, Spain

Javier Pagonabarraga
CIBER de Enfermedades Neurodegenerativas (CIBERNED), Barcelona, Spain
Neurology Service, Hospital Sant Pau, Barcelona, Spain

Chin-Chang Huang
Department of Neurology, Chang Gung Memorial Hospital and Chang Gung University College of Medicine, Taipei, Taiwan

Tzu-Chen Yen
Department of Nuclear Medicine, Chang Gung Memorial Hospital and Chang Gung University, Taiwan

Chin-Song Lu
Department of Neurology, Chang Gung Memorial Hospital and Chang Gung University, Taiwan

Efrosini Z. Papadaki
Department of Radiology, University of Crete School of Medicine, Heraklion, Greece

Dimitrios T. Boumpas
Internal Medicine and Rheumatology, University of Crete School of Medicine, Heraklion, Greece

Shahina Bano
Department of Radio diagnosis, G.B. Pant Hospital & Maulana Azad Medical College, New Delhi

Vikas Chaudhary
Department of Radio diagnosis, Employees' State Insurance Corporation (ESIC) Model Hospital, Gurgaon, Haryana

Sachchidanand Yadav
Department of Radio diagnosis, Dr. Ram Manohar Lohia Hospital & PGIMER, New Delhi, India

Zhaoda Zhang and Anna-Liisa Brownell
Athinoula A. Martinos Biomedical Imaging Center, Massachusetts General Hospital Harvard Medical School, Charlestown, Massachusetts, USA

Eva-Maria Ratai and Paul Caruso
Department of Radiology, Massachusetts General Hospital, Harvard Medical School, Boston, MA, USA

Florian Eichler
Department of Neurology, Massachusetts General Hospital, Harvard Medical School, Boston, MA, USA

Peter Brust and Winnie Deuther-Conrad
Helmholtz-Zentrum Dresden – Rossendorf, Research Site Leipzig, Germany

Printed in the USA
CPSIA information can be obtained
at www.ICGtesting.com
JSHW011408221024
72173JS00003B/467

9 781632 411860